Christina Schües (ed.)
Genetic Responsibility in Germany and Israel

Bioethics / Medical Ethics | Volume 4

Christina Schües is a professor for philosophy at the Institute for the History of Medicine and Science Studies at Universität Lübeck and titular professor for philosophy at the Institute for Philosophy and Art Sciences at Leuphana Universität Lüneburg. Her research focuses on political ethics, the power of time, the phenomenology of relationality, inter-corporeality and life, as well as the philosophy of medicine, especially with regard to reproductive and gene diagnostic technology.

Christina Schües (ed.)

Genetic Responsibility in Germany and Israel

Practices of Prenatal Diagnosis

[transcript]

This research was supported by the German Research Foundation (Deutsche Forschungsgemeinschaft, DFG), Grants No. RE2951/3-1 and Schu2846/2-1.

Bibliographic information published by the Deutsche Nationalbibliothek
The Deutsche Nationalbibliothek lists this publication in the Deutsche Nationalbibliografie; detailed bibliographic data are available in the Internet at http://dnb.d-nb.de

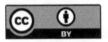

First published in 2022 by transcript Verlag, Bielefeld

© Christina Schües (ed.)
https://www.transcript-verlag.de/

https://doi.org/10.14361/9783839459881
Print-ISBN 978-3-8376-5988-7
PDF-ISBN 978-3-8394-5988-1
ISSN of series: 2702-8267
eISSN of series: 2702-8275

Contents

III. Comparative empirical bioethics of reproductive practices and their social contexts

IV. Intertwining knowledge practice, epistemology and ethics

Introduction – How Prenatal Diagnosis is Entangled in Historical and Social Contexts

Christina Schües

When reproductive medicine introduced prenatal testing and when genetics began to transform diagnosis and general prognoses into predictive genetics, genetic responsibility was introduced into bioethics and became the concern of (future) parents and affected persons. A country's biopolitics included these biomedical practices and became concerned with how states can evaluate and regulate genetic testing, and related questions of risk management. In order to better understand social and technological changes in the field of prenatal genetic diagnosis, their implications for the individual and society, and their cultural, philosophical and ethical meanings, a research project was funded by the Deutsche Forschungsgemeinschaft (DFG). Entitled *Meanings and Practices of Prenatal Genetics in Germany and Israel (PreGGI):*[1] *A comparative empirical and prospective study of the views and ethical concerns of users, non-users and providers of prenatal genetic services in their social and cultural contexts*, the project was conducted in 2017–2021 and led by Aviad Raz, Christoph Rehmann-Sutter and Christina Schües. The researchers thought that the emerging biomedical and social practices could best be studied through a comparative study of Israel and Germany. Such a cross-cultural approach is suited for giving insight into prac-

---

1   From 2017–2021, the PreGGI project was funded by the Deutsche Forschungsgemein-
     schaft (DFG, RE2951/3-1 and Schu2846/2-1). As one of the principal investigators of
     the project, as the editor of this book, and on behalf of the members (Aviad Raz,
     Christoph Rehmann-Sutter, Yael Hashiloni-Dolev, Hannes Foth, Tamar Nov-Klaiman,
     Anika König, Stefan Reinsch) of the research project, I would like to thank the DFG for
     their financial support of this research and publication. Furthermore, I am very grateful
     to Monica Buckland and Jackie Leach Scully for their careful language editing and help-
     ful comments. Lena Steimle deserves my thanks for her great assistance in handling
     the manuscript.

tices of prenatal genetic testing as well as differences and similarities in how they are implemented and understood.

This book about genetic responsibility grew out of that research project, using its results as the basis for further reflection to gain a deeper insight into the complex issue of prenatal genetics and how it is understood and implemented differently in Israel and Germany. The issues discussed include how innovations in prenatal diagnosis affect social relationships, and how prenatal genetic tests address moral questions and touch upon themes of eugenics and selection. Thus, the book assembles observations, interpretations and conversations from interdisciplinary angles across the social sciences, bioethics and philosophy, and with a comparative view of Israel and Germany.

The rise of new concepts and conditions

In modern medicine of the 20th and 21st centuries life, and elements of the beginning of life, are subject to a discourse of risk and security, as well as decision-making about who would be welcomed or who, prospectively, might be too burdensome for the parents, the family, or society, or considered to suffer too much. Since the notion of risk, and especially genetic risk, is at the centre of prenatal care, the guiding thread of this book is how issues of genetic responsibility are discussed in Germany and Israel. Considering these questions means opening up bioethics or biopolitics beyond the focus of prenatal genetic testing, to the ontology of the life sciences, the historical and cultural horizon of social norms and general values, and the perceptual practice and epistemic understanding that are equally, yet often only implicitly, involved in considerations and discussions.

Within the history of philosophy, responsibility is a rather young concept that has become more common from the 19th century. The growing complexities of the interrelation between humans, society and technology make responsibility an interesting and important notion because of its temporal, relational and multidimensional structure, which involves at a minimum the responsible person who performs an action or task with regard to another person, the addressee, according to prescriptive, normative criteria, within a particular realm of responsibilities and a certain time frame.

In the context of this book responsibility is taken mainly as a futural concept, yet it includes questions about retrospective responsibility, that is a responsibility directed toward the past and present. It is a question of how we care about the past, and so also about the future; how we care about other people, our offspring, and so also about society. The question of responsibility is traditionally directed at the shaping of interpersonal relationships and social conditions, at questions of the past, such as guilt, or questions of the future.

In the 1970s and '80s, prenatal genetic testing was established as part of pregnancy care, and with it the idea of genetic responsibility. Generally, responsibility as well as the more specific form of genetic responsibility concerns three areas: the legal area, which is the most strictly regulated and the narrowest, since it concerns the different laws and regulations. The political area of responsibility is the broadest, as besides policy making it also addresses the biopolitical discourses that are usually rather vigorous in Germany, for instance considering the question of whether non-invasive genetic testing should be financed by health insurance, and much calmer in Israel. The third area is ethics, probably the most difficult to understand. In addition to the very complex ethical concept of the responsibility to care for someone or something, the notion of genetic responsibility is already established in bioethical discourses of genetics and predictive genetic testing.

Relationships and the family are embedded in political, social and cultural practices, and norms of responsibility. Responsible acting is thus an ethical and political practice that is not simply there, but is characterised by a normative order and its dynamic transformation within a social and historical context. As well as the normative order of society, biomedical reproductive practices concern the social-ontological dimension of relationality, and the existential and temporal dimensions of plurality. These three dimensions are underpinned by the conviction that children are conceived within a particular normative, relational context, and that pregnancy and birth are not just a biomedical procedure but are shaped by a particular social, cultural, scientific and economic situation. Thus natality, the fact that humans are conceived and born by someone else, a woman, is central to the practices of reproduction and responsibility. Furthermore, natality is shaped according to the specific situations, relationships and society in which reproductive decisions take place. These dimensions inhere in all decisions concerning the foetus that may develop towards being born or being aborted during pregnancy.

Today's reproductive technologies and genetics show "what is about to be born" in advance (Löwy 2018: 1). The genetic disposition of the foetus can be tested and, according to genetic responsibility, *should* be tested. In prenatal diagnosis, invasive and non-invasive testing is differentiated. Invasive examinations involve intervening in the woman's body to take samples of the placenta (chorionic villus sampling), amniotic fluid (amniocentesis), or embryonic blood (cordocentesis). These samples are then examined for chromosomal defects or serious hereditary diseases. Invasive prenatal diagnostics are associated with risks to the pregnant woman or the foetus.

In contrast, with non-invasive prenatal diagnostics the risk to the pregnant woman or the foetus is much lower. Non-invasive prenatal diagnostics include ultrasound examinations, nuchal fold transparency measurement, and molecular genetic blood tests known as non-invasive prenatal tests (NIPT). This development in prenatal genetic testing – in particular the introduction and societal implementation of NIPT for chromosomal variations such as trisomies 13, 18 and 21 – change a morally and culturally complex practice of prenatal diagnosis in a variety of ways. These changes touch on fundamental ethical and philosophical questions about intergenerational relationships, pregnancy, and who should be born and why. With the introduction of NIPT in the Western world, medical testing of foetuses became even easier and more morally defensible for the (future) parents. Most of all, there is no risk to the foetus during the procedure.

In the course of NIPT, 10 ml of blood is drawn from the pregnant woman, containing the genetic information of the foetus in the form of cell-free DNA chromosome fragments as well as the DNA of the mother in her own cells. Subsequently, foetal and maternal blood components are detected, and the foetal components are isolated and analysed for trisomies 13, 18 and 21. It is also possible to determine the sex of the foetus. Further development of NIPT aims, for example, to detect microdeletion syndromes, i.e. the absence of small pieces of chromosomes. This condition can lead to heart defects and developmental delays. In 2012, the PraenaTest®, one of the first non-invasive molecular genetic blood tests, was introduced in Germany. NIPT has also been available in Israel from June 2013. Many other tests from different companies followed. In the meantime, the tests have become firmly established in Europe and the USA. The aim of all these examinations is to obtain the most accurate knowledge possible about diseases, such as heart defects, genetic predispositions to disability such as trisomies 13, 18 or 21, and other genetic mutations, such as Klinefelter syndrome. The examinations also reveal the sex of the foetus.

In view of these various test options, pregnancy care increasingly focuses on risk aspects and the possible termination of wanted pregnancies (Steger/ Orzechowski/Schochow 2018: 15). Since NIPT requires confirmation by amniocentesis, it is considered a "test" in Germany; in Israel it is included in the standard medical practice during pregnancy and can be chosen as part of the prenatal screening programme.

In Germany, prenatal diagnosis is differentiated into standard and additional examinations, some of which are not covered by health insurance and are considered something that should be a private expense. Standard examinations include three ultrasound examinations at the 10th, 20th and 30th weeks of pregnancy, as well as an examination of the abdomen and a blood sample to determine the normal course of the pregnancy (TAB 2019).[2] Additional tests include first-trimester screening with nuchal translucency measurement, NIPT, and the confirmatory and invasive procedures of chorionic villus sampling and amniocentesis, which can result in miscarriage in approximately 4 out of every 1000 tests. In Germany, it is estimated that more than 85 per cent of pregnant women with a positive test for trisomy 21 decide to have an abortion (TAB 2019: 12; Schidel 2020).

Shortly after the introduction of the first molecular genetic blood tests in Germany, the German Ethics Council gave its evaluation of the future of genetic diagnostics and its clinical application (Deutscher Ethikrat 2013; Steger et al. 2018). This evaluation states that the scope of genetic diagnostics is expected to expand in the future, and that the associated rapid increase in genetic information of each human being born will continue. The rapid and cost-effective availability of NIPT means that these tests are increasingly being considered as part of standard prenatal diagnostics. It is interesting to see that in Israel, NIPT is only one option within standard pregnancy care, yet it is not covered by health insurance. In general, critics warn about the medicalisation of pregnancy, which may lead to an increasing focus on the risk aspects of prenatal care and the termination of wanted pregnancies (TAB 2019: 168f.; Remennick 2006). Despite all the criticism, the use of NIPT in fact represents no risk for the pregnant woman, and prenatal detection of trisomies 13, 18 and 21 is improved. This leads to a reduction in invasive testing and, consequently, of miscarriages.

---

2   Bundesministerium für Gesundheit. Bekanntmachung eines Beschlusses des Gemeinsamen Bundesausschusses über eine Änderung der Mutterschafts-Richtlinien: Aufnahme einer Versicherteninformation zur Durchführung der Nicht-invasiven Pränataldiagnostik zur Bestimmung des Risikos autosomaler Trisomien 13, 18 und 21 mittels eines molekulargenetischen Tests (NIPT-Trisomie 13,18, 21) für die Anwendung bei Schwangerschaften mit besonderen Risiken vom: 19.08.2021, (https://www.bundesanzeiger.de/pub/de/amtliche-veroeffentlichung), accessed 10 July 2022.

Therefore, NIPT may be seen as a game changer in the field of prenatal genetic testing.

The social implementation of NIPT[3] as a technology that allows the testing of foetal DNA by testing the blood of the pregnant woman as early as 9 weeks after conception raises a series of different and difficult questions. With accuracy and scope of the tests improving, and costs decreasing, the German and Israeli healthcare systems are both currently implementing it in certain defined situations and for some conditions, yet they differ in how NIPT is implemented and also in the framework of reasoning used to justify it.

The focus on Germany and Israel

In recent decades, practices of and debates about prenatal genetic testing have resulted in heated controversies, an awareness of new routines and of aspects of producing a child that are now taken for granted. These controversies and normalities can best be brought out in a comparative study. When differences and similarities are brought to light, their conditions and implications, understandings and norms can be studied and evaluated. Israel and Germany are interesting countries for such studies because they take opposite directions in terms of what is permissible, how reproductive medicine and tests during pregnancy are experienced and viewed, and how practices are established and evaluated. The comparative setting of these two nations has already been established by Yael Hashiloni-Dolev (2010), Aviad Raz and Silke Schicktanz (2009, 2016). The two countries differ not only in moral and political terms but also in their geographical and historical situations. The juxtaposition of their painfully entangled histories and their different – almost opposite – regulations and politics on biomedicine at the beginning of life presents unique opportunities and challenges for sociological, bioethical and philosophical research in the 20th and 21st centuries.

The lessons learned from history are still an implicit or explicit part of bioethical and biopolitical discussions. In the German discourse, references to the historical dimension dominate – often implicitly – in public deliberation, in the form of a need to establish a distance from the inhuman practices of the National Socialist period and to avoid any resemblance to "selection" or

---

3   Now also referred to as Non-Invasive Prenatal Screening (NIPS) or cell-free DNA testing (cfDNA).

"eugenics", while emphasising the individual role of the pregnant woman and her right to an informed choice (Foth 2021). Meanwhile, in Israel's practice the different prenatal tests are well established, and are understood as empowering woman's choices, securing the life of the family, and enhancing the "health" of the Jewish collective body.

Israel and Germany are both countries with cutting-edge technology and very advanced healthcare systems; yet, to foreshadow a general thesis, Germany follows a *discourse of norms* that takes the notion of dignity as central. Different, and disputed, understandings of dignity and its role in different areas also provide the ethical legitimation of constitutional state democracy, including ideas of participation and freedom. Thus, ethical controversies and biopolitical questions about genetic tests are based on ongoing political and bioethical dispute about norms and their implementation in the practices of prenatal genetic testing. Israel, on the other hand, implements a *practice of normalisation* and holds the conviction that genetic diagnostic techniques may help to balance the responsibilities of human life and society's goods and qualities. The distinction between Jewish ethical positions, which are partially based on the hermeneutic of Jewish religious texts, and state regulations, is not perceived as being controversial. Here we see a genetic practice that is well established and normalised; therefore, there does not seem to be a reasonable basis for controversy.

It can be argued that both inclinations – the discourse of norms for Germany and the discourse of normalisation for Israel – follow a lesson learned from the 20th century's history and the atrocities of the Shoah: Never Again! The German Jewish political theorist Hannah Arendt tried to understand the Holocaust and, in 1961, reported on the trial of Adolf Eichmann in Jerusalem. This trial is generally seen as a significant moment in the public perception of the Holocaust. The eight-month trial, which ended with Eichmann's death sentence, was part of growing attention being paid to German crimes during National Socialism and, in particular, to the intention to exterminate European Jews. For the first time, a worldwide public was confronted with Jewish victims and witnesses of the Holocaust and their traumatic experiences. The focus of the trial in Jerusalem was not primarily the person of Eichmann and his deeds, but the history of the Jews under National Socialist rule itself. Both Israel and Germany adopted the conviction that this history must not be forgotten. "Politically speaking, the death factories did constitute a 'crime against humanity' committed on the bodies of the Jewish people" (Arendt 1946; see also Arendt 1965: 267f.). Arendt's report led to highly emotional disputes with Jewish intellectuals and was discussed beyond the Jewish community. In Arendt's understanding, the Holocaust could be interpreted in two ways: it was either a crime against the Jewish people, or a crime against humanity committed on the body of Jewish people. The second interpretation is the more universal one and includes the first one, but not the other way around. The distinction is important because the meaning of the famous dictum "Never Again!" changes depending on the interpretation. A "'Never again' crimes against the Jewish people" is different from "Never again crimes against humanity".

The concrete interpretations of "Never Again" are contrasting. Germany's concern is never again to be a perpetrator (*Täter*), which in the context of prenatal diagnosis means never-again-doing anything close to eugenics. The avoidance of biopolitical regulations or practices that could be connected to eugenics as pursued by the Nazi state still draws Germany's policy-making and bioethical discourses into normatively ambivalent regulations that avoid any reasoning on the basis of the foetus' wellbeing. In Israel however, "Never Again" usually means never again being a victim. Never being a victim again drives the urge to have power over one's own reproductive possibilities and, hence, a rather affirmative handling of reproductive technologies. Even though Israel is considered a secular state, biomedical ethics and bioethics are mainly considered within Jewish religion and traditions: more than half the population belong to Judaism, and one third describe themselves as religious. Overall, there is a pro-natal attitude anchored in religion (as in the book of Genesis: "be fruitful and multiply") as well as in the historical background of *society*: the intended extermination of the Jewish people during the time of Shoah, as well as the ongoing Arab-Israeli conflict, has produced the aspiration to secure the nation and promote a child-friendly policy. Having a large family compensates for the search for the Jewish homeland and for feelings of being uprooted. Family creates belonging and children mean life. Children are "the attempt to build a bridge to a better future," as psychologist Tali Gogol-Ostrowsky explains.[4] Thus, a birth rate of 3.1 among Israeli women, which is more than twice as high as in Germany, is not surprising. It is very common for Israeli women to use prenatal diagnostics when pregnant, not least because it is easily accessible and seen as part of "normal" prenatal care (Ravitsky et al. 2021; Zlotogora 2014).

---

4   Münch, Peter (2017) "Warum in Israel so viele Kinder geboren werden." For a different view about reproductive technological practices in Israel, see also Boas et al. (2018); Granek et al. (2017).

In one way or another, some chapters of this volume implicitly or explicitly refer to the observation that technological advances are approved of by the Jewish religion and by Israel's society because they are a means to an end: the preservation of Jewish values and family. Science may be used to overcome resistance from nature, in this case the occurrence of foetal diseases or of infertility. Biotechnological procedures such as prenatal diagnostics and IVF are also acceptable because of the ontological belief that a foetus only acquires the status of a human being after birth. According to the Talmud, before the 40th day of gestation the foetus is no more than "clear water".[5] As Larissa Remennick (2006: 46) points out, the central place of reproduction in the public agenda makes Israel an ideal "laboratory" for studying the social implications of reproductive and genetic technologies. Yet Germany could likewise also be described as a "laboratory" because of its anxieties and responsibilities for the past and its concerns about reproductive practices and options. Its regulations and bioethical concerns are distinctly different from those of other European countries. In Germany, some feminist and disability activists, conservatives and Roman Catholics are concerned that the use of technology leads to a blasphemous attempt to "play God", going against nature, discriminating against people with disabilities, or using eugenic methods that resemble the Nazi past. Thus, the individual decision, based on values and norms such as the value of life, dignity or free will, is the focus of bioethical discourses.

About the book and its four parts

Taking the countries' distinct differences and similarities as a point of departure, this book analyses the philosophical horizon, socio-cultural contexts, religious backgrounds, ethical and political key issues, and implications of the reproductive practices of both countries. Compiled as an interdisciplinary study, it presents a comparison between Israel and Germany from an empirical bioethical perspective and offering a transnational philosophical reconsideration of the historical, social and biomedical contexts. Combining comparative empirical bioethics with systematic philosophical reflection, this book introduces an interdisciplinary and transnational *conversation* to the field of biomedical ethical research. Looking at two very different cultural settings, biopolitical practices and social imaginaries, we find the distance needed to

---

5   For an empirical study see Rimon-Zarfaty et al. (2011).

understand both the other and ourselves, the unfamiliar and our own practice. Taking the specific topic of NIPT as our focus allows us to start a conversation between the experiences and observations, disciplines and backgrounds of these countries. Using conversation as a method enables the researchers to do comparative empirical work but also share their observations and self-reflections with each other, and to communicate and reflect across disciplinary and national boundaries. Conversation has thus created a third space within which ideas, experiences or arguments are addressed from different personal, philosophical, cultural or social perspectives.

The book is organised into four dimensions, presenting different methodological themes and approaches, and allowing for different ways of having conversations and different levels of abstraction. The first, rather theoretical dimension addresses historical and philosophical perspectives in terms of the entanglement between forms of the *biomedical rationalisations of "life", reproduction and responsibility*. In his chapter *Biological reproduction, offspring, and radical otherness, Burkhard Liebsch* explores the shaping of "life" by the biomedical approach of the life sciences, and considers the claims of responsibility within their epistemic horizons. The practice of genetic testing of the foetus focuses sharply on the biological substrate, the carrier of the genetic information. The biologisation of the foetus, human reproduction, and human generativity, as current reproductive technology presupposes, has particular prerequisites, such the focus on humans as organisms, that we all come from living cells, and also that questions of reproduction and risk are thought in terms of the recombination of cells. But then, how can we understand the "future"? As an irreversible future of mother and child, or a "radical future"? Or a future of "Never Again" (as Natan Sznaider thematises in his commentary)? Considering the future and reproduction in modern medicine leads to *Christina Schües*'s chapter on the *Origins and practices of genetic risk and responsibility*. This concerns the historical and social entanglement of genetic risk and genetic responsibility, and re-evaluates the political and ethical understanding of responsibility, non-responsibility and irresponsibility in light of the biopolitical regime and perceptual practices in Israel and Germany.

The second, more concrete dimension of *Governance and biopolitics* compares Israel and Germany in a straightforward way in terms of their policies, regulations and norms. In both countries, as *Tamar Nov-Klaiman, Hannes Foth* and *Yael Hashiloni-Dolev* show in their policy analysis, key decisions related to NIPT were made only recently. In 2019, NIPT was submitted to the Israeli "health basket" committee to be considered for public funding, where it competed against other technologies and drugs in the context of a limited budget. Following evaluation of all submitted items, funding for NIPT was rejected. Consequently, NIPT has not been adopted by the statutory health insurance and is not publicly funded. Since 2019, all invasive tests in Israel have been coupled with chromosomal microarray analysis, which enables a high-throughput analysis of genotyping and gene expression, and has a higher detection rate than standard karyotyping that provides only a genome-wide snapshot of an individual's chromosomes. In 2021, the German Federal Joint Committee (*Gemeinsamer Bundesausschuss GB-A*) developed new regulations for the coverage of NIPT in health insurance, and the officially recommended procedures in prenatal care (*Mutterschaftsrichtlinie*). The result is that from spring 2022 NIPT has been covered by health insurance (although only on a case-by-case basis, taking into account the situation of the pregnant woman and not of the foetus); yet its implementation has been accompanied by concerns and criticism.

The authors of the next two chapters present the individual positions of the two countries, before meeting for a conversation about their respective insights. In *Health services and uptake in cultural context* in Israel, *Aviad Raz* discusses the different health services that are available and how they are embedded in the cultural and historically influenced horizon. *Moral concerns and consumer choice* in Germany is the theme of the chapter by *Kathrin Braun* and *Sabine Könninger*. They discuss the ambivalence of German discourse between public concern about preproductive practices that involve selective decisions about which children should be born, on the one hand, and the increasing routinisation of genetic testing, on the other. Both the details of *Policymaking in Germany and Israel* they describe and the jointly written comment by *Braun, Könninger* and *Raz* on the different concerns show that in many respects, the regulation of and cultural attitudes towards genetic and reproductive medicine in Israel and Germany are contrary to one another. The general idea of presenting the chapters in this specific order and inviting the authors to comment on each other led to conversations between the authors, and should also inspire implicit conversations with the readers.

The third section focuses on themes from the angle of comparative empirical bioethics. Each chapter of this section discusses one particular thematic area and presents a particular methodological approach to comparing the social context of Israel and Germany. The comparative empirical study conducted a total of 42 semi-structured interviews in Germany and 52 in Israel. Interviewees included health professionals specialising in obstetrics and gynaecology and/or genetics, disability activists, women without unusual medical family history, and parents or other close family members of children with Down syndrome. The interviews were conducted in Hebrew and in German. They were transcribed, and key parts were translated into English, so they could be interpreted and discussed by the Israeli-German team.

For the cross-cultural comparative work, it was important to focus empirically on a set of more narrowly defined questions. Working from the Israeli and German interviews, *Tamar Nov-Klaiman, Marina Frisman, Aviad E. Raz* and *Christoph Rehmann-Sutter* brought out the different views and concerns of families with Down syndrome, their understanding of discrimination, and the attitudes of parents of children with Down syndrome towards NIPT. One commentator from Israel and one from Germany was invited to discuss, from their specific social context, the meaning of prenatal diagnosis for people with disabilities. The perspective of disability studies, contributed by *Swantje Köbsell* from Germany, is very hesitant about genetic testing, while the Israeli disability activist *Rachel Lishansky* tells her personal story of having a child with Down syndrome. These approaches stand as examples of the different social and cultural contexts that need to be taken into account when considering prenatal diagnosis and disability.

The Israeli and German researchers *Christoph Rehmann-Sutter, Tamar Nov-Klaiman, Anika König, Stefan Reinsch, Yael Hashiloni-Dolev* and *Aviad Raz* ask: what does prenatal testing mean for women who used the test? This question involved extensive discussion in the team about the interviews and how they can be understood from the different cultural and social angles of the research. The aim of this chapter is to bring out the different ways of making sense of genetic testing, and to show how the women who had used it interpreted their own choice. For example, one German woman said that she had NIPT/PND in order to be prepared for the birth of a child with special needs, while an Israeli woman wanted to do everything right and according to her physician's suggestions.

These concrete empirical insights show that pregnancy and the beginning of life has become a morally challenging project that demands many decisions from the parents-to-be, each of which must be made with careful deliberation and moral reflection. The distinct national laws and cultural contexts therefore demand a specific type of "genetic responsibility", as well as care responsibility from expectant parents and pregnant women. Israel and Germany are seen as two political entities, as cultures and as constellations of practices, and each is a melting pot of secular or religious, national or international ethical discourses.

Although Israel is considered to be a Jewish state, both Israel and Germany can also be considered non-religious states. Yet religion still plays an important role in policy-making, public opinion, and the personal decision-making of (future) parents, although the roles are different with respect to pregnancy, family, and matters of life and death. All this results dynamically in concrete, yet very different, cultural settings, medical practices and social understandings of what constitutes responsible prenatal care.

Regardless of whether a pregnant woman tests or not, she always has her social context. This context, as well as the overall discussion about prenatal genetic testing, is framed by religious traditions, beliefs and authorities. In order to find out more about the different religious horizons, *Anne Weber* and *Christina Schües* initiated a conversation between the German Catholic theologian and philosopher *Hille Haker* and the Israeli ethnographer and anthropologist *Tsipy Ivry*, whose research focuses on the interrelation between Jewish religion and new reproductive technologies. They share their insights into different socio-cultural and religious views in Israel and Germany, and the social and religious practices and reasonings, concerning the use of reproductive or reprogenetic technology, taking into account the different histories, political circumstances and religious beliefs about the family, relationships and children. The question of who is or is not allowed into the human community highlights the importance of the Christian church and the rabbis. The following chapter turns the conversation to another setting. In a review of two films, the Israeli film *Week 23* (שבוע) and the German film *24 Wochen*, *Christoph Rehmann-Sutter* and *Christina Schües* discuss the familial and social contexts of prenatal genetic testing and, most importantly, female intuition and ambivalence towards medical knowledge.

Conversations about sense-making, about different beliefs, religious, social or cultural settings, and the comparison of the two films show that it is necessary to examine the *intertwining of knowledge practice, epistemology and ethics*. Thus, the fourth dimension of the book reconsiders particular historical and philosophical horizons of prenatal genetic testing in Israel and Germany and shows how the empirical sciences work together, thematically and methodologically. An overall aim of several chapters of the book is to understand how diverging meanings of medical practices of prenatal genetic testing are entrenched in familial and social settings, the human condition, and understandings of responsibility. If, traditionally, when children are born, their physical traits are accepted unconditionally, and if it was – at least implicitly – assumed that the parent-child relationship is characterised by unconditional bonding, then the question arises of whether such "unconditionality" will be transformed by prenatal genetic diagnosis. This is discussed by *Hannes Foth* through concrete prenatal genetic practices in Israel and Germany. He shows how philosophical scrutiny may interact with concrete observations in a way that can lay the ground for future questions. There are urgent questions to address about whether human life, value or dignity should depend on bio- logical disposition or social performance. More and more children are born on condition that prenatal genetic tests are negative and that other people, at least the parents – of course without having obtained the child's consent – already know their genetic disposition, at least partially. Meanwhile, scientists are discussing the expansion of NIPT to NIPW – whole-genome sequencing. This seems possible technically, although not yet economically feasible, and philosophically it opens up a new shift in the paradigm of genetic testing.

There are women who do not want to know and who do not want to test. This observation prompts us to reconsider the concept of not-knowing, a concept that, philosophically and scientifically, has a bad reputation. Yet for prenatal genetic practices, it is not only interesting but also philosophically stimulating to sort out the "other side" of choice, of normality, or of routine. *Christina Schües*, *Stefan Reinsch*, *Aviad Raz* and *Christoph Rehmann-Sutter* discuss conceptually and empirically the phenomenon of not wanting to know, and whether it is irresponsible not to know genetic risks in advance (which one Israeli woman clearly suggested in her interview). Not-knowing is not simply the opposite of knowing, but has its own rational structure and ontological, epistemic and social status. As several conversations seem to suggest, in Israel prenatal testing is normal and standard, and may even be considered a social requirement, whereas in Germany such assurance and "normality" of NIPT seems less common. Thus, the meaning of not-knowing oscillates culturally and socially, changing with the communicative and social context.

Towards the end of the "PreGGI" project, some members of the research team felt a strong urge to write about what they had actually done. The last chapter is therefore devoted to questions of the methodological approaches, interdisciplinary and transnational conversations, and what it means to think through different differences. Readers of this book may find our paths of doing so an enrichment for their own future studies or observations.

This book about responsibility contributes to an ongoing philosophical, so- ciological and ethical discussion about the prenatal genetic diagnostics and in- tergenerational responsibility.

Thus, it will enrich and inspire a range of debates in bioethics, social philosophy, sociology of biomedicine, and medical anthropology. It shows that concepts of ethics and epistemics are not absolute, but dynamic, socially contextualised, historically inspired, and formed by technically produced paradigms of perception. Ultimately, it may well be that it is not the application of a particular technology that reveals differences between practices, cultures or countries, but how they are justified and what is considered good reasons for their use.

References

Arendt, Hannah (1946): "The Black Book: The Nazi Crime Against the Jewish People; and Hitler's Professors, by Max Weinreich." Book reviews. In: Commentary Magazine, September, (https://www.commentary.org/artic les/hannah-arendt/the-black-book-the-nazi-crime-against-the-jewish-p eople-and-hitlers-professors-by-max-weinreich/), accessed 10 July 2022.

Arendt, Hannah (1965): Eichmann in Jerusalem: Report on the Banality of Evil, New York: Viking Press.

Boas, Hagai/Hashiloni-Dolev, Yael/Davidovitch, Nadav/Filc, Dani/Lavi, Shai J. (eds.) (2018): Bioethics and Biopolitics in Israel: Socio-legal, Political, and Empirical Analysis, Cambridge: Cambridge University Press.

Deutscher Ethikrat (2013): "The future of genetic diagnosis – from research to clinical practice." Opinion. Berlin: Deutscher Ethikrat, (https://www.ethik rat.org/en/publications/kategorie/opinions), accessed 10 July 2022.

Foth, Hannes (2021): "Avoiding 'selection'? – References to history in current German policy debates about non-invasive prenatal testing." In: Bioethics, 35/6, pp. 518–527, (https://onlinelibrary.wiley.com/doi/full/10.1111/bioe.12 880), accessed 10 July 2022.

Granek et al. (2017): "Women and health in Israel." In: The Lancet 389/10088, pp. 2575–2578.

Hashiloni-Dolev, Yael (2010): A Life (Un)Worthy of Living. Reproductive Genetics in Israel and Germany, Dordrecht: Springer.

Löwy, Ilana (2018): Tangled Diagnoses: Prenatal Testing, Women, and Risk, Chicago: University of Chicago Press.

Münch, Peter (2017) "Warum in Israel so viele Kinder geboren werden." In: Süddeutsche Zeitung, 6 January 2017, (https://www.sueddeutsche.de/leb en/geburtenrate-warum-in-israel-so-viele-kinder-geboren-werden-1.332 0566), accessed 10 July 2022.

Ravitsky, Vardit/Roy, Marie-Christine/Haidar, Hazar/Henneman, Lidewij/ Marshall, John/Newson, Ainsley J./Ngan, Olivia M.Y./Nov-Klaiman, Tamar (2021): "The Emergence and Global Spread of Noninvasive Prenatal Testing." In: Annual Review of Genomics and Human Genetics 22, pp. 309–38 (https://doi.org/10.1146/annurev-genom-083118-015053), accessed 10 July 2022.

Raz, Aviad/Schicktanz, Silke (2009): "Lay perceptions of genetic testing in Germany and Israel: The interplay of national culture and individual experience." In: New Genetics and Society 28/4, pp. 401–414.

Raz, Aviad/Schicktanz, Silke (2016): Comparative Empirical Bioethics: Dilemmas of Genetic Testing and Euthanasia in Israel and Germany, Dordrecht: Springer 2016.

Raz, Aviad/Nov-Klaiman, Tamar/Hashiloni-Dolev, Yael/Foth, Hannes/Schües, Christina/Rehmann-Sutter, Christoph (2021): "Comparing Germany and Israel regarding debates on policy-making at the beginning of life: PGD, NIPT and their paths of routinization." In: Ethik in der Medizin, pp. 1–16, (h ttps://link.springer.com/article/10.1007/s00481-021-00652-z), accessed 10 July 2022.

Remennick, Larissa (2006): "The Quest for the Perfect Baby: Why Do Israeli Women Seek Prenatal Genetic Testing?" In: Sociology of Health & Illness 28/1, pp. 21–53.

Rimon-Zarfaty Nizan/Raz Aviad E./Hashiloni-Dolev Yael (2011): When does a fetus become a person? An Israeli viewpoint. In: J Fam Plann Reprod Health Care. Oct. 37/4, pp. 216–24.

(https://srh.bmj.com/content/37/4/216), accessed 10 July 2022.

Schidel, Regina (2020): "'Disabled lives matter' – Diskriminierung behinderter Menschen durch Pränataltestung?" (https://www.praefaktisch.de/diskri minierung/diabled-lives-matter-diskriminierung-behinderter-mensche n-durch-praenataltestung/), accessed 10 July 2022.

Steger, Florian/Orzechowski, Marcin/Schochow, Maximilian (eds.) (2018): Pränatalmedizin: Ethische, juristische und gesellschaftliche Aspekte, Freiburg/Munich: Alber.

TAB (Büro für Technikfolgen-Abschätzung beim Deutschen Bundestag) (2019): "Aktueller Stand und Entwicklungen der Pränataldiagnostik." Arbeitsbericht 184 (https://www.tab-beim-bundestag.de/projekte_aktueller-sta nd-und-entwicklungen-der-praenataldiagnostik.php), accessed 10 July 2022.

Zlotogora, Joël (2014): "Genetics and genomic medicine in Israel." In: Molecular Genetics & Genomic Medicine 2/2, pp. 85–94.

I. Biomedical rationalisations of "life", reproduction and responsibility?
Historical, social and ethical perspectives

1. Biological Reproduction, Offspring, and Radical Otherness

Burkhard Liebsch

Today we are confronted with a huge mass of literature on bioethics, biomedicine, biopolitics, and biotechnical issues – rubrics under which problems of human reproduction are regularly treated as the epistemological object of the life sciences. The technical term "reproduction" refers by way of abstraction to the complex of human sexuality and gender, fertility, pregnancy, birth, parenting and the forms of life in which offspring are taken care of (cf. Almond 1988; Liebsch 2001; Boelderl 2006; Schües 2008, 2016/17; Liebsch 2016). The life sciences are therefore at least indirectly related to human relations between persons, their love, their successive, interconnected and divergent filiations and histories.

In view of the fact that the human species evolved over thousands of years from its pre-human predecessors, it is astonishing that key factors of human reproduction such as the fertilization of sperm and egg cell were not discovered until the late 19th century, when Oscar Hertwig demonstrated (in 1876) how it works in sea urchins. Since then, the life sciences have had a largely uncontested authority in matters of human reproduction. Today, they seem to have the final say when it comes to the question of how exactly human reproduction "works," how it can fail and how it could be optimized, and so on.

This holds true in spite of the obvious fact that the life sciences often present themselves in unfamiliar terms which, consequently, must be translated to the public, who are normally incapable of understanding sophisticated bio-technical concepts adequately. While – for example – the abbreviation DNA (deoxyribonucleic acid) and the term *genetic code* are well known, the public associates them with more or less naïve ideas about human heredity, about genes as bio-chemical mechanisms of "encoding" or determining parental "traits," and about the technical devices for rearranging them in order to enhance or prevent expected outcomes... In contrast to what most people may think, DNA is not "written" in a linear fashion so as to be "readable" and to be "edited" like a book (cf. Blumenberg 1986; Kay 2005). Only in very specific cases do genes predetermine phenotypic outcomes. Even an identical set of genotypic material normally unfolds into quite different histories of individual human beings... In spite of obvious problems in adequately "translating" concepts and results of the life sciences into lay understandings of human reproduction, ordinary people are left with the task of uncovering how our current knowledge works, fails, or misleads.

This raises the question of where philosophical reflection on human reproduction can (and perhaps must) make a distinctive contribution (cf. Canguilhem 1974 [1942/1996]: 150). Must it, too, succumb to the authority of the life sciences, acknowledge and recognize that authority without qualification (cf. Böhme 1980; Feyerabend 1981)? Should it confine itself to problems that arise in the application of biomedical and biotechnical knowledge to the life world of human beings who, in their more or less naïve way of "reproducing" themselves, have at best an inadequate understanding of their fertility? Or should it assist them in their resistance to the "colonialization" of the life-world through the supreme power of biological and medical knowledge, that demands that such knowledge must be properly applied and thus that our generative relations should be rationalized in every respect – in spite of the fact that "c'est hors des laboratoires que les vivants croient vivre d'une vie dont ils ne savent pas tous qu'au laboratoire elle a perdu sa vie avec son secret. C'est hors des laboratoires que l'amour, la naissance et la mort continuent à présenter aux vivants, enfants de l'ordre et du hasard, les figures immémoriales de ces questions que la science des vivants ne pose plus désormais à la vie" ("It is outside laboratories that the living continue to believe they live a life, not all of them being aware that life itself has lost its life and mystery in the laboratory. Outside the laboratory, love, birth and death continue to present to the living, these children of order and chance, the timeless figures of these questions, which the science of the living today no longer poses to life" (Canguilhem 1971: 25).

To be sure, the relations between knowledge and the life-world, epistemology, and being in the world are not that simple. They do not simply pose the question of mere application or of subjugation... This becomes obvious when we take into account the readiness with which many people are willing to understand themselves and their offspring as biological creatures who should abide by the laws that seem to determine the *lógos* of human forms of life (*bíoi*) everywhere. In this respect, Aldous Huxley's dystopic vision of a despotic government that controls the reproduction of its underlings misses the point, insofar as people are willing to submit, paradoxically, to the "self-chosen diktat" that human fertility should be the object of willed, biologically rationalized production and reprogramming (Bernard 2014: 443).

In the following discussion, I confine myself to identifying basic ontological assumptions that are implicitly at work in the lay understanding of human reproduction, insofar as it orients itself to a (more or less naïve) concept of what people believe to be the "laws" of the biological realm.

The fact that we can and (ultimately) must understand ourselves as biological beings goes without saying for almost everybody. However, biology is a neologism that did not come into use in Europe until the first decade of the 19th century, when it was adopted by authors such as Jean B. Lamarck, Gottfried R. Treviranus, and Friedrich Burdach (Klein 1954; Canguilhem et al. 1960; Jacob 1972; Lepenies 1978). Prepared by forerunners of Charles Darwin and Alfred R. Wallace (Glass, Temkin and Straus 1959), a biological and evolutionary understanding of human life in every respect rapidly began to dominate even political and especially state-centred thought – at times with disastrous consequences (Engels 1995; Claeys 2000). While it seemed to *become "self-evident"* that we *are* biological beings, it was forgotten that this is a matter of human self-understanding. In the preface to his *Phenomenology of Perception* (1945) Maurice Merleau-Ponty drew his readers' attention to this basic insight: We can be *interpreted as* biological beings, but we *are* not *"in fact"* to be equated with such creatures (Merleau-Ponty 1945: v). While several philosophers – from Wilhelm Dilthey and Helmuth Plessner to Hans Jonas – have rightly insisted that we need a hermeneutics of life that pays tribute to the contestable understanding of human beings *as* biological organisms, we find that the significance of the hermeneutic latitude indicated by this "as" is very often simply forgotten (Jonas 1973; Plessner 1975; Rodi and Lessing 1984).

Here, I cannot try to uncover the profound reasons for this result. Instead, I presuppose that we have to start by accepting that it is now largely uncontested that we are biological beings and that our generative relations must be conceptualized, possibly reconstructed, and even eventually refigured as biological relations in keeping with the laws of life. Seen this way, it is *the result of our cultural history* that a biological self-image of human beings is prevalent today.

This is not to say this self-image is exclusively dominant. On the contrary: there are many signs of dissension, contradiction, and conflict. Some bemoan that intervening in human generativity will eventually dethrone God as the supreme creator. Others claim that such an endeavour is "against nature", and anticipate the horrors of the planned, serial fabrication of human beings (Bernard 2014: 197). Less frightened, others ask sensitively and mournfully – as if already remembering a past that is lost forever – whether there is no difference between the "cool" fusion of cells in a laboratory and the passionate intercourse between human beings in their direct, personal encounters (ibid: 378, 435).

Ironically, it is precisely this seemingly "romantic" understanding of human generativity that ultimately puts it down to "dialogical" relations, normally heterosexual, between human beings, which has gained support in at least one important respect from modern biology. In striking contrast to former conceptions of creation such as Nicolas Malebranche's (cf. Liebsch 1997: ch. 3; Bernard 2014: 37), modern epigenetic theories from the late 18th century onwards (Blumenbach 1830: 14; Bernard 1878: 316; Temkin 1950) have made it plain that fertilization and the ontogenetic development that it engenders does not simply make visible a preformed entity; rather, it must be understood as the *original production* of a new living being (Needham 1934; Löw 1980: 101; Lenoir 1981, 1982; Gould 1985; Bernard 2014: 42, 50).

Each time, we are dealing with a new creation – out of biological material, to be sure, provided by a human couple who instigate the unforeseeable production of a new human being whose future possibility cannot be reduced to what seemed to be possible before (Richards 1987). Thus, this human being is "made possible" (*ermöglicht*) without ever being simply the result of causal predetermination or of a plan, as the template of the future of one *another*. It was primarily Henri Bergson who heralded the philosophical implications of this specifically modern understanding of the emergence of the *irreducibly new* (Bergson 1907), closely related to American pragmatism (Charles S. Peirce, William James, James M. Baldwin, etc.) and to the genetic epistemology upon which, in turn, Jean Piaget predicated his biological theory of knowledge (Liebsch 1992), before Emmanuel Levinas referred to Henri Bergson in his conception of a "radical" future that cannot be anticipated as it irreversibly divides parents and offspring (Levinas 1947: 63).

This connection between the notion of a "radical" future that cannot be de-futurized is closely linked to the history of modern biology. At the same time, it has changed our understanding of human generativity in an unforeseen manner which is relevant to our present situation. Taking this connection into account warns us not to believe that the aforementioned challenges to a comprehensive biologisation of the human self-image that has recourse to

God, nature or the dialogical character of human relations could simply draw on a previous non-biological model.

The same objection that advocates of the "primacy of the social" have to face when they contest the authority of the life sciences in all respects also has to do with human generativity. No clear-cut notion of "the social" was available before modern biological thought launched its astounding career, reaching a climax in the 20th century (Röttgers 1996; Liebsch 2018: ch. 1). If the authority of the life sciences regarding human generativity is nevertheless not indisputable, the question arises as to what alternatives could otherwise be considered.

I propose here to draw on the resources of human negativity. While the hegemony of biological, bioethical and biotechnical thought cannot be denied, it would be an exaggeration to claim that it dominates us with no resistance. The triumph of the biological, bioethical and biotechnical is not yet complete. In spite of the widespread eagerness to understand problems of life and living, death and dying, primarily as matters of biology, in the life world it collides with heterogenous understandings of what it means to live, to be alive, to live a liveable life, and to promise others such a life. By "others" I have in mind offspring who cannot (before their conception) be asked by their progenitors whether or not they would accept being "thrown" into the world as it currently presents itself.

For Immanuel Kant, and many others who follow the same lines today, this most basic insight acts as a gatekeeper for any debate about human generativity. Every debate circling around related questions will concern future human beings who cannot be asked for their agreement or consent as regards their future existence under conditions that to a great extent are inevitably unforeseeable. According to Levinas, the "grand scandale de la condition humaine" ("the great scandal of the human condition") is "que nous n'avons pas choisi notre naissance" ("that we have not chosen our birth" Levinas 2009: 109, 156). In a Kantian perspective it directly follows that every person directly or indirectly responsible for the future existence of others is accountable (Habermas 2002). Paradoxically, this accountability refers to others who do not yet exist and cannot hold anyone accountable at all. When this becomes possible, many others who in turn would have to give account to them can no longer be called to account for what they have done or refrained from doing...

I cannot go into the details of the complicated time-structure of human responsibility and accountability in terms of human generativity here (cf. Abe 2017). Instead, I shall focus on several implications of the widespread biologisation of human generativity that seem particularly to provoke objections – thus indicating how human negativity resists the hegemony of a biological, bioethical and biotechnical mentality – without relying on a notion of God, nature or society that was allegedly previously available.

The *biologisation of human generativity* rests on the following *basic tenets*:

(1) Human beings are organisms and, thus, composed of cells, the basic units of biology.

(2) *Omnis cellula e cellula* (Bernard 2014: 68). The origin of cells is the division of pre-existing cells. In other words: *Omne vivum ex vivo* – at times translated as follows: "Every living thing comes from a living thing." The physiologist Rudolf Virchow and his predecessors extended this to state that the only source for a living cell was another living cell.

(3) Consequently, as regards sexual reproduction, modern biology confines itself once and for all to the level of organic material that is capable of fusion, fertilization, division and multiplication. Thus, sexual reproduction and descent are understood as a question of recombination of biological "things" (ultimately, chromosomes, triplets of nitrogenous bases...) – severed from sexual relations between persons and their generative, familial and generational perspectives such as motherhood, fatherhood, childhood.

Consequently, the recombination, manipulation and quasi-industrial handling of human reproduction has become possible. *Reproduction itself seems to be reproducible* via willed, biochemical intervention by "third" subjects, who are technically able to produce human beings in test tubes *in vitro...* so that "partners" as subjects of human generativity are no longer necessary. The production of human beings in laboratories is simply a matter of transforming infrastructures of "something," i.e. cells (determined by chromosomes), into living beings.

Human life, however, can only be *initiated* in laboratories. Its inevitably historical "development" can only take place in forms of life where it is taken care of as the life not of "something" but, rather, of *somebody*. Therefore, any previous biological "abstraction" from the context of social forms of life where motherhood, fatherhood and childhood take shape must be re-embedded in their generative horizons.

Currently, any such attempt to re-embed a biological understanding of human reproduction faces serious difficulties since the destabilization of traditional concepts such as begetting (*Zeugung*) with the necessity of heterosexual relations, of their fertility, of their community and of the very relatedness that was commonly held to manifest itself in familial relationships of motherhood, fatherhood, and childhood.

This destabilization does not lend itself to the "rehabilitation" of a traditionality that would simply reject the modern biologisation of human reproduction altogether. On the contrary, it forces us to take human reproduction seriously by negating what seems to be "unacceptable," to the extent that this biologisation amounts not just to a reduction but rather to a downright *reductionism* of human generativity.

It cannot be denied that it is possible to understand human beings *as* organisms, that is, as living "things" determined by chromosomes, self-regulatory homeorhetic mechanisms etc. Unacceptable reductionism, however, results from this if we forget the hermeneutic "as" that inevitably comes into play here. Something that can be understood "as" something else, is, precisely for this reason, not identical with this something else.

The denial of a reductionist understanding of human generativity leads us, by way of negation, to the following propositions:

(1) Biological cell theory, prenatal testing of chromosomes and genes, and techniques of fertilization refer directly to "living things"; indirectly, however, they refer to the future of children, that is, of others whose otherness proves to be unforeseeable. The "authentic future" (Levinas) of others cannot validly be subjected to defuturisation.

(2) It is nevertheless reasonable to expect that these future children will normally be able to relate to their own life as the life of somebody (not something), and to those people who are directly or indirectly responsible for its inception (Esposito 2017: 15) in order to "check back" about the origin and causes of and reasons for their conception, their "being welcomed" (or neglected...), their being cared for (more or less adequately...), being acknowledged and accepted, etc. (or abandoned...).

(3) These and related questions pivot around the central problem that confronts the unforeseeable life of an "other": whether or not it is possible to live a life that proves to be really *"liveable"*. What counts as a "liveable life" (Butler 2009) depends on every individual's own judgement. (Kant was already keenly aware of this. The most basic question regarding human generativity, he wrote in his *Critique of Judgement* (1977: 394), is whether or not a future human being will be "content" with his or her existence – in spite

of its very finitude and mortality, that is [we could add], in spite of being exposed to pain, injury and vulnerability, to misfortune and violence of all sorts.)

(4) Seen this way, the yardstick of any decision to "have a baby," to "reproduce" oneself in one's offspring, to augment one's people, to strengthen its biopolitical potential, and therefore to intervene in someone's biological constitution, etc. is an anticipated responsibility in the retrograde perspective of somebody who does not yet exist and who will be an "other" – in the most radical sense philosophy has to offer, to be sure, that is, in the sense of a *radical otherness* that is paradoxically "other than itself" without remaining the same and without being sublatable in a dialectics of identity (Ricœur 1990: ch. 10).

(5) That every human individual is an "other" in this "strong sense" cannot, however, be demonstrated or proven. We can only *testify to* this (cf. Ricœur 1994 [1972]; Liebsch 2012) – and how the promise to vouch for the radical alterity of the other in practical life is kept or betrayed – thus objecting to any "appropriation" of human life through the seemingly sovereign power of progenitors, peoples or the state that wants to capitalize on its biopolitical resources.[1]

---

1   Cf. Birenbaum-Carmeli (2010). The author draws attention to "the outstanding importance that the state [of Israel] attributes to genetic reproduction. Additionally, the admission of practically every woman, without any screening, to funded care conveys the state's view that any genetic family formation is solid and competent enough to comprise a favourable living environment for the baby that it helps to create. This inclusive policy has often been attributed by researchers to the Biblical commandment 'Be fruitful and multiply' and to the impact of the Holocaust trauma and the state's demographic interest in Jewish growth. However, these motivations to expand the local Jewish population could in principle be fulfilled by social kinning as well. After all, adopted children, including ones adopted abroad, are converted into Judaism and count as full Jewish Israeli citizens. This line of argumentation thus provides no explanation for the state preference for genetic relatedness" (2010: 81). Birenbaum-Carmeli then offers an explanation for this discrepancy in political terms: "[The] blood-based definition mythically connects contemporary Jewish Israelis to Biblical times. As such it can be tacitly embedded into political territorial claims to *eretz avotenu*, the 'land of our forefathers.' Now, if the pursuit of genetic kinship is an element in substantiating the state's geopolitical claims, then the import of genetic kinship transcends the domain of family relations, to the survival of the historical/mythical collectivity as a political vehicle. Possibly, it is an interest in this 'resource,' the genetic 'essence' of the Jewish collectivity, that may account for the sharp dichotomy between full state support to technologies that aim to accomplish genetic kinship and complete denial of state sup-

(6) That we feel obliged to testify to the radical otherness of any other must be understood as a lesson to be learned from the biopolitical power that reached its zenith in Nazi ideology (cf. Liebsch 2019). The negativity of this historical experience motivates our objections to any reductionist treatment of human life as a matter of technical reproduction. It might be helpful for limited purposes to *understand* human life *as* reproducible. In doing so, however, we run the risk of "forgetting" that this may amount to a fatal reductionism that would ultimately eliminate any radical alterity (Esposito 2017: 58) between generations, generative subjects and offspring.

In a thesis like this, the assertion that "we" feel obliged to testify to the radical alterity of the other may appear highly contestable. Therefore, in the final section of my outline of relations between biological reproduction, offspring, and radical otherness I wish to briefly draw attention to a couple of questions that such a claim raises.

Who is this "we"? To whom does it refer? Only to those of us who keep in mind the history of Nazi biopolitics in a way that arouses such a feeling of obligation? Or does an obligation to testify to the radical alterity of the other exist irrespective of our remembrance and our feelings? Is it plausible to maintain that decades of intense historiographic documentation of this type of biopolitics have led to the conclusion that the radical alterity of the other "in fact" evades any access and denies any appropriation? If this were the case, any demand to respect the alterity of the other would seem superfluous. To insist on such a demand would – in contrast – imply that the otherness of the other cannot itself effectively resist any form of violence (cf. Liebsch 2017).

These questions refer to a crossover of history and social philosophy – implying either that historical experience teaches us which consequences should be drawn in terms of a theory of alterity, or that we have to gather from a social philosophy of alterity how the documented historical experience should be interpreted. However, it is quite clear that there is no well-established area of cooperation between social philosophy and history. The two disciplines follow

---

port from those routes that breach the genetic paradigm and aim for social kinship" (ibid: 82). – Yael Hashiloni-Dolev offers a historical explanation for the stark interest in strengthening the "essence" of the Israeli people: "[C]enturies of living in hostile societies led to a strengthening of family ties and obligations," and "fears of extinction translate[d] into pro-natalism" that seeks to secure the "essence" by way of biological multiplication (2018: 123).

largely different tracks – even though, to look only at the philosophical side, the work of many authors – from Hannah Arendt, Günther Anders, Emmanuel Levinas, Maurice Blanchot, Hans Jonas, and Sarah Kofman to Zygmunt Bauman and Edith Wyschogrod (to mention only a few) – appears to be imbued with the dark negativity of a historical disaster from which human reason has not yet recovered and from which it may well never recover completely. In this way Levinas seemed to read Blanchot's *L'écriture du désastre* as a form of writing at the crossroads of philosophy and history that remains forever wounded by the very darkness to which it testifies (Blanchot 1980; Levinas 1993; Liebsch 2020).

In his reference to human testimony that is devoted to the infinity of the other and thus opposes the enduring reign of this darkness, Levinas refrained from theological argumentation. Although he never made a secret of his "Jewish inspiration," he avoided any appeal to the alleged evidence of a religious revelation. "The religious," he claimed instead, must forever "remain suspicious" (Levinas 1937: 194). Whether or not he was consistent in this respect or simply took a random "theological turn" in his social philosophy is another question (Janicaud 2009, 2014). The central impulse of his thought was motivated by the attempt to uncover a binding-back or reconnecting (*religio*) to the appeal of the other as a radical (though not absolute) "other", who establishes our responsibility in such a way as to resist a biopolitics that ultimately denies any unconditional ethical relation to others at all. Initially, most of the victims could not believe that a genocidal form of biopolitics was even possible, and would indeed happen to them. But what does the undeniable possibility and historical reality of this form of excessive violence really prove? In Levinas' perspective it did *not* make it plain that the victims were "successfully" reduced to an "ethical nothing," to say the least. The mass murder was "ethically impossible," Levinas claimed, insofar as it had to try to breach a demand that strictly prohibited murder. The Nazi genocide was doomed to failure insofar as it was impossible to eliminate the injunction not to treat others that way. This injunction becomes obvious, Levinas tried to make his readers believe, *vis-à-vis* the other, any other, in view of his/her very otherness even when he/she is no longer able to speak.

As far as I can see, Levinas made no attempt to relate the ethical consequences he expected of any philosophy that deserves this name "after the genocide" (Levinas 1980) to problems of reproductive medicine and bioethics. This will disappoint readers who expect instructions from his work on what to do in relation to others yet to come into the world, who may well have to face all sorts of violence. Levinas' first seminal work, *Totalité et infini* (1961), ascribes to the alterity of the other an exteriority that withdraws it from any conceptual and practical comprehension and appropriation, so that it also evades any war-like or genocidal violence (Levinas 1990 [1961]: 5). He then links this exteriority with the generative conception of filiations from which others emerge, who in turn will be handed over to surviving *other* others who cannot sublate the past of their predecessors in their own present. In this perspective on human alterity and generativity (which at first sight seems to have nothing to do with violence in general, or with genocide and war specifically), Levinas at least suggests normative conclusions such as the following: We *should respect the radical alterity* of the child even when it is not yet born; we *should never reduce it to any identity* (*mêmeté* or *ipséité*); and we *should release it again to its very otherness* if it temporarily runs the risk of falling prey to questionable genealogical, ethnic, historical or other identifications.

This way, Levinas appeals to the generative self-image of parents and any other persons who adopt or otherwise take care of children. But he refrains from any direct normative injunction to do this or that in the practice of responsibility. Nothing of this sort follows definitively from Levinas' social philosophy of alterity. He insists only on what he takes to be the most radical ethical "fact": that the alterity of the other is never at anyone's disposal. This holds true, he claims, in the darkness of the most extreme, excessive and radical forms of violence and in human generativity as well. Even when parents, educationalists of all sorts, and biopoliticians take this into account, they must, however, acknowledge their responsibility for embryos, children and any offspring in terms of their own identity. It is up to them to decide how it might be possible (*if at all*) to do justice to the radical otherness of descendants – and especially how they might protect it from "identitarian" identifications in contexts of social, cultural and political forms of life that raise complex questions of distribution, of equality, of neighbourhood, juridical integration etc.

It will never be enough to refer to the alterity of the other in order to find out what to do in given circumstances – as suggested by Hans Jonas, who maintains with respect to parental responsibility: "Look and you know [what you have to do]" (1982: 235). These rather cryptic words do *not* imply: "you know without any further consideration what you have to do in a given situation if you only notice what is already obvious" – namely: the other as radically "other". Not even *vis-à-vis* a single child is it immediately evident by way of careful "looking" what we have to do in order to do justice to this child (cf. Schäfer 2007).

Rather, Jonas calls to mind what is at stake *face à l'autre*: namely, one's own responsibility as such in view of this other' and his/her very singularity (*Diesheit*) which was completely unforeseeable beforehand. One's responsibility refers to precisely *this* being in its "wholly contingent uniqueness" – which has in this case nothing to do with a normative claim that this single human being *deserves* to be treated responsibly, and nothing to do with a *previously existing contract* from which corresponding obligations would follow, Jonas adds.[2]

The "knowledge" to which Jonas refers does not arise from a normative and comparative judgment about what one has to do in a given situation, but emerges from the *páthos* (*Widerfahrnis*) of the ethical appeal of the child, which cannot be severed from its very bodily existence. It suffices that it is simply there in order to "give" us our responsibility; and this is a responsibility that we can deny or otherwise contest only afterwards. Jonas refers to this basic ethical "fact" as the "archetype of all responsibility," (1982: 98) which he deems to be realized *par excellence* in human parenthood. At the same time he knows very well how questionable such an appeal to alleged "evidence" must appear in many readers' eyes. It seems that instead of evidence in the strict sense he can offer only hypothetical considerations that suggest crosschecks such as: Where would it lead if we were to presuppose that in ethical terms literally nothing follows from the sheer presence of an other – especially nothing that would imply our responsibility *to* or *for* the other as such? Neither Jonas nor Levinas convincingly refers to uncontested and uncontestable evidence in this respect. They offer quite different concepts, such as *unicité*, singularity, and uniqueness in order to grasp the practical significance of the otherness of the other. Uniqueness is probably the most commonly known of them, whereas *unicité* and singularity raise complex problems of interpretation that cannot easily be pinned down in normal language (cf. Waldenfels 1995: 303).

From a biological point of view, human uniqueness can be explained through reduction to singular combinations of genes. The number of possible gene combinations far exceeds the number of real existing human beings in the world, says the biologist Peter Medawar (1969: 162). In this perspective,

---

2   "*Dieses* [...] in seiner absolut kontingenten Einzigkeit ist es, dem jetzt die Verantwortung gilt – der einzige Fall, wo die 'Sache' nichts mit einer Beurteilung der Würdigkeit zu tun hat, nichts mit einem Vergleich, und nichts mit einem Vertrag" ("this in its wholly contingent uniqueness is that to which responsibility is now committed – the only case where the 'cause' one serves has nothing to do with appraisal of worthiness, nothing with comparison, and nothing with a contract" Jonas 1982: 241).

however, human uniqueness seems to be only a matter of biological *diversity* that fulfils the evolutionary function of preventing every species from running into a biological impasse (ibid: 194).

In contrast to this biological perspective taken by a theoretical observer outside evolution, philosophers such as Levinas and Jonas ground their notions of uniqueness, *unicité* and individuality *on the relation* to the other as such. We are not related to this other as a contingent objective occurrence in a neutral world of things and its earthly future, but rather by way of our being affected by his/her claim calling for our "dialogical" response. The idea that such an appeal to our response emerges from the very otherness of the other even when he/she cannot say a word (like the newborn infant [*infans*]), and even when he/she is not yet present in the world as a distinct being, makes no sense from a biological point of view. But this does not mean that uniqueness and radical otherness cannot be related. It only means that "biology" cannot do justice to this relationship.

Biology has no monopoly on the conceptualization of life *as* life. In fact, biology is the result of a *biologisation of a previous non-biological understanding of life* that rests on social interrelations of human beings who are – now more than ever – confronted with problems of the interpretation of (human) life *as (human) life*. In what sense does it deserve the attribute that it *is* human life? In what sense is a living being *"alive"*? How do living beings, from the very moment of becoming conscious of their life, *relate to their life as such*? How can they deem their *own* life to be truly *liveable*? These questions obviously transcend any biological concept of life – which we must regard *as a reduction* of previous, richer conceptions. Such a reduction may appear to be legitimate for scientific purposes – at least as long as the reduction is recognized as such. But if we forget that it is a reduction, the consequence will necessarily be a colonialization of the life world where we first experience our being related to others as such. And this consequence may finally amount to a far-reaching *forgetting of the differences between biological and social life* – so that ultimately the reduction is longer recognized at all. This may well be a dystopia. But what makes us sure that it does not loom ahead of us? Does the social philosophy of radical alterity promise sufficient resistance to the triumph of a biologistic culture that blurs the border between legitimate reductions and violent reductionisms of the meaning of life? Serious doubts in this respect cannot be denied. On the one hand, as indicated above, this social philosophy insists on a meaning of uniqueness that cannot be reduced to biological diversity. But on the other hand, insofar as it fails to draw normative consequences from this insight, it runs the risk of playing into the hands of biopolitical positions that claim to demonstrate how one can deal with the genetic potential of every individual in order to secure the future of a family, a people or a nation – without any "residue" that deserves to be taken seriously. Is radical otherness ultimately to be regarded as such a "residue" – void of any concrete social and political significance that would make calls on our responsibility?

During the Third Reich the worst extremes of reductionist biopolitics became obvious. It was claimed that complete belonging to one's people (without "residue") is the only thing that "counts"[3] – in other words, there is no radical otherness to be taken seriously at all. From this historical experience we can draw the conclusion that the only form of biopolitics that can enjoy legitimacy is one that does not assume complete power over individuated human life. Life in this sense, however, cannot evade subjugation under totalitarian biopolitics simply by virtue of its uniqueness, or *unicité*, as Levinas would have it. To this day, it is open to question how the *withdrawal* of the other into radical otherness can be connected with a *relation* of others to forms of medically, ethically and politically motivated care. We move back and forth between *withdrawal of* and *relation to* the other as such – and no dialectical sublation of this tension has yet appeared. Not only can a "bad ambiguity" (in Merleau-Ponty's sense) be seen in this movement, but it can also enhance our consciousness of two forms of violence that linger before us: on the one hand, the biopolitical subjugation of everybody, irrespective of radical otherness, and on the other hand, the absolute retreat of the other into the darkness of a strangeness which ultimately fails to give us the least hint about how to do justice to others as such. In both respects we fail to come to terms with a world that calls for caring for others as such in complex contexts of forms of life.

References

Abe, Hiroshi (2017): "Apel and Locke on our Duty to Future Generations." In: Metodo 5/2, pp. 47–56.

---

3   This seemed to follow directly from Hitler's dictum: "Nur eine Grenze kennen wir: Wer nicht zu unserem Volke gehört, für den rühren wir keinen Finger [...], von uns hat er nichts zu erwarten." ("We know only one border: we do not lift a finger for those who do not belong to our people [...], they can expect nothing from us," cited in Hamann 2002: 301).

Almond, Brenda (1988): "Human Bonds." In: Journal of Applied Philosophy 5/1, pp. 3–16.

Bergson, Henri (1907): L'évolution créatrice, Paris: Alcan.

Bernard, Andreas (2014): Kinder machen: Samenspender, Leihmütter, Künstliche Befruchtung, Frankfurt: Fischer.

Bernard, Claude (1878): Leçons sur les phénomènes de la vie communs aux animaux et aux végétaux, Paris: J.-B. Ballière.

Birenbaum-Carmeli, Daphna (2010): "Genetic relatedness and family formation in Israel: lay perceptions in the light of state policy." In: New Genetics and Society 29/1, pp. 73–85.

Blanchot, Maurice (1980): L'écriture du désastre, Paris: Gallimard.

Blumenbach, Johann F. (1830): Handbuch der Naturgeschichte, 12th ed., Göttingen: J.C. Dietrich.

Blumenberg, Hans (1986): Die Lesbarkeit der Welt, Frankfurt: Suhrkamp.

Boelderl, Artur R. (2006): Von Geburts wegen: Unterwegs zu einer philosophischen Natologie, Würzburg: Königshausen & Neumann.

Böhme, Gernot (1980): Alternativen der Wissenschaft, Frankfurt: Suhrkamp.

Butler, Judith (2009): Frames of War: When is Life Grievable? London and New York: Verso.

Canguilhem, Georges (1971): "La logique du vivant et histoire de la biologie." In: Sciences 71, pp. 20–25.

Canguilhem, Georges (1974 [1942/1966]): Das Normale und das Pathologische, Munich: Hanser.

Canguilhem, Georges/Lapassade, Georges/Piquemal, Jacques/Ulmann, Jacques (1960): "Histoire de la biologie: Du développement à l'évolution au XIXe siècle." In: Thalès 11, pp. 3–63.

Claeys, Gregory (2000): "The 'Survival of the Fittest' and the Origins of Social Darwinism." In: Journal of the History of Ideas 61/2, pp. 223–240.

Engels, Eve-M. (ed.) (1995): Die Rezeption der Evolutionstheorien im 19. Jahrhundert, Frankfurt: Suhrkamp.

Esposito, Roberto (2017): The Origin of the Political: Hannah Arendt or Simone Weil? New York: Fordham.

Feyerabend, Paul (1981): Erkenntnis für freie Menschen, 2nd ed., Frankfurt: Suhrkamp.

Glass, Bentley/Temkin, Owsei/Straus, William L. (eds.) (1959): Forerunners of Darwin 1745–1859, Baltimore: Johns Hopkins University Press.

Gould, Stephen J. (1985): Ontogeny and Phylogeny, Cambridge: Cambridge University Press.

Habermas, Jürgen (2002): Die Zukunft der menschlichen Natur: Auf dem Weg zu einer liberalen Eugenik? 4th ed. Frankfurt: Suhrkamp.

Hamann, Brigitte (2002): Hitlers Wien: Lehrjahre eines Diktators, 5th ed., Munich, Zurich: Piper.

Hashiloni-Dolev, Yael (2018): "The Effect of Jewish-Israeli Family Ideology on Policy Regarding Reproductive Technologies." In: Hagai Boas/ Yael Hashiloni-Dolev/Nadav Davidowitch/Dani Filc/Shai J. Lavi (eds.), Bioethics and Biopolitics in Israel: Socio-legal, Political, and Empirical Analysis, Cambridge: Cambridge University Press, pp. 119–138.

Jacob, François (1972 [1970]): Die Logik des Lebenden: Von der Urzeugung zum genetischen Code, Frankfurt: Fischer.

Janicaud, Dominique (2009): La phénoménologie dans tous ses états, Paris: Éditions de l'éclat.

Janicaud, Dominique (2014): Die theologische Wende der französischen Phänomenologie, Vienna: Turia + Kant.

Jonas, Hans (1973): Organismus und Freiheit: Ansätze einer philosophischen Biologie, Göttingen: Vandenhoek & Ruprecht.

Jonas, Hans (1982): Das Prinzip Verantwortung: Versuch einer Ethik für die technologische Zivilisation, 3rd ed., Frankfurt: Suhrkamp.

Kant, Immanuel (1977): Kritik der Urteilskraft, Complete works vol. VIII (ed. W. Weischedel), Frankfurt: Suhrkamp.

Kay, Lily (2005): Das Buch des Lebens: Wer schrieb den genetischen Code? Frankfurt: Suhrkamp.

Klein, Marc (1954): "Sur les résonances de la philosophie de la nature en biologie moderne et contemporaine." In: Revue Philosophique 144, pp. 514–543.

Lenoir, Timothy (1981): "Teleology without regrets. The transformation of physiology in Germany: 1790–1847." In: Studies in the History and Philosophy of Science 12/4, pp. 293–354.

Lenoir, Timothy (1982): The Strategy of Life, Dordrecht: Reidel.

Lepenies, Wolf (1978): Das Ende der Naturgeschichte: Wandel kultureller Selbstverständlichkeiten in den Wissenschaften des 18. und 19. Jahrhunderts, Frankfurt: Suhrkamp.

Levinas, Emmanuel (1937): "Lettre à propos de Jean Wahl." In: Bulletin de la Société française de philosophie 37, pp. 194–195.

Levinas, Emmanuel (1947): Le Temps et l'Autre, Paris: PUF.

Levinas, Emmanuel (1980): "Un langage pour nous familier." In: Le Matin hors série consacré à Sartre).

Levinas, Emmanuel (1990 [1961]): Totalité et infini: Essai sur l'extériorité, Paris: Kluwer.

Levinas, Emmanuel (1993): Dieu, la mort et le temps, Paris: Grasset & Fasquelle.

Levinas, Emmanuel (2009): Parole et silence et autres conférences inédites. Œuvres 2, Paris: Grasset-Imec.

Liebsch, Burkhard (1992): Spuren einer anderen Natur: Piaget, Merleau-Ponty und die ontogenetischen Prozesse, Munich: Fink.

Liebsch, Burkhard (1997): "Das Spiel des Lebens und der Tod des Anderen." In: Burkhard Liebsch, Vom Anderen her: Erinnern und Überleben, Freiburg and Munich: Alber, pp. 92–119.

Liebsch, Burkhard (2001): Zerbrechliche Lebensformen: Widerstreit – Differenz – Gewalt, Berlin: Akademie.

Liebsch, Burkhard (2012): Prekäre Selbst-Bezeugung: Die erschütterte Wer-Frage im Horizont der Moderne, Weilerswist: Velbrück Wissenschaft.

Liebsch, Burkhard (2016): In der Zwischenzeit: Spielräume menschlicher Generativität, Zug: Die Graue Edition.

Liebsch, Burkhard (ed.) (2017): Der Andere in der Geschichte: Sozialphilosophie im Zeichen des Krieges, 2nd ed., Freiburg and Munich: Alber.

Liebsch, Burkhard (2018): Einander ausgesetzt: Der Andere und das Soziale, vols. I/II, Freiburg and Munich: Alber.

Liebsch, Burkhard (2019): "Unconditional Responsibility in the Face of Disastrous Violence. Thoughts on *religio* and the History of Human Mortality." In: Journal for Continental Philosophy of Religion 1, pp. 191–212.

Liebsch, Burkhard (2020): "Maurice Blanchots Schrift des Desasters und die Historizität menschlicher Sterblichkeit." In: Zeitschrift für Genozidforschung 18/1: Todeszonen, pp. 92–127.

Löw, Reinhard (1980): Philosophie des Lebendigen, Frankfurt: Suhrkamp.

Medawar, Peter (1969): Die Einmaligkeit des Individuums, Frankfurt: Suhrkamp.

Merleau-Ponty, Maurice (1945): Phénoménologie de la perception, Paris: Gallimard.

Needham, Joseph (1934): A History of Embryology, Cambridge: Cambridge University Press.

Plessner, Helmuth (1975 [1928]): Die Stufen des Organischen und der Mensch: Einleitung in die philosophische Anthropologie, Berlin: de Gruyter.

Richards, Robert J. (1987): Darwin and the Emergence of Evolutionary Theories of Mind and Behavior, Chicago: Chicago University Press.

Ricœur, Paul (1990): Soi-même comme un autre, Paris: Seuil.

Ricœur, Paul (1994 [1972]): "L'herméneutique du témoignage." In: Lectures 3. Aux frontières de la philosophie, Paris: Seuil, pp. 105–138.

Rodi, Frithjof /Lessing, Hans-U. (eds.) (1984): Materialien zur Philosophie Wilhelm Diltheys, Frankfurt: Suhrkamp.

Röttgers, Kurt (1996): "Konzepte von Sozialphilosophie im Spannungsfeld von Neukantianismus, Soziologie und Kulturphilosophie." In: Martina Plümacher, Volker Schürmann (eds.): Die Einheit des Geistes. Probleme ihrer Grundlegung in der Philosophie Ernst Cassirers, Frankfurt, Berlin, Bern: Lang, pp. 233–255.

Schäfer, Alfred (ed.) (2007): Kindliche Fremdheit und pädagogische Gerechtigkeit, Paderborn: Schöningh.

Schües, Christina (2008): Philosophie des Geborenseins, Freiburg and Munich: Alber.

Schües, Christina (2016/17): "Natality: Philosophical rudiments concerning a generative phenomenology." In: Thaumazein no. 4/5, pp. 9–35.

Temkin, Owsei (1950): "German Concepts of Ontogeny and History around 1800." In: Bulletin of the History of Medicine XXIV/3, pp. 227–246.

Waldenfels, Bernhard (1995): Deutsch-französische Gedankengänge, Darmstadt: WBG.

Commentary – The Ethics of Never Again

Natan Sznaider

After reading Burkhard Liebsch's paper about *Biological reproduction, offspring, and radical otherness*, the first question that came to mind was whether we as sociologists have anything to say when it comes to ethics in our times. Is it better to leave ethics to the philosophers, and care intellectually only about what is and is not rather than what should or could be? In the following remarks, I try to suggest sociological ethics, in connection with the idea of this book and Christina Schües's invitation to contextualise the different perspectives of Israel and Germany. I will attempt to do this and at the same time do justice as far as I can to Burkhard Liebsch's reflections. If sociology is indeed about what is or even what was, how do we at the same time connect to an openness that reaches towards something new, undetermined by the past and unpredicted by the present? This is especially true in a country and within societies that are so shaped by the past. What is the relationship between our being "biological beings" and simultaneously historical ones? This also applies to people whose definition as biological people had disastrous consequences, as discussed clearly in Burkhard's paper. Let us stop for a moment at the point of the "radical future", in relation to Emmanuel Levinas.[1] Levinas has always fascinated me, and I can relate to the idea of "radical future" as absolute surprise, defining our responsibility to people who are not yet born. It connects in some ways with my own work on Hannah Arendt. At the end of her report of the Eichmann trial, she stated: "Every generation, by virtue of being born into a historical continuum, is burdened by the sins of the fathers as it is blessed by the deeds of the ancestors" (*Arendt* 1963: 298).

This brings us to the future. As Arendt has shown, the German and French words for "future" (*avenir* and *Zukunft*) mean something quite distinct from the

---

1   The translator Richard A. Cohen summarised Levinas' approach concerning "Time and the Other" (1987 : 11) under the heading of the "radical future".

English word "future". They mean something coming toward you rather than lying ahead of you like some kind of progress. The future does not emerge out of the past, nor is determined by it, and there is a radical freedom involved in constructing it. We know that the future is unforeseeable. It will have different categories of reality accompanied by different categories of thought. We will not be able to understand how it works until we or even our children get there. It will emerge out of the present like a *gestalt* that is more than the sum of its parts. But until it does – and it never does for us – we are always facing a future that is beyond us. Living in the transition between the present and the future, we have to continuously keep guessing what will best capture the future that might possibly be. These are precisely the visions of horror and hope articulated by Franz Kafka, who once claimed that there is "infinite amount of hope in the universe ... but not for us".[2] And it is no coincidence that these very words are quoted by Walter Benjamin in his essay honouring Kafka. Hope is precisely what you need when you do not know what the future will bring, and a world order collapses. Thus, we need a new starting-point, one that continues the present but that also recreates it and understands its newness by maintaining a dialogue between present and past.

This is where I believe a sociological ethics comes in. Hannah Arendt (1958) called this "natality". I see this as similar to Levinas' radical future, as mentioned in Liebsch's paper. In *The Human Condition*, Arendt defines "natality" as the condition of having been born. She asserts that our natality is the "source" or "root" of our "capacity to begin", by which she means the capacity to break with the status quo and initiate something new. Only human beings possess this capacity, she says. Arendt is therefore claiming that our capacity to begin springs from our condition of having been born.

I have been busy in my work to translate this into a sociological ethics, and I hope it will make sense to you. We do have a powerful formula that provides us with moral certainty within a temporally organised world. I call this formula very simply *Never Again*. Never Again can mean many things to many different actors. As an apparent neologism, it has been surprisingly under-conceptualised. Are we talking politics? If so, what kind of normative implications does a politics of Never Again have? Are we talking aesthetics that imply a kind

---

2 Max Brod (1921, 1213) was a friend and a biographer of Franz Kafka. In 1921, he published a piece titled "Der Dichter Franz Kafka" ("The Poet Franz Kafka") in the literary journal "Die Neue Rundschau". Brod repeats this sentence "Oh, Hoffnung genug, *unendlich viel Hoffnung* – nur *nicht für uns.*" from a conversation he held with his friend in 1920.

of Never Again sentiment – a feeling without great political consequence? We need to explore the question of a globally relevant ethics in a world full of risks and uncertainties.

While in philosophy, morality often needs to be universal to be considered valid, in sociology other rules apply. Sociology is about social groups, particular experiences, and about how people, embedded in space and time, make sense of their lives and give meaning to their world. It deals with power, interests, and the social bases of our experiences. Morality, on the other hand, is about human beings in general, irrespective of temporal or spatial references, not about territorially confined groups and their frontiers. Moral rules are supposed to be inviolable and to apply to humanity as a whole. Morality is about dignity and the abstract human being, and does not need any kind of sociological garb. We need to inquire into the interface between particular actions and universal explanations of those actions by looking at a complex picture that combines cultural meanings and social structures of the sociological phenomenon. A first suggestion could be a moral perspective based on the actors' historical experiences and horizons. I would like to call it an "Ethics of Never Again."

The logic of *Never Again* tells those who use it that an event is already over; that the past, the catastrophe, has already passed. By embracing the Never Again paradigm, social actors construct a new temporal framework that represents the past and the present as radically different and antagonistic. However, while the catastrophe is placed behind us, it is situated in the future as well as a ghastly possibility. The future does not emerge out of the past, nor is it determined by it, but there is rather a radical freedom involved in constructing it. This is not the usual social-scientific lamentation, but a renewed effort to write the *Book of Lamentations*, wherein the destruction of the Temple in Jerusalem is lamented, but where hope is always on the horizon:

> How lonely sits the city
> that once was full of people!
> How like a widow she has become,
> she that was great among the nations!
> She that was a princess among the provinces
> has become a vassal!
> (Lamentations 1:1, NRSV)

We are back in place and time and historical memory, which is situated, constructed, constantly evolving and reframing and reinterpreting events of the

past. It is a book about memory, but memory as an anxious ethics of anticipation. Those Judeans who remained after the destruction of Jerusalem composed the book around 2500 years ago. Worshippers are still reading it every
year, on the day that commemorates the destruction of the temple and the city
by the Babylonians. It is both a book about violence and grief in general, and a
book about the violence and grief done to us at a certain point in time. You may
recall Rembrandt's depiction from 1630 of Jeremiah lamenting the destruction
of Jerusalem, which hangs in the Rijksmuseum in Amsterdam. As a sociologist,
I am interested, for instance, in understanding how people choose between a
universal standpoint or a communitarian identity with their own group, and
how they negotiate between the two. On the one hand, we can judge political
ideas and practices according to a universal standard of reason; on the other,
we are bound to lived experience and its intricacies. The politics of memory
is no exception to this. Thus, the ethics of Never Again is a theory of morality
based on particularity and on identity. And thus, we can read *Lamentations* as a
general story or an historical one; we are back to square one of my comment. I
certainly do not want to dismiss the roots of responsibilities in identity as particular ideologies, but to understand them as the basis of a sincere attempt to
think morally. There is a communitarian argument at work here as well. This is
a point not only about personal identity but also about who you are as a member of a community. However, membership of a community is the beginning,
not the end. Thus, we will argue that a value-free description of the political
world is not wrong, but is useless because the *Ought* is immanent in the *Is*. The
notion that the basis of morality lies in identity, and that the basis of personal
identity lies in collective identity – or in overlapping collective identities – is
one possible answer to the question of how to maintain a tension between the
universal and the particular. I am not arguing that all morality is based on identity but that some of it is, and that it is an essential part, because it is the part
that makes us who we are. This part gives people moral motivation because it is
the basis of their passions and themselves. Thus, we speak with different voices
depending on the circumstances. Moral knowledge is knowledge in flux. Historical experience does separate us from others, but the question is how to deal
with this separation. Public memory – even when institutionalised by education and regulated by law – is embedded in an affective matrix of "anxiety",
which at one and the same time is capable of creating the conciliatory conditions of political virtue – Never Again – and of fuelling the terror of political passion – Again and Again. Never Again is not, however, merely a mental
attitude. It starts with the body and its vulnerability – its mortality. Thus, it

seems that we are back to "biological beings", but this is certainly not enough. It also demands that people recognise this vulnerability and feel the need to act upon it. Vulnerability becomes one of the new global conditions, which is constantly mediated by direct access to the sight of suffering across the world. People become witnesses to the violation of others. They need to react in some way or other, considering that not doing anything is one of the possible reactions. Thus, the questions are: How and why do people react and how do they feel and think about the past in this connection? How do specific past catastrophes – whether of local or global significance – condition our understanding and reactions towards current forms of violence and human rights violations?

Universalist understandings of an Ethics of Never Again may conflict with particular interpretations. The array of meanings and lessons of Never Again can be not only diverse but also incompatible: for instance, present-day Germany's *Never Again*, which tries to be universal ("Never again war"), stands in contrast to Israel's *Never Again*, which tries very much to be particular ("Never again Us as victims!"). Here, the concept of "Negative Symbiosis" is very pertinent for this analysis. The Holocaust has bound "Germans" and "Jews" forever to the past, opening an insurmountable gap that conditions their mutual relationship, as well as the passing on of the group identity of victims – and in the German case also of perpetrators stuck in a permanent position of culpability – to succeeding generations.

Moreover, this also means different founding moments when we look at Germany and Israel. Here is a quote from the late Tony Judt that I would like you to consider for a moment:

> The problem with Israel [. . .] is not – as is sometimes suggested – that it is a European "enclave" in the Arab world; but rather that it arrived too late. It has imported a characteristically late-nineteenth-century separatist project into a world that has moved on, a world of individual rights, open frontiers, and international law. The very idea of a "Jewish state" – a state in which Jews and the Jewish religion have exclusive privileges from which non-Jewish citizens are forever excluded – is rooted in another time and place. Israel, in short, is an anachronism (Judt, 2003: n.p.).

Thus, more 16 years ago, Tony Judt declared Israel to be an anachronism, an entity refusing to move on to the next stage, to a kind of imagined transnational modernity. An anachronism means that there is a chronological inconsistency in which Israel is caught up, of its own volition. Israel is the past, while Europe is the future. Clearly, Judt's comment was also the *cri de coeur* of a disappointed

Leftist Zionist, but is it true at all? Like many proponents of a new transnational perspective, he like many others who look at Israel conceive of modernity as falling roughly into two phases. First is a nation-centred stage that began with the French revolution. Second is a cosmopolitan stage, the arcs of which begin at many different times after the Second World War. In this view, these various trends have recently begun to converge into visibly different paths of economic and cultural development, where the nation state is beginning to recede behind the increasingly transnational reality of our social, economic and cultural life. Now, in Israel this is not the case at all, but can you place this development on a past-present-future axis? I think we need to take into account the concept of "Non-Contemporaneity of the Contemporaneous" (better said in German as *Ungleichzeitigkeit der Gleichzeitigkeit*). I suggest a very banal sociological point here, namely that at every moment in time, various historical epochs and styles exist simultaneously and next to each other. They are not distinct and closed historical units. Looking at Israel and Germany, I would like to argue against a notion of historical time according to which one epoch replaces another, following the logic of evolution or progress. The radical break between tradition and modernity does not allow us to grasp today's realities in Israel. These worlds do exist here in Israel simultaneously and nothing seems simpler than to call Israel's pre-modern formations the traditional remnants of a world now past. Rather, what you have here are radically different descriptions of the same reality. Moreover, if we define modernity as the capacity to contain different descriptions of the same reality at the same time, we can easily define Israel as a hyper-modern society. The liberal credo of the "autonomous individual" is therefore just one of the many descriptions we have available to describe our humanness in this society.

Thus, imagine for a moment what would happen if Israel applied for membership of the European Union. What would be the response? Its application would either be deferred or flatly rejected. Why? Is Israel not European enough? Does it belong to Europe even though it is geographically located in Asia? Although it was founded in Europe, Israel is out of Europe but not in Europe. It lies in Asia and, like Turkey, connects Asia to Europe. Those who share the European continent, but do not share its Christian heritage, are seen as Europe's Other. Israel is certainly not a Christian country. One can almost claim that it is the opposite, with its particularistic and ethnic self-definition as a Jewish state. Israel arose out of the Ottoman Empire and constantly has to balance processes of Europeanisation, Americanisation, the expectations of international institutions, and the pressure of local groups and traditions.

Israel defines itself ethnically and its criteria of citizenship are exclusive. Wouldn't the term "European" imply, at least politically, a demand to change the basis of the Israeli national definition and found it on the conventional territorial principle – equality before the law of all citizens living within Israeli territory, irrespective of ethnic origins, race, community, religion or sex? Shouldn't Israel first "Europeanise" and stop opposing those who think that nations are either "imagined" or "invented" and as a consequence, live with the illusion that nationalism will disappear when it is shown and "proven" that the nation is a creation of the mind? Questions asked, demands made, from outside Israel but also from within, especially from the social and cultural circles we all move in.

However, the continuation of the Israeli-Arab conflict and the persistence of antisemitism will resist these kinds of tendencies. Israel attempts to be universally democratic and particularly Jewish at the same time, and thus reaches its limits of universality. Israel suggests a different reading of European history, undermining the project of reconciliation between former enemies enabled by the breakdown of the socialist regimes. Israel's alternative reading of European history keeps alive the memory of destruction for which Nazi Germany and its allies were responsible. Its existence presents a challenge to the European, especially Western European, countries, who see transnationalism as almost self-evident. Clearly, there are challenges to this ethics of Never Again and these are challenges facing society as well as the science of society: sociology.

Sociology is a child of that national gaze, and more than that, it provides the tools for understanding and legitimising the nation. Following the historical route of the universalist philosophical tradition from Hellenism via Christianity to the modern Western world makes the idea of universalism open to criticism from outside the Western traditions. People are doing it all the time. Nothing new here. However, we can do better, I believe. In the sociological ethics of Never Again, the universal means what it does because the particulars are its background, and are where the particulars mean what they do because the universal is their background. So that when one changes, the other changes – but neither disappears.

So, where does that leave us, looking at the notion of a radical future? Israel's legitimacy to exists as an ethnic nation state for the Jews rests partly on the Holocaust and, therefore, on the memory of that tragedy. Understood in this sense, the memory of the Holocaust is not just a monument to Europe's sense of the tragic. It is a memorial specifically to the European barbarism that was made possible by the marriage of modernity and the nation state. Europe and within it Germany took a different path. Europe's collective memory of the Holocaust recalls the basis of the EU. It is a warning sign that when modernity develops exclusively in the grooves of the nation state, it builds the potential for a moral, political, economic and technological catastrophe, without limit, without mercy, and even without any consideration for its own survival. That is how the memory of the Holocaust was understood in Europe's own self-image. But it also laid the foundations for Israel's existence as a particular ethnic nation state where the Jews can feel protected after the Holocaust. An altogether European project. It is what enables Europe to find its continuity at the very point at which it breaks from the past. It allows it to establish future-oriented forms of memory, against national founding myths and myths of warfare and with a cosmopolitan self-critique. However, this is not how the memory of the Holocaust is perceived in Israel. Just the opposite. For Jews, the Holocaust took place because the Jews did not exercise political sovereignty. Protecting the Jews at all costs became one of the pillars of Israel's identity. Thus, Israel was founded at the very same moment when the new Europe arose out of the ruins of the Second World War. Both entities were formed on the same background, but former perpetrators and former victims drew very different conclusions from the memory of the Holocaust. To sum up: we should talk about a radical future, about an absolute surprise; otherwise, we could not sit here and talk. Nevertheless, we need to keep in mind the radical past as well, and there are less surprises there.

References

Arendt, Hannah (1963): Eichmann in Jerusalem: A Report on the Banality of Evil, London: Faber & Faber.

Arendt, Hannah (1958): The Human Condition, Chicago: Chicago University Press.

Benjamin, Walter (1934): "Franz Kafka: Zur zehnten Wiederkehr seines Todestages." In: Gesammelte Schriften 2.2, ed. Rolf Tiedemann and Hermann Schweppenhäuser, Frankfurt: Suhrkamp, 1977, 409–438.

Brod, Max (1921): »Der Dichter Franz Kafka« In: Die neue Rundschau, Nr. 11, 32,1210–1216.

Judt, Tony (2003): "Israel: The Alternative." In: New York Review, 23 October. (https://www.nybooks.com/articles/2003/10/23/israel-the-alternative/), accessed 06 January 2022.

Levinas, Emmanuel (1987): Time and the Other, translated by Richard A. Cohen, Pittsburgh: Duquesne University Press.

2. Origins and Practices of Genetic Risk and Responsibility
Is it Irresponsible Not to Test?

Christina Schües

The beginning of life as a human being has historically been discussed and handled in very diverse ways. It was seldom an arbitrary thing to decide whom
to admit and welcome as a fellow human being into a community, a collective or a society. One traditional way to become part of the community as a
fellow human is through procreation and birth. Procreation has always fascinated people. There is also a fascination in using techniques and practices to
improve one's own species, to guide society, i.e. to pursue population policy,
to eliminate or even improve the "bad genetic material" for future generations
– all these developments in biology, medicine and genetics clearly reveal an
inherent entanglement of knowledge and values, of science and politics. The
"sciences" aimed to improve heredity – race theory, eugenics and racial hygiene were particularly promoted in the 19th and 20th centuries. At its peak,
this fascination turned into a cruel selection regime during the Nazi era. After the Second World War genocide of Jews and other ethnic groups, people
with disabilities and political prisoners, the discourses in Israel and Germany
about prenatal genetic testing and its associated responsibilities were still influenced by this historical event. In the first two decades of the 21st century,
state-promoted eugenics as pursued under the Nazi regime, or other forms
of systematically excising "unworthy life", has no official approval from health
ministries, human rights advocates, politicians or ethicists.

Today, a strong concept of responsibility pushes the quest for individual
and autonomous choice to the centre of the praxis of pregnancy. Under the
"rhetoric of the 'right to know' and 'informed choice'" (Petersen 1998: 64), the
pregnant woman bears the responsibility for her pregnancy and her child; depending on the context, she alone is considered to have this responsibility, per-

haps with her partner, with the aid of the medical staff, or in some Jewish religious contexts with support from a rabbi (Ivry/Teman 2019; see chapter 7 of this book). With the emergence of reproductive technologies and genetic testing, the concept of genetic risks became established, and a general responsibility of care during pregnancy essentially became *genetic* responsibility. This chapter therefore focuses on both terms, genetic risk and genetic responsibility, looking at their relationship and the different ways they have been conceptualised in the last two decades of prenatal care for mother and child.

The question is not how a pregnant woman might share or assume responsibility; I want instead to understand the motives and the object of being responsible and how these correlate with the perception of genetic risk. What is the aim of being responsibility in "responsible motherhood" or "irresponsible motherhood" (Ivry/Teman 2019: 861)? The general message seems to be finding what is best for the children (Ruckdeschel 2015). Is the main objective, for instance, the well-being of the child or the family, their health, avoiding unworthy life, or producing healthy offspring? In any case, it seems that the burden of responsibility can be heavy, and sometimes involve a decision about life and death; it certainly involves a decision about how much and what should be genetically tested and known about the foetus.

The increasing availability of genetic tests and the capacity to decide about the child's life in light of genetic findings corresponds with the genetic responsibility to test, to know and to act accordingly. Women who do not want to know about the genetic make-up of their offspring may face accusations of irresponsibility, as we found, for instance, in interviews conducted in Israel (cf. chapter 7 of this book). Reproaching a mother for irresponsibility about the future child is a strong attack on her moral integrity and affects her close family and social relationships. German interviewees mostly emphasised that genetic testing is a decision for the individual or couple. Even though the debate about NIPT is much more publicly driven in Germany, interviewees explicitly refrained from judging other decisions or opinions within the field of genetic testing. Yet it does not follow that parents who have a child with a disability always receive understanding and sufficient support.

The historical background of Nazi cruelty and atrocities still forms an underlying reference in both countries: the discourse in Germany cannot refrain from a restrictive approach towards genetic testing and research; the influence of guilt alternates between collective trauma that is perpetuated through generations (Bar-On 1989) and a "historic responsibility" (Zimmermann 2016) that

is also propagated by the state.[1] This leads to a balanced objection against prenatal practices that are implemented as a standardised routine that "selects"
life. If prenatal genetic testing is *not* done on an individual and deliberate case-
by-case basis, then at least in the German context, it may give the impression
of a eugenic strategy (cf. Rubeis 2018; Braun 2021; Foth 2021).

Israel's culture still includes the memory of the Shoah in its discourse. As
a consequence of this victimisation, it emphasises the survival of the Jewish
people. This emphasis is supported by, as stressed by Weiss (2004), Jewish culture and the Zionist movement, both of which have an historical objective of
producing strong and healthy Jewish bodies. Distinct from Protestant or Roman Catholic ethics, which emphasise the dignity of the foetus, Jewish religion
does not have a concept of personhood or dignity of the foetus and is open to its
physical improvement; hence, Israel's permissive genetic testing is supported
by these historical, religious and cultural motives. Reproductive institutions –
whether offering genetic testing, IVF or other reproductive technologies – provide the means for exercising one's responsibility towards the collective body of
Israeli society (Prainsack 2006: 242). Germany hesitates to be permissive about
prenatal genetic testing, and if anything, the discourse emphasises individual
reproductive self-determination, with the focus especially on "the balance between the 'right to know' and 'not to know'" (Perrot/Horn 2021), and not on the
Volkskörper ("body of the people") or the improvement of a race; these concep-
tualisations are not part of the discourse either semantically or structurally.

The complexity of the situation and questions at stake make it easy to categorise an action as irresponsible. For example, in Germany, aborting a foetus
diagnosed with trisomy 21 for embryopathic reasons is sometimes condemned
for "selecting life"; likewise, the parents of a child with Down syndrome may
receive critical looks or comments that a child like that is not "necessary any
more". On the other hand, several campaigns that fight for the rights of people
with Down syndrome use the slogan "Don't screen us out!"[2] Consequently,
in Germany, several religious and non-religious organisations and groups,
such as the *Bundesvereinigung Lebenshilfe* (2015), that formulate a rather critical
stance towards NIPT, arguing that these genetic tests discriminate against

---

1   https://www.germany.info/us-en/welcome/03-Jewish-Life-Germany, accessed 02
    June 2022.
2   For instance, the British campaign "Against making chromosomes count" (https://ma
    kingchromosomescount.co.uk/dont-screen-us-out-2/ or https://dontscreenusout.org/
    or rambazamba-theater.de), accessed 26 July 2022.

people with disabilities and the parents who have not prevented the birth of such children (Schidel 2020). At the same time, parents of a child with disabilities face discrimination, and pregnant women who learn that their foetus has a trisomy will include fear of such discrimination in their deliberations about genetic testing and abortion. At least in Germany, critical positions can be found for both the decision to genetically test or not to test, and parents are stuck between a duty towards health (meaning aborting foetuses with trisomy) and their reproductive autonomy (Primc 2018). Psychologists Philipp et al. (2000: 26f.) observe that "particularly the divided social attitude towards giving birth to a disabled child, but also towards terminating a pregnancy, puts couples under pressure and creates a sense of vulnerability and attackability."

In Israel, the question of genetic testing has largely been answered on the basis of a well-established prenatal care practice that includes a choice of invasive and non-invasive genetic tests. Where there is a positive finding of a genetic variation linked to disability, the reason for abortion is generally based on the possible "suffering" of a disabled child and whether her life would be "worth living" (Hashiloni-Dolev 2007; Remennick 2006). While the Israeli abortion law includes embryopathic reasoning, in Germany it is only the burden on the mother of having a child with disability that legally counts as reason to end a pregnancy. Thus, the Israeli and German discourse with regard to the main reasoning behind abortion shows very different groundings. Even more fundamentally, the difference between Israel's and Germany's practice and discourse on prenatal genetic diagnosis is based on different understandings of genetic responsibility and genetic risk. Working from this idea, I will introduce some historical background on the concepts of responsibility and risk. Both are rather recent concepts with histories predominantly in non-medical areas.

Responsibility and risk have distinct origins. After bringing out their diverging lines, I want to show how they merge with the establishment of genetic practice and how they are transformed into *genetic* risk and *genetic* responsibility. These historical and systematic observations will lay the ground for drawing a distinction between genetic responsibility and care responsibility in the contexts of pregnancy, the foetus, and the future of the child. Furthermore, I will introduce three types of moral conduct with reference to the genetic testing and care relationships: *responsibly, irresponsibility* and *non-responsibility*. The delineation of dissimilar thematic orientations of responsibility will support diverse paths of decision-making and acting in the realm of pregnancy care and genetic testing.

Era of responsibility

In the shadow of the Second World War and the atomic bombs dropped on Hiroshima and Nagasaki that killed more than 200.000 people – children, women, men – the concept of responsibility and care for the future and the human condition was brought to the fore by Hans Jonas, Emmanuel Levinas, Hannah Arendt and Günter Anders in the 1960s. Jonas, in his 1979 work *The Imperative of Responsibility*, presents a future-oriented responsibility concerned with the life of the next generation, the protection of humanity and nature, and a warning against large-scale technologies in general. One of his insights is that when we act, we cannot pretend not to know the meaning of this particular action, and we should be cautious if we do not know what the outcome of our action might be.

Hans Jonas' ethics of responsibility is an attempt to propose an ethics of global co-responsibility. Humans have the power to invent science and technology, and are therefore responsible for these inventions. Jonas primarily wrote about ecological ethics, calling for the protection of human life on earth. The context of this ethical need is the observation that technical and medical possibilities could endanger the lives of future generations because scientists *have the ability to* invent more than they are able to control. Since we, as humans of the 20th century, have the power to invent technologies whose effects are unforeseeable, far-reaching, and irreversible, and that might potentially endanger future generations, we must take responsibility. A "heuristic of fear" should guide decisions on which technology may be used and which we should refrain from using (Jonas 1984: 35). Thus, Jonas' concept of responsibility has a rather pessimistic overtone.

In this primary phase of the concept of future responsibility, warnings were issued against the new gene technologies and the possible biological hazards, in addition to other chemical industries and atomic technologies. This debate continued to be dominated by the growing awareness of limited resources, overpopulation and the looming ecological crisis, as discussed in the Club of Rome report (Meadows 1972; Leefmann/Schicktanz 2016). The recommendation was for society, and especially scientists and other experts, to adopt a political responsibility towards the next generation. An individualised concept of future responsibility that correlated with the concern about reproductive technologies very soon steered the discourse and practice of pregnancy and the beginning of life.

In the 1970s, pregnancy became increasingly medicalised; yet it was also criticised and the hope for a healthy child romanticised (Illich 1975; Conrad 2007), Later, in the 1980s, this attitude changed to a demand for comprehensive medical care during pregnancy. As a responsible person, and in consultation with her physician, the woman's concern had to be for her pregnancy and the foetus. Her responsibility was directed primarily toward good behaviour: eating healthily, avoiding drugs and alcohol. If a pregnant woman was not behaving "properly", she was considered irresponsible. Responsibility was primarily seen as a way of living and behaving according to particular social norms. Accordingly, Linda McClain (1996) critically discussed three paradigms of irresponsibility that were used to propagate social stigmatisation in the name of care: the single mother, the welfare mother, the teenage mother. This is the period in which the child (to be) became central to motherhood; the terms "responsible motherhood" and "responsible parenthood" appeared, and became a central part of the discussion and of the self-understanding of a mother (to be) (Haker 2001; Ruckdeschel 2015).

More specifically, since the 1970s and '80s a pregnant woman has been expected to pursue a particular medical and social practice of care and control, in which the foetus has become the strong focus of biomedical and social attention. Accurate genetic testing became the key to evaluating the "health" of the foetus from the point of view of the future parents. For the prenatal phase, the general responsibility for the health of the (expectant) mother was transformed into a *special responsibility* for the child to come: *genetic* responsibility. In the 21st century, *genetic responsibility* in pregnancy is central, focusing on genetic aspects of the foetus that may lead to physical or mental phenotypic variations.[3] These different options demand a set of *personal responsibilities* of the (expectant) parents, because as well as aspects of care, which may also be provided by family members, they demand a focused attitude towards consideration of the *genetic risk* associated with the genetic disposition of the foetus and the (biological) parents.

The term "genetic responsibility" became part of the discussion in genetic counselling contexts. The term "genetic responsibility" was used explicitly as

---

3   Currently, in addition to the wide range of reproductive services available, we can also observe a trend towards including non-medical practices of birth preparation and childbirth aimed at the health and well-being of mother and child (Matthew/Wexler 2000). And ultrasound provides images of the baby, located in the exciting ambivalence between "(bio)medicalisation" and "demedicalisation" (Ullrich 2012).

early as a 1972 symposium on "choosing our children's genes" (Lipkin/Rowley 1974). Here, genetic responsibility was seen in a collective perspective of acting "responsibly" towards the next generation. An ethics of responsibility was supposed to be one "which at once releases our hope and restrains our injustice," and avoids hereditary disease (Fletcher 1974: 94).

Ultrasound made the foetus visible and, hence, measurable; amniocentesis showed whether it is "genetically healthy". More and more tests are being introduced into prenatal diagnostics. The establishment of prenatal genetic tests signifies that responsibility is having a strong impact in bioethical and biopolitical discourse. This impact is particularly supported by neo-liberal tendencies of brash marketing in the form of "fertility fairs", which are actively accepted by inquiring consumers, and which increase individualisation and introduce a variety of genetic tests.[4] The conceptual linkage between genetic diagnosis, genetic knowledge and genetic responsibility is becoming a fixed parameter of *risk procedure* in the biomedical care of pregnancy and the beginning of life.

Silke Schicktanz states broadly: *"where there is risk there is responsibility"* (2018: 236), and describes how responsibility emerges in situations where a risk awareness is raised by the information about genetic risks (e.g. biological disposition of pregnant woman, genetic testing), is considered in decision-making, and is central to different practices.[5] She and Aviad Raz introduce the relationship between responsibility and risk as an "epistemic turn" (2016: 38f.) that takes place in the context of a socially implemented upheaval caused by the rising importance of paying attention to genetic risks.

With the epistemic and normative introduction of genetic risk into the practice of pregnancy and into the bioethics of prenatal genetic testing, the relationship between genetic responsibility and genetic risk is strong. However, responsibility and risk have different historical backgrounds. Having addressed the socio-historical horizon of responsibility, I now turn to the concepts of risk and security. Then I will consider the conjunction between genetic responsibility and genetic risk and observe some aspects of how it works in the respective socio-cultural contexts of Germany and Israel.

---

4   "Fertility fears" have also become socially relevant in the contexts of egg-freezing and vaccines, e.g. COVID-19, or breast cancer treatment.

5   To refer to Hans Jonas in this matter is rather misleading because he does not, as I explain above, derive responsibility from risk but from human power. In addition, he is alluding not to risk but to the possible dangers of technology.

Risk, security and genetic responsibility

The modern concept of risk has its origin in the maritime insurance of the European Middle Ages and is therefore relatively young in terms of its linguistic history. From the Italian *rischio*, the term was introduced into German as *Risiko* and into English as "risk". [6] In the Romance languages, it is a Latin loanword from the Greek root *rico* (cliff), and probably originally referred to navigation round a cliff. In the merchant language of the Middle Ages, "risk" designated uncertain commercial transactions. In German-speaking countries, the term remained a technical economic one until the 19th century and only then found its way into other sciences and everyday life.

The German sociologist Ulrich Beck combines Jonas' observation that scientists have a power of knowledge that has potential for technological and industrial catastrophes with the thesis that, in the context of the 1980s, we live in a *risk society* which is organised in response to risks. [7] "Risk may be defined as a systematic way of dealing with hazards and insecurities induced and introduced by modernization itself" (Beck 1992: 21). Beck has global, environmental, industrial and gene technology risks in mind, and observes prenatal testing practices to be a "quality control of embryos" with reference to "a socially and ethically 'desirable', 'used' or 'healthy' genetic substance" (Bräutigam/Mettler 1985, quoted in Beck 1992: 206). Giddens emphasises that such a risk society is "increasingly preoccupied with the future (and also with

---

6   In Hebrew the word for risk is סיכון (sikun).

7   What is the difference between danger and risk? In referring to the atomic or chemical industry and gene technology we often speak about dangers and risks. Since the 1980s the triangle of danger, security and risk has become the focus of discussion. Although these terms have different meanings and objectives, they are often used interchangeably. Since our focus here is on genetic risk, I would like to distinguish it from danger. The perspective of system theory may help us to understand this distinction. Danger is a form of possible damage that is considered to be externally caused, i.e. attributed to the environment that lies outside one's own social system. If the cause of damage is attributed to one's own realm of decision-making then we speak of risk, and if it is outside our realm of decision-making then we speak of danger. This makes it possible to distinguish responsibilities from damage. In summary, the main difference between risk and danger is that in the case of a danger, the damage is caused externally and the system (or subject) does not know what decision it should or could make to avoid the damage (Luhmann 2003). This demarcation makes the decision into an immanent part of the risk. Thus, decisions and their consequences, i.e. risks and their consequences, are directly attributable to the decision-maker.

safety), which generates the notion of risk" (Giddens/Pierson 1998: 209; see also Giddens 1990), and answers to the problems of modernity insofar as it introduces a new concept of risk.[8] In a conversation with Pierson, Giddens goes on to explain that "[e]ssentially, 'risk' always has a negative connotation, since it refers to the chance of avoiding an unwanted outcome. But it can quite often be seen in a positive light, in terms of the taking of bold initiatives in the face of a problematic future. Successful risk-takers, whether in exploration, in business or in mountaineering, are widely admired" (1998: 209). As soon as dangers are transformed into risks, the range of possibilities for influence expands. Technology transformed dangers that were given by nature into risks, and perhaps in doing so has created new risks (Rosa et al. 2014: 103). In contrast, a genetic variation is given as a statistical calculation, and the concept of genetic risk is described not only in medical terms but also in terms of its social consequences and the difficulties it may bring for daily life. Genetic risks in pregnancy care are considered with regard to the foetus, and are described as being more or less severe according to particular criteria, such as the age or genetic heritage of the pregnant woman. Generally, within every pregnancy, there are genetic risks which call for technologies that make the genetic disposition of the foetus visible.

When it comes to "genetic risks", the prevention or avoidance of the consequences of certain genes that may result in particular conditions is seen as a heroic act, as exemplified by the tabloids' reporting about Angelina Jolie and her mastectomy. Thus, the concept of *genetic* risk as introduced into prenatal care implies a normative duty of the pregnant woman to be concerned about the foetus in terms of what behaviour is appropriate. It implies a responsibility to retrieve genetic information about the foetus and to decide on the basis of informed choice to minimise as far as possible the insecurity with respect to the risk. From a Foucauldian view of governmentality, the concept of risk has now become established in the field of prenatal genetic diagnostics and is part of society's concern and vocabulary, and leads to "genetic responsibilisation"

---

8   Beck and Giddens approach the concept of risk in the horizon of modernity and the traditional class structure of society. Contrary to Beck, Giddens defines risk more optimistically as also providing possibilities of empowerment and self-activity. He distinguishes two types of risks: external risks and manufactured risks. Manufactured risks depend on human agency and allow for both producing and mitigating risks. The Chernobyl disaster was one motive to think about risk. Genetic risks as we know them today were touched upon but not explored.

(Lemke 2000, 2004, 2006). Likewise, the notion of "genetic risk" is embedded politically in both modern liberal capitalism and the discourse on selection and eugenics that emerged in the 19th and 20th centuries. While the first is directly linked to the economic history of risk and the present social and economic order of society, the second is connected to the medical discourse on risk factors that developed during the early 20th century with regard to social hygiene, and in the late 20th century as a reaction to an increase in diseases typical of Western civilisation (e.g. heart attack, particular forms of cancer). Furthermore, genetic risk can be traced back to the 19th and 20th centuries' history of genetics, eugenics and racial hygiene.[9] Certainly, the late 19th and early 20th century was a period of vivid discussions about different understandings of the biological foundations and mechanisms of heredity. For instance, in researching the basis of heredity, the zoologist August Weismann was able to show that the biologisation of social contexts has no hereditary equivalent. Nevertheless, a fear of the danger of social degeneration, as it was perceived, stirred by the unholy alliance of Darwin's and Lamarck's theories, developed further in the 20th century and became a major source of the eugenic movement before and during the National Socialist regime (Weingart et al. 1992).

In 1909, the physician Archibald Garrod set a milestone in the history of genetics. He noticed that there were diseases with a family history whose characteristic, for example, could be found in both father and son at the same time. Further, he noticed that the disease is inherited as a Mendelian autosomal recessive trait. His work made him into a founder of medical biochemical and molecular genetics and established the study of genetic disease (Perlman/ Govindaraju 2016). By 1909 the Danish botanist Wilhelm Johannsen, who first used the word "gene" as an empirical working concept, was well aware of the vagueness of the collective term. In the early 20th century, the notion of "gene" nevertheless increasingly became – first in the natural sciences and then in public perception – a central concept for denoting questions of the biology of heredity (Paul 2006: 343; Keller 2002). Later, heredity, which is related to medical human genetics, focused on cancer research and tumour development in somatic mutations. However, the international upsurge of eugenics and, later on, National Socialist race politics (*Rassenpolitik*) overshadowed the results of

---

9   The term "racial hygiene" (in German: *Rassenhygiene*) denotes a special and dehumanising interpretation of eugenics in the German-speaking countries (for further reference, see Schües 2021a). It is important to mention this background in this context because it still overshadows the discussion of prenatal genetics (see Foth 2021).

molecular genetic research into the functions of the hereditary substance. The intertwining of medical, genetic and social concerns is described in, for instance, the *Reichsgesetzblatt* of 3 July 1934, which speaks of looming "dangers" for the health of the *Volkskörper* (body of the people) (Fangerau/Noack 2006; Fuchs 2008: 195, 197).[10]

The population and racial policies of the Nazi regime meant that after the Second World War the field of genetics was challenged to position itself in a new way. Eugenics had come under general suspicion after the recent inhumane and horrific selection procedures. Scientific genetics found it difficult to free itself from this suspicion. While "eugenics" became taboo in Germany (Foth 2021), the improvement of the "gene pool" of the population nevertheless continued to be propagated under the heading of "reform eugenics", especially in the USA (Paul 2006: 346) and also in Israel. In the USA, improving the genetic basis of human existence was also supposed to lead to an improvement in human living conditions. In Israel, eugenics was much discussed between 1930 and 1955. "Psychiatrist [Arie] Kochinsky, for one, argued in 1938 in the journal *Harefuah*[11] that the findings of a census of the mentally ill in Palestine should serve primarily as 'a basis for methods to improve the [Jewish] race'", as the journalist Yotam Feldman reported in the newspaper *Haaretz* (Feldman 2009). Later, in 1942, with the aim of strengthening the Jewish race by means of controlling births, Kochinsky focused on "population policy and psychopathology" at the second conference of the Neuro-Psychiatric Society. In August 1952, a decision was passed by the World Congress of Jewish Physicians to establish a scientific institute dedicated to issues of eugenics in Israel (ibid.). The institute was never established.[12]

Jewish physicians and psychiatrists who escaped from Germany to Israel stirred the debates about population policy, racial hygiene, and eugenics. The basic question was, as Yosef Meir, the head of a health fund, wrote in 1934

---

10   In the horizon of this research and in the year 1949, Linus Pauling, for example, described sickle cell anaemia as a "truly molecular disease with its origin in the change of gene structure and function" (cf. Paul 2006: 345).

11   The journal Harefuah is the medical-scientific periodical of the Israeli Medical Association. It was founded in 1920 (https://www.ima.org.il/eng/ViewContent.aspx?Categor yId=11081), accessed 26 July 2022.

12   In 2009 the daily newspaper Haaretz also reported on a 1958 letter by Golda Meir, then foreign minister of Israel, to the Israeli ambassador to Poland. Golda Meir raised the possibility of preventing handicapped and sick Polish Jews from immigrating to Israel (Galili 2009).

in *Ha'em Vehayeled* ("Mother and Child"): "Who is entitled to bear children?" (quoted in Feldman 2009). The focus of this question particularly concerned the psychiatric community, whose members were often immigrants from Germany; they included Kurt Löwenstein (Levinstein), originally a German psychiatrist and neurologist and president of the neuropsychiatric society in Israel, who promoted eugenics at a 1944 medical conference in Tel Aviv (Feldman 2009). In his lecture, he argued against allowing those with mental disorders to bear children. He was not alone in this view, yet it was important to him that he be understood as distancing himself from Nazi ideology. He certainly knew about eugenic ideology's political connotation and close connections to the Nazi regime and its systematic atrocities against Jews and other groups. I presume these thoughts should be seen in the historical context and as an attempt to understand mental disorder and to find a social-moral order to alleviate human suffering. The historian Rakefet Zalashik (2012) wrote about the history of psychiatry in Palestine during the Mandate and following the founding of the State of Israel. She explains that eugenic social engineering was not only part of the ideology of Israeli/German psychiatrists, but was also central to the Zionist vision of Israel and to the idea of a Jewish body which should be born under the "condition" of being healthy (cf. Weiss 1994). Thus, the question: Who is entitled to be born?

In 1962, the CIBA Foundation organised the symposium "The Biological Future of Man" in London. Not only was so-called "reform eugenics" discussed at this meeting, but also the view, spurred on by the discovery of the double helix in 1953, that genes were essentially building blocks of biological information. Genetics became an information-based science. The idea that "genetic information" was present in the chromosomes as a biological "code" was born[13] (cf. Kay 2000). This scientific activity inspired the expansion of genetics and acceleration towards the human genome project.

Research into human genetics has not only advanced into knowledge of the structural instability of a gene and even the decoding of the human genome, but has also provided the basis for a radical expansion of the concepts of health and disease. Once genetic prognoses, or at least statistical probabilities, are

---

13   Terms like "information", "message" or "code" did not appear in the language of biologists until the 1950s. This way of thinking basically goes back to the scientists of the Cold War, e.g. John von Neumann's game theory, because during that period many physicists, mathematicians and cyberneticists who had previously been involved in war-related activities moved into biology. They brought this metaphor with them.

possible, methods of prenatal genetic testing can be used to diagnose diseases or disabilities (such as trisomies, Huntington's disease, cystic fibrosis) before they become symptomatic. Biomedicine now includes the search for genetic dispositions and risks for disease or disability. This not only expands the concept of disease and makes new legal, economic or insurance policy issues relevant, but also shifts the responsibility to those who are confronted with genetic testing of their foetus (or of their own genetic disposition).[14]

By 1978 the maternity guidelines (*Mutterschaftsrichtlinien*) in Germany mentioned "genetic risk", which at that point referred primarily to the recommendation that the doctor should offer counselling (Fuchs 2008: 306). In addition, the guidelines spoke of a "genetic age risk", which is why "high-risk pregnant women" should "make use of prenatal diagnostics" (Fuchs 2008: 299). The paradigm of genetic risk was born. Today, pregnancy care is understood, experienced and guided by the concept of genetic risk. It is thus assumed that the pregnant woman has a genetic responsibility towards the foetus, the family or society according to the perceived genetic risk, i.e. whether this risk is socially or culturally perceived as being low or high. She has a responsibility to determine the genetic risks and to take steps to control them with the help of her gynaecologist. These steps include taking genetic tests and subsequent action should a test be positive.

NIPT, genetic risk and genetic responsibility

Prenatal genetic testing has been under discussion for several decades, and NIPT has been offered since 2012 as a prenatal genetic test in Germany and as a screening test in Israel.[15] If NIPT is positive, it has to be confirmed through

---

14 *Prediction* is both a medical and an everyday concept, even a utopian ideal, aimed at reducing health risks and preventing disease. It is firmly anchored in the individual consciousness as well as at the societal level. The prediction of individual health risks that ideally corresponds with prevention and a therapeutic intervention is of great interest to the individual patients and to the social perception of health and disease.

15 Principally, diagnostic testing is used when there is cause for concern, i.e. a risk; screening tests are performed in order to find out whether there are reasons to be concerned, i.e. whether there is a genetic risk to be followed up. (https://www.healthknowledge.org.uk/public-health-textbook/disease-causation -diagnostic/2c-diagnosis-screening/screening-diagnostic-case-finding), accessed 02

amniocentesis, a genetic test. Strictly speaking, the positive result of a chromosome variation found by amniocentesis, such as trisomy 13, 18 or 21, is not a risk but a medical diagnosis which, however, does not say all about the severity of the symptoms in real life. Thus, the notion of risk is firstly formulated on the side of the pregnant woman who may transmit a genetic risk based on predefined criteria, for instance being aged over 35 years, which means that statistically she has a higher risk of having a foetus with a chromosomal variation. Secondly, risk is considered on the side of the foetus before any test or diagnosis is done and, furthermore, a risk is perceived as the result of a positive outcome of a genetic test. Such risk includes the question of how the genetic variation will become symptomatic as a phenotype. For example, some children with trisomy 21 develop heart problems or malformations of the gastrointestinal tract (Guedj/Bianchi/Delabar 2014), while others do not.

Most disabilities or health problems associated with chromosomal variations cannot be treated. Some families, as reported by interviewees in Germany, say they took the test result as a chance to prepare themselves better for a child with disability, socially, psychologically and practically (Philipp et al. 2020: 27f.; cf. chapter 8). However, most parents respond to a positive finding by ending the pregnancy. It is worth mentioning that some of these pregnancies are terminated without confirmation of a test result. This should probably be understood as an expression of the enormous psychological stress under which the pregnant woman finds herself in the case of an "abnormal finding" (Kagan/Hoopmann 2020: 22).

The recommendation to verify a positive NIPT with amniocentesis indicates the risk of false positive results. The clinical geneticist Christian Netzer (2022) has investigated the test security of NIPT. Companies advertise NIPT as having a sensitivity (false positive) of 99 per cent and a specificity (false negative) of 99.9 per cent with regard to trisomy 21. However, these numbers depend upon the frequency of trisomy in the investigated group. In 20-year-old pregnant women, trisomy is less likely to be found in the foetus, which is why accuracy is reduced to 48 per cent (sensitivity), compared to 93 per cent in 40-year-olds. NIPT is considered a quantum leap compared to first-trimester screening, with a false positive rate of only 3 per cent in 20-year-old pregnant women. If a test result is positive, what can women do? Usually, they feel a strong insecurity. Now they *must* decide: once the positive result is known, the "risk" is

---

June 2022. In our interviews, some women perceived NIPT as a diagnostic test because the first-trimester nuchal fold scan revealed a risk of trisomy.

no longer on the side of the pregnant women (e.g. her age), but on the side of the biomaterial of the foetus. The risk can no longer be suppressed. This situation leads to further diagnostics, possibly to an abortion or to a constant uncertainty about whether the child, once it is born, might have something that has turned out to be a false diagnosis. In this context women feel that they are caught in a testing "spiral" (Schöne-Seifert/Junker 2021: 962). Society, politics and the market push the genetic responsibility onto the woman. She knows the risk and has to deal with it, yet she may not be fully aware of the complexity of the personal and social issues at stake. Even though she may not be fully aware of it, the ethical discourse defines her as a person with reproductive autonomy, which does not release her from genetic responsibility – especially not when NIPT strongly indicates a genetic risk. In view of these various genetic options, pregnancy care increasingly focuses on risk aspects and the possible termination of the pregnancy (Steger et al. 2018: 15).

Overall, prenatal genetic tests are well established in Germany, Israel, and throughout the countries of the Western world. Genetic knowledge obtained by prenatal testing conveys either the possible statistical distribution of genetic differences in the population, or the assurance of a genetic variation that leaves it more or less open how severe this variation, e.g. trisomy 21, will turn out. The idea of "genetic responsibility", which may be ascribed to the (future) parents/pregnant mothers, shows that the content and goal of medical and genetic consultation may include the entire family as well as any future offspring (Remennick 2006). For Israel in particular it has become a social norm to "equate 'good mothering' in pregnancy with taking 'genetic responsibility' for future offspring and the entire family" (Hashiloni-Dolev 2018: 126).

The results of testing always affect the individual, the family and perhaps others who are close, and they reflect different debates in public health (Ravitsky 2017). In the context of human genetics and genetic testing, the separation of individual and public health issues is increasingly blurred.

The genetic risk status within a pregnancy may be low or high depending, among other aspects, on the age of the woman and the family history. Risk determination as part of genetics is not just about an individual, but about biological connections that become socially relevant. The geneticisation of life, and of foetal life, supports the social development of genetic responsibility and risk management practices that normalise and institutionalise prenatal genetic testing practices, such as NIPT, amniocentesis or chorionic villus sampling (CVS). These practices are being implemented in both Israel and Germany, with different meanings, patterns and regulation (Raz et al. 2022; see chapter 3 of this book).

Paid for privately as in Israel or, since spring 2022, in individual cases by insurance companies as in Germany, the availability of genetic tests and the associated promotional information has strengthened the perception of genetic risk and pushed the way in which people respond to it. If a woman is pregnant she will have to respond to the practice of prenatal genetic testing and its availability – but how she responds to it will show whether she is acting with genetic responsibility. With regard to general risks, it is first of all important to state the obvious: whereas amniocentesis includes the small risk of miscarriage, any description of NIPT mentions that there is no risk of this kind, since it is performed on a blood sample from the pregnant woman (Holloway et al. 2022). NIPT is provided by private companies that publish advertising information about the tests, their use and aims.[16] Such advertising information sets an epistemic and emotional context for the meaning of genetic responsibility and its connection to the perception of genetic risk. Looking at different websites can also illuminate some differences between Germany and Israel.

An overview of company websites in Germany shows that the advertising and information leaflets about NIPT focus on the *security* of the test, the *feelings* of the woman, and her overall *responsibility*. For instance, information about the Harmony® Test promises: "Gain certainty", "Be unburdened", "Be reassured" ("*Gewissheit erlangen*", "*Entlastet sein*", "*Beruhigt sein*"),[17] "Three steps to clear answers" ("*Drei Schritte zu klaren Antworten*"). The pages convey the sense that the test provides quick and easy assurance and soothes the anxiety. This is accompanied by pictures showing a happy mother with her big belly. Clearly, a private company is advertising its product. The focus on safety and security prevails: "safe method, secure result" – this is the promise of the Harmony® Test.[18] The counter-notions are "risk" and "insecurity". Women with a so-called risk pregnancy are particularly targeted. When they search for information, they quickly find *genetic* information and the picture of a young woman with trisomy

---

16   Representatives of genetic prenatal diagnostics argue that the close link between reproductive medicine and selective abortion prematurely conflates the two and ignores the possibility that parents may wish to prepare for a child with special needs (Löwy 2018: 147, with reference to the CEO of the company *Natera*). The fact that over 95 per cent of foetuses tested with a genetic defect are aborted is concealed by this company.

17   https://lifecodexx.com/fuer-schwangere, accessed 02 June 2022.

18   http://www.cenata.de/der-harmony-test/, accessed 02 June 2022.

21. Her picture is more reminiscent of police mugshots than of pregnancy websites. All in all, the site seems to play on the worries of the parents-to-be and emotionally suggests avoiding the "result" shown on the picture.[19] The *Gemeinsamer Bundesausschuss* (G-BA) in Germany first published its patient information as recently as 2021.

In Israel, the information about prenatal genetic testing is provided by the health ministry, clinics and companies. The tenor is informative. NIPT is described as a screening test, alongside ultrasound, and as something done prior to amniocentesis. The concept of risk with regard to bearing a "Down syndrome baby" is part of this information; it is explained statistically: "In Israel, the risk of Down syndrome is considered high if it is greater than 1:380 (0.26 per cent). Women with this risk level (or higher), are recommended to undergo an amniotic fluid test. This risk level of bearing a child with Down syndrome is equivalent to that of women in the general population who were aged 35 at the time of becoming pregnant. When the risk is lower than 1:380, it is considered low."[20] The message is clear: the risk level lies on the side of the woman and the object of the risk is a Down syndrome baby. Thus, the reader understands that the only responsible thing to do is have the test in order to avoid such a "result".

Another Israeli website informs its readers about replacing amniocentesis, and lists the common tests, such as MaterniT21, the Harmony® Test, and NIFTY, states which company is marketing and manufacturing them, and provides information about their advantages and shortcomings, e.g. they do not endanger the pregnancy, but on the other hand they are expensive and the accuracy of the test is unclear.[21] Mostly, NIPT is presented as one test option among others as part of prenatal care. When it comes to company advertising, accuracy is the major selling point: "Harmony is the most precise test of its kind, whose accuracy has been proven in dozens of scientific studies," promises Fugene Genetics.[22]

---

19   http://www.downsyndromenipt.info/genetik/?lang=de, accessed 02 June 2022.

20   https://www.health.gov.il/English/Topics/Genetics/checks/during_pregnancy/Pages/screening_tests.aspx, accessed 02 June 2022.

21   https://www.genes.co.il/%D7%91%D7%93%D7%99%D7%A7%D7%94-nipt/. An example from the information site of a clinic: https://hospitals.clalit.co.il/soroka/he/med-units/ob-gyn-division/pages/prenatal-diagnosis.aspx; https://iw.lifehealthdoctor.com/prenatal-screening-tests-25423, accessed 02 June 2022.

22   הרמוני בדיקת | Harmony בדיקת הרמוני דם לגילוי תסמונות – Fugene Genetics, accessed 02 June 2022.

It seems that the information provided for future parents varies widely in style. General information is basically always given, but the framing of responsibility seems a bit different: safety and security in Germany, normal procedure in prenatal care in Israel. Looking at this advertising information suggests that genetic testing does not just concern medical practices but is embedded in a social setting that varies in policy regulation, normative consideration, and emotional understanding.

Furthermore, the concern of genetic testing – illness or disability – despite its genetic factors, is a complex multifactorial event involving the interplay of genome, environment and behaviour, and is also a social phenomenon from the perspective of the (future) parents. This fact seems rather underemphasised in the bioethical debate on genetic information. It seems that the "genetic risk" is largely absent from the discourse on social risk and, accordingly, from strategies of coping with risk which may develop in connection with the parents' social circumstances and individual environment. Put practically, the life of a family with a child (or an adult) with Down syndrome may be very different according to how this genetic disposition is realised. In addition, such realisation is developed according to social support, institutional structures, and emotional acceptance, among other things. Thus, the feeling that there is a social risk in having a child with a disability depends upon the concrete social context. However, accepting a child regardless of whether she has a disability is often something the parent(s) have to do even beyond any feeling of taking a "risk". If the intertwinement of the genetic and social context is disregarded, the individual – whether the pregnant woman or the affected person with health risks – is left alone with her decision. In practice, genetic risks and the question of how to deal with them are individualised by transforming the rational category of risk probability into a non-social category of a biological risk-body, which is determined in disregard of its ascribed social complexities. But it conveys as biological fact a specific social calculation that functions in the logic of prevention and mitigation.[23]

The idea that a pregnant woman should have genetic testing in order to retrieve genetic knowledge about the physical material of the foetus and to en-

---

23   Since about the early 1990s, insurance companies have also included the logic of prevention and mitigation, especially in the health sector, in their calculations. This form of logic does not work in the old way of insurance companies trying to predict the statistical possibility of events in order to calculate sums of capitalisation and compensation.

sure that there is no genetic risk of a trisomy (or other genetic variation) implies that she is supposed to take genetic responsibility. Even more so if a pregnant woman fulfils certain criteria, such as being older than 35 or already having a genetic condition, she should take particular genetic responsibility. The stronger the perception of genetic risk, the more important genetic responsibility becomes. Is taking *genetic* responsibility the only way to be responsible as a (future) mother?

Assuming genetic responsibility correlates with perceiving genetic risk

Generally speaking, responsibility is a relational and temporal concept which is interpreted within a concrete situation, and which includes several poles and aspects. A *prospective relational intergenerational concept of responsibility* is most suitable for questions posed in the context of pregnancy and birth, children and family. This concept of responsibility is oriented towards the future, is based on a relationship context, and is directed towards both the well-being of individuals and the success of relationships. These relationships are intergenerational, i.e. between parents and children or grandparents and grandchildren, or they exist within one generation, i.e. between a couple, siblings and others. These familial and social relationships may of course be very different, such as relationships of care, neglect, attention, disregard; they can be broken or close. Very concretely, during pregnancy (future) mothers especially are asked to assume genetic responsibility. But perhaps care responsibility, irrespective of any genetic check-ups, is equally appropriate? Care responsibility has a much broader focus than genetic responsibility; it extends beyond individual ethics because it is not only attentive and responsive towards the general well-being of the foetus, but also towards the familial context and social relationships, which can be more or less supportive and caring. Focusing on care responsibility acknowledges that the vulnerability and well-being of someone (also) depends upon the kind of care relationships in which that person lives. This table depicts the different structural elements of genetic responsibility and care responsibility.

Responsibility	Genetic responsibility	Care responsibility
subject	pregnant woman + partner	pregnant woman + partner
object, content	bio-material of foetus; testing?	(future) child, family, relationship
addressee	future child, family, or society	future child, family, or society
legitimating instance	society, family, authorities, religion, conscience, medical perspective	society, family, authorities, religion, conscience, feelings of humanity
value, norm	humanity, dignity, health, sanctity of life, benefit	humanity, dignity, health, sanctity of life, well-being
motive	standard procedure, specific risk awareness, fear, or concern	general concern and care for the individuals and the relationships
intention and aim	prevention, mitigation of risk, knowledge for decisions, care, family planning	care, good relationships, well-being, family planning
consequences of the action	personal life, avoidance of discrimination, benefit of family	general well-being of individuals and family (provided the care succeeds)

Elements of prenatal genetic responsibility and care responsibility.
Inspired by Lenk/Maring 1993: 229; Schicktanz/Schweda 2012: 142.

Prenatal genetic responsibility and care responsibility are forms of prospective responsibility and related to prenatal care. They are similar with regard to the question of who the subject and the addressee of the responsibility are. For each type of responsibility, it is mostly the (future) parents or the family who are part of the decision-making process; but it seems that in the end it is still the pregnant woman who takes responsibility for the foetus/child. For both forms of responsibility, the legitimating social instances are similar, but in addition, genetic responsibility is strongly supported by a medical perspective. In Israel and Germany, the obstetricians or gynaecologists are legally requested to mention prenatal genetic testing, and they often even recommend it as part of parental responsibility (Ravitsky 2021: 320; Schmid et al. 2015: 508).

Although both types of responsibility generally focus on pregnancy and the (future) child, each form has a specific thematic content and a specific motive. However, I argue that in contrast to genetic responsibility, (future) mothers can assume a *responsibility of care* that does not include a responsibility for the genetic disposition of the foetus. The motive of genetic responsibility is based on risk perception, whereas care generally focuses on the well-being of a person regardless of particular concerns about needs, illness, special vulnerabilities or general problems – or genetic risks. I will first describe how genetic responsibility relates to genetic risk perception and then turn to the question of whether not to test would be irresponsible. By arguing that (future) mothers/parents may have "good reasons" not to have genetic testing, I will introduce the concept of non-responsibility as well as the notion of care responsibility, which is broader than genetic responsibility.

Genetic responsibility in pregnancy is directed toward detecting genetic variations of the body material of the foetus on the basis of perceiving genetic risks, or even just fearing them. It focuses on getting to know the genetic dispositions of the foetus. The motive to test is thus mostly wondering or fearing that there may be something "wrong" with the "child" (Remennick 2006: 21; Schicktanz 2018). Genetic prenatal testing provides genetic information that is intended to give pregnant women knowledge so that they can reduce "risk", and to help them to exercise their "reproductive autonomy". However, it is not always clear what exactly women perceive and understand when they are informed about the genetic disposition of their foetus. In bioethical discussions, some authors understand genetic information as empowering (Beauchamp/ Childress 2008; Schicktanz 2018: 237), while others see the women's insecurities and uncertainties, since it is sometimes difficult for them to really understand the outcome of prenatal genetic tests because there is no prognosis about how, for instance, trisomy 21 will be realised in life and in the family.

The object of genetic responsibility is the foetus under genetic consideration. The genetic testing concerns the body material and the biological substance: genetic tests, statistical probabilities, and genetic prognosis. Genetic testing needs a strong focus on the biological substrate, the carrier of its genetic information. The foetus is subjected to biomaterial technology, whether in testing or subsequent selection. Prenatal genetics does not address the individual as a whole, but is a practice that targets the genotype of the species.

Biopolitically speaking, in the age of "making life" (Foucault 2008) genetic tests are not about someone. They omit the person (cf. Gehring 2006: 175). The focus on the "biological substrate" leaves the person outside the consideration and leads to a "biologisation of everyday life"; and prenatal genetics become an "everyday biology" (Gehring 2006: 182). This description can even be extended further: the biological substrate, the material, is understood as being inherent to the human being. It certainly does not simply determine behaviour or characteristics in their entirety; to assume this would be to adopt an unfounded naturalisation of persons. Nevertheless, this biological substrate, decoded as genetic determination and biological disposition, is like a promise implanted in the body and radiating into the future. It is a transmitter of coded information containing species characteristics that can be separately judged as "inconspicuous" or "conspicuous", "desirable" or "undesirable" (Schües 2016a: 287).

From the perspective of genetic responsibility, the child will be born (or not born) precisely under the conditions of the biological substrate. As Löwy (2018: 1, 147) argues, prenatal genetic diagnosis allows us "to see *what* is about to be born" (my emphasis). The reference to "*what* will be born" implies, on the one hand, a vision of "what" will happen – "life" with a disability or without – and on the other hand, technical insight into a biological substrate whose characteristics may reveal a particular vision to be interpreted beyond medical statistics. Because it is bound to the biomedical perspective, the test result cannot mean a person in her social entirety; but later, after birth, it will be possible to tell the person in retrospect that her genetic disposition has been tested. The "what" is understood differently depending on the temporal perspective and personal attitude. The biomedical discourse itself does not simply mean a human being or biological substrates. But once a person is born, the genetic check has been carried out; from the point of view of biomedical laboratory practice, only the biological material of a foetus is examined. But from the everyday point of view, the issue is understood differently: if genetic prenatal tests had produced the desired outcome, i.e. a "negative" result, then a genetically non-disabled – "healthy" as most parents would say – child is born.

In contrast to genetic responsibility, care responsibility may include concern about genetic risk but is primarily attentive to a wider range of themes, such as care and support. Care responsibility is understood as an ethics of relationship (*Beziehungsethik*) that considers the well-being of all persons involved and their relational practice of care, attentiveness, support and responsiveness (Schües 2016b; see also Tronto 1993: 127 ff.). Responsibility of care and concern can be grounded on very different facts, such as empathy, needing or wanting to help, but perhaps also risks. In other words – and this is the main difference – the observation of risk is only *one* possible motive for being concerned and of responding with care, but care responsibility is not just guided by a risk paradigm. It may therefore include genetic responsibility, but it can still be valuably exercised without it. Not acting according to genetic responsibility presupposes a different set of motives, intentions and aims, as mentioned in the table.

How not testing may yet be considered as a form of responsibility will be discussed in the next section.

Genetic irresponsibility, non-responsibility, and care responsibility

When we look at the practice of NIPT, in society as well as in our interview study, some people judge a woman or future parents *as being irresponsible* if they do not follow up a perceived genetic risk in pregnancy, and if they do not want to know the genetic disposition of their child (cf. chapter 11). It seems these reproaches assume that if she had known about a trisomy she would surely have aborted the foetus. At this point I do not want to discuss the question of whether a woman would or should terminate a pregnancy if a diagnosis is positive. I ask whether a woman who does not test is necessarily irresponsible.

Most generally, a (future) mother is considered morally irresponsible if she is capable of reflecting, deliberating and thinking ahead, yet makes insufficient effort to do so,[24] and she is unconcerned about the future of her child (or her family) and the consequences of her decisions. We might furthermore refer to a violation of norms and values as well as the observation that she is acting in a field of knowledge that she should have considered.

Andre et al. (2000) argue that acting wrongly and acting irresponsibly should be distinguished morally and philosophically, and that this distinction should be applied to the question of what it means to reject prenatal testing. They argue that responsible care for a child does not necessarily mean having genetic testing. Parents may have reasons not to question the future

---

24   The condition of sufficiency is context-sensitive and depends on medical practice and cultural and social norms. Generally speaking, children or people with intellectual disability, i.e. people who do not think ahead or reflect sufficiently because they lack the capacity to do so, can be considered non-responsible but not irresponsible.

existence of this one child they have conceived. If they reflect on their reasons and "if they make a conscientious decision not to control genetic outcomes they are *exercising* their responsibility, not evading it" (Andre et al. 2000: 145). This argument takes the presence of moral reflection and a conscientious decision as testimony against the accusation of irresponsibility. By showing that irresponsible action can be taken without the action itself necessarily being judged as wrong, it separates a person's attitude from the decision or action, which can come out good or bad. Thus, in this approach, the concept of irresponsibility is aimed at the attitude of the persons acting and not at their actual choice. Andre et al. define irresponsibility as an attitude that leads to imprudent decisions or actions. I agree with their argument that responsible care in pregnancy does not necessarily involve genetic testing but I disagree that responsibility is *just* a matter of the attitude of the person in question. Surely, irresponsibility describes an attitude of a person but in light of the relational concept of responsibility laid out above, and the fact that irresponsibility structurally involves the same elements as responsibility, the evaluation of a person's decision-making or action does not depend just on the attitude of the person whose responsibility is under scrutiny. An ethics of responsibility is not *just* bound to the attitude of the actor, nor *just* to the morality of the action. Rather, in light of the different elements that structure responsibility and irresponsibility, we have to consider elements in addition to the pregnant woman's attitude, such as the addressee, the motive, the intention, and the thematic realm.

In order to explain my approach, I would like to emphasise the following: the criteria for responsibility concern both the future child and the future of the child. While the former idea denotes the characteristics of the child (i.e. genetic dispositions) in relation to seeing *what* is about to be born, the latter concerns the future of whoever is born in the context of care, relationships and the environment. If a test is positive, the biological material of the foetus is associated with a possibly disabled future body; and a future is often imagined depending on possible health problems, suffering, or special need for care. The mother's possible life is also considered in terms of whether she is willing or able to care for a child with a disability. After such a test result, the question of abortion is raised. *Genetic* irresponsibility means that even though the pregnant woman, her partner, obstetrician or gynaecologist, or society's accepted medical discourse perceive a genetic risk for the foetus, the woman does not want to know its genetic disposition and denies any considerations to act accordingly.

Is not wanting to have genetic testing necessarily irresponsible? Is the charge of "genetic irresponsibility" necessarily applicable to all non-users?[25] Or can we find the preference of not-knowing irresponsible within a discourse of biologisation but socially still consider it a responsible option? To address these questions, I introduce three different forms of morality of how to deal with the scope of genetic knowledge and care in pregnancy and for a child: genetic responsibility, irresponsibility, and non-responsibility. I would like to advocate that the conscious and justified rejection of genetic responsibility can also be acknowledged and respected as a form of genetic *non*-responsibility looking at the future of the child and not only at the "future child". Those who choose not to know and not to be concerned about genetic dispositions can still – for better or for worse – be responsible for the care of the child (and the family) in the future. Prenatal genetic diagnostics gives them the option to decide which foetus to select on the basis of a genetic disposition. This option is based on a genetic risk discourse and comes with genetic responsibility. However, this option and the idea of being guided by the paradigm of genetic risk can be rejected without therefore being considered irresponsible.

Generally defined, the term "non-responsibility" refers to a situation or action in which responsibility is rejected with "good reasons"; for example, in cases where we cannot do anything, in fields we do not know anything about, for which, clearly, someone else is responsible (Heidbrink 2017). The practice of pregnancy is very much governed by a genetic risk discourse and (future) mothers are more or less expected to assume this perception of risk and the associated genetic responsibility. But if a woman decides against testing, with "good reason", I call this *responsible genetic non-responsibility*. It is a decision that involves declaring oneself not responsible for the area of genetic decision-making, but nevertheless assuming responsibility of care for a child with whatever genetic disposition.

The thesis of responsible genetic non-responsibility can be understood in terms of two different positions: one, opting out of testing, and the other, opting in. The first would argue that typically and according to standard procedure (unless there are "good reasons"), care responsibility includes genetic responsibility. The burden of proof, i.e. having "good reasons" not to do genetic testing,

---

25   One reason for not-testing, as Jackie Leach Scully has mentioned (personal communication, 2022), could be that the parents themselves have the disability and consider life with that disability to be normal. From that perspective discourse of testing and abnormality is irrelevant.

lies with the pregnant woman. The other position, opting in, reverses the burden of proof: this position of responsible genetic non-responsibility is found when genetic testing is not standard practice. It argues that women who want to have the foetus genetically tested need to express "good reasons" to do so. Thus, the burden of proof lies on the side of the women (and the gynaecologist) and their view that genetic testing is necessary. Whereas the former reasoning practice regards genetic testing as normal and standard, and, hence, asks the women not willing to test to give reasons for opting out, the latter considers the individual cases and finds reasons to opt into the practice of genetic testing.

Having considered the different status of the positions of opting out and opting in, we now need to consider the difficult question "What are good reasons?" They are "good" if they are convincing. But whether they are convincing depends quite strongly on social and cultural norms and values that differ according to context and country. For example, "good reasons" may be religious reasons, respect for the genetic privacy of the future child, or the refusal to connect social care to the perception and calculation of risk. Certainly, responsibility for the genetic testing of the biological substrate and responsibility for the future life of a child are by no means the same thing; however, they are often implicitly equated. Even though it is not possible for one person to find "good reasons" that are convincing for all, I nevertheless want to argue that not wanting to know the genetic dispositions and not wanting to think and decide on the basis of risk-considerations might not necessarily be regarded as irresponsible. If the parents confirm that for them any genetic test result would be irrelevant to the continuation of the pregnancy and the future care of the child, then the issue of irresponsibility is questionable in relation to their intention. However, social normative orders might not be on their side.

If a genetic practice is socially and culturally normalised, self-evident and firmly established, as in Israel, and refusing a genetic test, opting out, would be only conceivable for religious reasons or perhaps for some "alternative lifestyles", then ultimately a woman who does not have her foetus genetically tested and who does not regard genetic risks as a basis for responsibility cannot find socially convincing reasons to reject *genetic* responsibility. A concept of genetic non-responsibility seems unacceptable even if parents decide to give full care to a child unconditionally, i.e. regardless of any illnesses or disabilities.

Germany has an ambivalent norm-oriented social context for genetic responsibility (cf. chapter 5). It seems that both positions, finding "good reasons" for opting in and opting out, must be brought to the consideration. The discourse on genetic testing still tries to maintain a balancing act between a normative critique of routinisation and case-by-case decision-making, and a normalising practice that is increasingly becoming established. If a woman finds "good reasons" and an accepted norm for not wanting to know the genetic disposition of her foetus and if she openly states that she cares unconditionally for the child, this attitude may be accepted under the acknowledged concept of individual decision-making. However, this does not mean that children with disability are necessarily welcomed in society. To phrase this ambivalence more optimistically, the German paradox is between social rejection and support: "It has never been so easy to identify a foetus with trisomy 21 in a society that approves of this chromosomal defect as a legitimate reason for abortion. And it has never been so easy to raise a child with Down syndrome in a society that is rightly proud of its efforts towards inclusion" (Schulz 2017: 198; TAB 2019: 157). Yet this optimistic view may not be shared by many women or families confronted with a positive test result. Although Schulz observes that the situation for people with disability has improved during the last decade, this does not mean that society – in Germany as well as Israel – is sufficiently supportive of people with disabilities and their families.

Theoretically, the difference between genetic irresponsibility and genetic non-responsibility comes down to the question of whether or not a woman has "good reasons", i.e. acceptable or convincing reasons, to reject genetic responsibility. Nonetheless, the distinction between genetic irresponsibility and genetic non-responsibility may not make sense in countries where genetic practice is seen as routine and is an integral part of prenatal care, i.e. it is considered prenatal risk management; there would be no "good reasons" not to test. All possible explanations would bounce off a firmly established reproductive medical practice that is taken for granted and perceived as normal.

Depending on the country's regulations, genetic practices and their social contexts, we may see inconsistencies, contradictions, dilatory compromises and dissents in interpretation, but we also see different tendencies in discourses in terms of what counts as good reasons or criteria for decisions or risk perception, and different understandings of responsibility and irresponsibility, security or insecurity. It appears that the constellation of responsibility and irresponsibility and the option of finding "good reasons" to refrain from genetic responsibility presupposes a concrete kind of care perception (that is not guided by genetic risk) and a particular normative order.

When it comes to the genetic disposition of the foetus, the narrower concept of genetic responsibility seems decisive; but when looking much more generally at the future of the child, a broader concept of responsibility would be in play, one that includes various health and societal aspects, the child's general welfare, and the life of the family. Today's transformation of the concept of responsibility in the social discussions of reproductive medicine practice appears in the fact that it is not just the question of what belongs to responsible parenthood that is relevant, but the question of *how responsible decisions* can be made in order to avoid irresponsible actions. Pregnancy and the beginning of life has become a morally challenging "project" that demands many decisions from the parents-to-be, and each decision has to be made with careful deliberation and moral reflection.

Ascribing genetic responsibility to expectant parents appears an attempt to translate a normative order of care into a specific cause-effect relationship. The irrationality of this translation consists in the assumption that, by analogy with contexts of social interaction, we can equally assume responsibility for our decisions in the context of genetic predispositions and the resulting consequences for the condition of the life in the future (Schües 2021b). If the broad notion of care responsibility is guided by reframing pregnancy into risk management and by reducing responsibility to genetic responsibility, the aspect of care may be lost in translation. Care responsibility extends more broadly over all structural elements and is mainly motivated by care for the other, the family, and social relationships.

Does responsibility of care, a responsibility that concerns the care of a child who is *entrusted* to someone, necessarily need genetic information as a prerequisite? How this question is answered is strongly correlated with the perception of genetic risk and whether prenatal genetic testing is perceived as a "standard procedure". If the general perception acknowledges genetic risks and perceives genetic testing as *standard*, this will influence how we evaluate what it means to be a responsible mother/parent. How the options of a responsible genetic non-responsibility are perceived and exercised might bring out central differences between prenatal care practices in Israel and Germany.

References

Andre, Judith/Fleck, Leonard M./Tomlinson, Thomas (2000): "On Being Genetically 'Irresponsible.'" In: Kennedy Institute of Ethics Journal 10/2, pp. 129–146, (https://doi.org/10.1353/ken.2000.0010), accessed 02 June 2022.

Bar-On, Dan (1989): Legacy of Silence: Encounters with Children of the Third Reich, Cambridge, MA: Harvard University Press.

Beauchamp, Tom. L./Childress, James F. (2008): Principles of Biomedical Ethics, 6th ed. Oxford: Oxford University Press.

Beck, Ulrich (1992): Risk Society: Towards a New Modernity, translated by Mark Ritter, London: Sage.

Bräutigam, Hans H./Mettler, Lieselotte (1985): Die programmierte Vererbung, Hamburg: Hoffmann und Campe.

Braun, Kathrin (2021): Biopolitics and Historic Justice: Coming to Terms with the Injuries of Normality, Bielefeld: transcript.

Bundesvereinigung Lebenshilfe (2015): "Gegen Diskriminierung von Menschen mit Trisomie 21: Lebenshilfe und Down-Syndrom – Verbände wenden sich gegen Reihenuntersuchung mit PraenaTest." Press release 17.3.2015, (https://www.presseportal.de/pm/59287/2974404), accessed 02 June 2022.

Conrad, Peter (2007): The Medicalization of Society: On the Transformation of Human Conditions into Treatable Disorders, Baltimore: Johns Hopkins University Press.

Fangerau, Heiner/Noack, Thorsten (2006): "Rassenhygiene in Deutschland und Medizin im Nationalsozialismus." In: Stefan Schulz/Klaus Steigleder/ Heiner Fangerau/Norbert W. Paul (eds.), Geschichte, Theorie und Ethik in der Medizin, Frankfurt: Suhrkamp, pp. 224–246.

Feldmann, Yotam (2009): "Eugenics in Israel: Did Jews try to improve the human race too?" In: Haaretz, 15 May, (https://www.haaretz.com/1.5052629), accessed 10 May 2022.

Fletcher, John C. (1974): "Genetics, Choice and Society." In: Mack Lipkin/Peter T. Rowley (eds.), Genetic Responsibility: On Choosing our Children's Genes, New York: Plenum, pp. 93–100.

Foth, Hannes (2021): "Avoiding 'selection'? – References to history in current German policy debates about non-invasive prenatal testing." In: Bioethics, 35/6, pp. 518–527, (https://doi.org/10.1111/bioe.12880), accessed 02 June 2022.

Foucault, Michel (2008): The Birth of Biopolitics: Lectures at the Collège de France, 1977–1978, translated by Graham Burchell, New York: Palgrave Macmillan.

Fuchs, Richard (2008): Life Science: Eine Chronologie von den Anfängen der Eugenik bis zur Humangenetik der Gegenwart, Berlin: LIT.

Galili, Lily (2009): "Golda Meir Told Poland: Don't Send Sick or Disabled Jews to Israel." In Haaretz, 9 December, (https://www.haaretz.com/1.5017879), accessed 7 May 2022.

Garrod, Archibald E. (1909): Inborn Errors of Metabolism, London: Frowde, Hodder & Stoughton.

Gehring, Petra (2006): Zwischen Menschenpart und Soft Eugenics. In: Petra Gehring (ed.), Was ist Biomacht? Vom zweifelhaften Mehrwert des Lebens, Frankfurt: Campus, pp. 154–183.

Giddens, Anthony (1990): Consequences of Modernity, Cambridge: Polity Press.

Giddens, Anthony/Pierson, Christopher (1998): Making Sense of Modernity: Conversations with Anthony Giddens, Stanford: Stanford University Press.

Guedj, Fayçal/Bianchi, Diana W./Delabar, Jean-Maurice (2014): "Prenatal treatment of Down syndrome: a reality?" In: Current Opinion in Obstetrics & Gynecology 26/2, pp. 92–103, (https://doi.org/10.1097/GCO.00000000000 00056), accessed 02 June 2022.

Haker, Hille (2001): "Präimplantationsdiagnostik und verantwortliche Elternschaft." In: Sigrid Graumann (ed.), Die Gen-kontroverse: Grundpositionen, Freiburg: Herder Spektrum, pp. 179–184.

Hashiloni-Dolev, Yael (2007): A Life (Un)Worth of Living: Reproductive Genetics in Israel and Germany, Dordrecht: Springer.

Hashiloni-Dolev, Yael (2018): "The Effect of Jewish-Israeli Family Ideology on Policy Regarding Reproductive Technologies." In: Hagai Boas/Yael Hashiloni-Dolev/Nadav Davidovitch/Dani Filc/Shai J. Lavi (eds.), Bioethics and Biopolitics in Israel: Socio-legal, Political, and Empirical Analysis, Cambridge: Cambridge University Press, pp. 119–138.

Heidbrink, Ludger (2017): "Definitionen und Voraussetzungen der Verantwortung." In: Ludger Heidbrink/Claus Langbein/Janina Loh (eds.), Handbuch Verantwortung, Wiesbaden: Springer, pp. 3–33.

Holloway, Kelly/Simms, Nicole/Hayeems, Robin Z./Miller, Fiona A. (2022): "The Market in Noninvasive Prenatal Tests and the Message to Consumers: Exploring Responsibility." In: Hasting Center Report 52/2, pp. 49–57.

Illich, Ivan (1975): "The Medicalization of Life." In: Journal of Medical Ethics, 1/2, pp. 73–77.

Ivry, Tsipy/Teman, Elly (2019): "Shouldering Moral Responsibility: The Division of Moral Labor among Pregnant Women, Rabbis, and Doctors." In: American Anthropologist, 121/4, pp. 857–869.

Jonas, Hans (1984 [1979]): The Imperative of Responsibility: In Search of an Ethics for the Technological Age, Chicago: University of Chicago Press.

Kagan, Karl Oliver/Hoopmann, Markus (2020): "Erweiterung des Anwendungsspektrums der vorgeburtlichen zellfreien DNA-Analyse." In: Zeitschrift für medizinische Ethik 66, pp. 17–23.

Kay, Lily (2000): Who Wrote the Book of Life? A History of the Genetic Code, Stanford: Stanford University Press.

Keller, Evelyn F. (2002): The Century of the Gene, Cambridge, MA: Harvard University Press.

Leefmann, Jon/Schaper, Manuel/Schicktanz, Silke (2016): "The concept of 'Genetic Responsibility' and its meanings: A systematic review of qualitative medical sociology literature." In: Frontiers in Sociology 1/18, pp. 1–22.

Lemke, Thomas (2000): "Die Regierung der Risiken: Von der Eugenik zur genetischen Gouvernementalität." In: Ulrich Bröckling/Susanne Krasmann/Thomas Lemke (eds.), Gouvernementalität der Gegenwart: Studien zur Ökonomisierung des Sozialen, Frankfurt: Suhrkamp, pp. 227–264.

Lemke, Thomas (2004): Veranlagung und Verantwortung: Genetische Diagnostik zwischen Selbstbestimmung und Schicksal, Bielefeld: transcript.

Lemke, Thomas (2006): "Genetic Responsibility and Neo-Liberal Governmentality: Medical Diagnosis as Moral Terrain." In: Alain Beaulieu/David Gabbard (eds.), Michel Foucault and Power Today: International Multidisciplinary Studies in the History of the Present, Lanham, MD: Lexington, pp. 83–91.

Lenk, Hans/Maring, Matthias (1993): "Verantwortung – Normatives Interpretationskonstrukt und empirische Beschreibung." In: Lutz H. Eckensberger/Ulrich Gähde (eds.), Ethische Norm und empirische Hypothese, Frankfurt: Suhrkamp, pp. 222–243.

Lipkin, Mack/Rowley, Peter T. (eds.) (1974): Genetic Responsibility: On Choosing Our Children's Genes, New York: Plenum.

Löwy, Ilana (2018): Tangled Diagnoses: Prenatal Testing, Women, and Risk, Chicago: University of Chicago Press.

Luhmann, Niklas (2003): Soziologie des Risikos, Berlin/New York: De Gruyter.

McClain, Linda (1996): "'Irresponsible' Reproduction." In: Hastings Law Journal 47/2, pp. 339–453.

Meadows Donella/Meadows, Dennis/Randers, Jørgen/Behrens, William W. (1972): Limit to Growth: A Report for the Club of Rome's Project on the Predicament of Mankind, New York: Universe Books.

Matthew, Sandra/Wexler, Laura (2000): Pregnant Pictures, London and New York: Routledge.

Netzer Christian (2022): "NIPT – medizinischer Sachstand und Perspektiven". Presentation at "Wissens-Wert? Zum verantwortlichen Umgang mit nicht-invasiven Pränataltests (NIPT)." Deutscher Ethikrat, Forum Bioethik, 23 February (https://www.ethikrat.org/forum-bioethik/wissens-wert-zum-verantwortlichen-umgang-mit-nichtinvasiven-praenataltests-nipt/?cookieLevel=not-set), accessed 8 May 2022.

Paul, Norbert W. (2006): "Humangenetik und Medizin: Geschichte Theorie, Ethik." In: Stefan Schulz/Klaus Steigleder/Heiner Fangerau/Norbert W. Paul (eds.), Geschichte, Theorie und Ethik in der Medizin, Frankfurt: Suhrkamp, pp. 341–367.

Perlman, Robert L./Govindaraju, Diddahally R. (2016): "Archibald E. Garrod: The Father of Precision Medicine." In: Genetics in Medicine 18/11, pp. 1088–1089.

Perrot, Adeline/Horn, Ruth (2021): "The ethical landscape(s) of non-invasive prenatal testing in England, France and Germany: Findings from a comparative literature review." In: European Journal of Human Genetics, (https://www.nature.com/articles/s41431-021-00970-2), accessed 02 June 2022.

Petersen, Alan (1998): "The new genetics and the politics of public health." In: Critical Public Health 8/1, pp. 59–71.

Philipp, Swetlana/Rodeck, Johanna/Strauss, Bernhard (2020): "Psychologische Aspekte der Beratung von Schwangeren über nicht-invasive Pränataldiagnostik (NIPD)." In: Zeitschrift für medizinische Ethik 66, pp. 25–36.

Prainsack, Barbara (2006): "'Natural force': The regulation and discourse of genomics and advanced medical technologies in Israel." In: Peter Glasner/Paul Atkinson/Helen Greenslade (eds.), New Genetics, New Social Formations, London: Routledge, pp. 231–252.

Primc, Nadia (2018): "Nicht-invasive Pränataltests und genetische Beratung zwischen dem Recht auf reproduktive Autonomie und der Pflicht zur Gesundheit." In: Florian Steger/Marcin Orzechowski/Maximilian Schochow (eds.), Pränatalmedizin: Ethische, juristische und gesellschaftliche Aspekte, Freiburg/Munich: Alber, pp. 33–53.

Ravitsky, Vardit (2017): "The shifting landscape of prenatal testing: between reproductive autonomy and public health." In: Hastings Center Report 47, pp. S34–S40.

Ravitsky, Vardit/Roy, Marie-Christine/ Haidar, Hazar/Henneman, Lidewij/ Marshall, John/Newson, Ainsley J./Ngan, Olivia M.Y./Nov-Klaiman, Tamar

(2021): "The Emergence and Global Spread of Noninvasive Prenatal Testing" *Annual Review of Genomics and Human Genetics*, 22(1), pp. 309–338, (https://www.annualreviews.org/doi/abs/10.1146/annurev-genom-083118 -015053), accessed 02 June 2022.

Raz, Aviad E./Nov-Klaiman, Tamar/Hashiloni-Dolev, Yael/Foth, Hannes/ Schües, Christina/Rehmann-Sutter, Christoph (2022): "Comparing Germany and Israel regarding debates on policy-making at the beginning of life: PGD, NIPT and their paths of routinization." In: Ethik in der Medizin 34, pp. 65–80, (https://doi.org/10.1007/s00481-021-00652-z), accessed 02 June 2022.

Raz, Aviad/Schicktanz, Silke (2016): Comparative Empirical Bioethics: Dilemmas of Genetic Testing and Euthanasia in Israel and Germany, Cham: Springer.

Remennick, Larissa (2006): "The quest for the perfect baby: Why do Israeli women seek prenatal genetic testing?" In: Sociology of Health & Illness 28/1, pp. 21–53.

Rosa, Eugene A./Renn, Ortwin/McCright, Aaron M. (2014): The Risk Society Revisited: Social Theory and Governance, Philadelphia: Temple University Press.

Rubeis, Giovanni (2018): "Das Konzept der Eugenik in der ethischen Debatte um nicht-invasiver Pränataltests (NIPT)." In: Florian Steger/Marcin Orzechowski/Maximilian Schochow (eds.), Pränatalmedizin: Ethische, juristische und gesellschaftliche Aspekte, Freiburg/Munich: Alber, pp. 102–130.

Ruckdeschel, Kerstin (2015): "Verantwortete Elternschaft: 'Für die Kinder nur das Beste'." In: Norbert F. Schneider/Sabine Diabaté/Kerstin Ruckdeschel (eds.), Familienleitbilder in Deutschland: Kulturelle Vorstellungen zu Partnerschaft, Elternschaft und Familienleben, Opladen/Berlin/Toronto: Barbara Budrich, pp. 191–206.

Schicktanz, Silke (2018): "Genetic risk and responsibility: reflections on a complex relationship." In: Journal of Risk Research 21/2, pp. 236–258.

Schicktanz, Silke/Schweda, Mark (2012): "The Diversity of Responsibility: The Value of Explication and Pluralization." In: Medicine Studies 3/3, pp. 131–145.

Schidel, Regina (2020): "Pränataldiagnostik als Instanz von struktureller Diskriminierung?" In: Zeitschrift für Praktische Philosophie 7/1, pp. 231–264, (https://doi.org/10.22613/zfpp/7.1.8), accessed 02 June 2022.

Schmid, Marianne/Klaritsch, P./Arzt, W./Burkhardt, T./Duba, H. C./Häusler, M./Hafner, E./Lang, U./Pertl, B./ Speicher, M./Steiner, H./Tercanli, S./

Merz, E./Heling, K S./Eiben, B. (2015): "Cell-Free DNA Testing for Fetal Chromosomal Anomalies in clinical practice: Austrian-German-Swiss Recommendations for non-invasive prenatal tests (NIPT)." Ultraschall in der Medizin, 36(5), pp. 507–510.

Schöne-Seifert, Bettina/Junker, Chiara (2021): "Making use of non-invasive prenatal testing (NIPT): rethinking issues of routinization and pressure." In: Journal of Perinatal Medicine 49/8, pp. 959–964.

Schües, Christina (2016a): Philosophie des Geborenseins, Freiburg/Munich: Alber.

Schües, Christina (2016b): "Ethik und Fürsorge als Beziehungspraxis." In: Elisabeth Conradi/Frank Vosman (eds.), Praxis der Achtsamkeit: Schlüsselbegriff der Care-Ethik, Frankfurt: Campus, pp. 251—272.

Schües, Christina (2021a): "'Ein Thier heranzüchten, das versprechen darf' – Eine paradoxe Aufgabe der pränatalen Diagnostik am Lebensanfang." In: Olivia Mitscherlich-Schönherr (ed.), Das Gelingen der künstlichen Natürlichkeit: Mensch-Sein an den Grenzen des Lebens mit disruptiven Biotechnologien, Berlin/Boston: de Gruyter, pp. 213–238.

Schües, Christina (2021b): "'Genetische Verantwortung' – was kann das heissen?" In: Claudia Bozzaro/Orsolya Friedrich (eds.), Philosophie der Medizin, Paderborn: Mentis, pp. 199–216.

Schulz, Sandra (2017): "Das ganze Kind hat so viele Fehler": Die Geschichte einer Entscheidung aus Liebe, Reinbek: Rowohlt.

Steger, Florian/Orzechowski, Marcin/Schochow, Maximilian (2018): "Einleitung." In: Florian Steger/Marcin Orzechowski/Maximilian Schochow (eds.), Pränatalmedizin: Ethische, juristische und gesellschaftliche Aspekte, Freiburg/Munich: Alber, pp. 13–31.

TAB (2019): "Aktueller Stand und Entwicklungen der Pränataldiagnostik." Alma Kolleck/Arnold Sauter, Büro für Technikfolgen-Abschätzung beim Deutschen Bundestag, TAB-Arbeitsbericht 184.

Tronto, Joan (1993): Moral Boundaries. A Political Argument for an Ethic of Care, New York: Routledge.

Ullrich, Charlotte (2012): Medikalisierte Hoffnung? Eine ethnographische Studie zur reproduktionsmedizinischen Praxis, Bielefeld: transcript.

Weingart, Peter/Kroll, Jürgen/Bayertz, Kurt (1992): Rasse, Blut und Gene: Geschichte der Eugenik und Rassenhygiene in Deutschland, Frankfurt: Suhrkamp.

Weiss, Meira (1994): Conditional love: Parents' attitudes toward handicapped children, Westport, CT: Greenwood.

Weiss, Meira (2004): The chosen body: The politics of the body in Israeli society, Stanford: Stanford University Press.

Zalashik, Rakefet (2012): Das unselige Erbe: Die Geschichte der Psychiatrie in Palästina und Israel, Frankfurt/New York: Campus.

Zimmermann Rolf (2016): "Historische Verantwortung." In: Ludger Heidbrink/Claus Langbein/Janina Loh (eds.), Handbuch Verantwortung, Wiesbaden: Springer, pp. 625–643.

II. Governance and biopolitics

3. Non-Invasive Prenatal Testing in Germany and Israel
A Matter of Course or a Matter of Discourse?

Tamar Nov-Klaiman, Hannes Foth, Yael Hashiloni-Dolev

Since its introduction into clinical practice in 2011, non-invasive prenatal testing/screening (NIPT/NIPS) has prompted concerns over its ethical, legal and social implications (Dupras et al. 2020; Haidar/Dupras/Ravitsky 2016). These concerns have intensified worldwide as many countries consider implementing NIPT in their national healthcare system, or have already done so (Ravitsky et al. 2021). Against the backdrop of this broad debate, we examine the local discourses of NIPT policymaking in Germany and Israel. These countries, related through a traumatic history, are both characterised by advanced medical technology and universal health coverage. Nonetheless, they are often opposed in terms of lay moralities, professional practice and healthcare policies, especially for genetic testing (Hashiloni-Dolev 2007; Raz/Schicktanz 2016). Israel is known as an early and enthusiastic adopter of biomedical technologies, whereas Germany is perceived as being relatively restrictive and cautious.

This study contributes to the comparative analysis of policymaking in healthcare. Cross-country comparisons are a powerful tool for understanding national variation in health policies and the moral and political assessment of biomedicine. Our focus on how NIPT policies are debated in Israel and Germany enables us to test the interplay of technological imperative in healthcare (McCoyd 2010) and cultural persistence/change. Raz (2018: 234) argues that in its genetic policies, "Israel is both reckless and pioneering – depending on one's perspective". Its early adoption of these technologies sometimes leads the way for other countries. Should we therefore expect the convergence of Israeli and German policies with the passing of time and advancement in techniques? Or rather, their divergence due to situated variables, such as previous approaches to screening for Down syndrome (Lôwy 2020)?

The case of NIPT highlights three major, inter-related challenges that are important for healthcare policy. First, NIPT policymaking provides a setting for considering various approaches to parental autonomy, selective abortion, embryo protection and disability rights (Haidar/Dupras/Ravitsky 2016; Heyd 1994). Second, it highlights different emphases in the context of care/prevention. While usually about prevention through abortion, NIPT may also be used to provide parents with early options of preparation (Kibel/Vanstone 2017; Lôwy 2020). Third, NIPT policymaking reflects different configurations of health governance that interconnect the State, the market, at-risk social categories, the family and the individual (Allyse et al. 2015; Lemke 2005; Ravitsky 2017).

These characteristics make NIPT a test case for stakeholder involvement. We compare the setting in which NIPT has been introduced in both countries: the legislative and regulatory framework as well as the socio-political context. This enables us to portray the discourses and stakeholders related to the use and potential implementation of NIPT in public healthcare in each country and their influence on decision making. Who is leading the debate? Which agendas drive the process? Do the decisions reached correlate with the legal and regulatory framework, and do they match former policies or take a new path?

Our analysis was done through systematic examination of policy documents and opinion papers issued by relevant stakeholders in Germany and Israel, such as medical organisations and advocacy bodies, in the period 2012–2021. It also involved an assessment of the legal framework with which this technology interrelates. Previous comparative studies between the countries, including in the field of biomedicine, were reviewed in order to establish the historical and social context in which the current debate takes place.

1.   Foundations of the comparison

Non-invasive prenatal testing (NIPT) is a genetic test that targets placenta-derived cell-free DNA present in maternal plasma. It is used at present mainly to detect certain chromosomal aberrations with high accuracy in the detection of trisomy 21, which results in Down syndrome (DS) (Gregg et al. 2016). However, NIPT also enables the detection of single gene disorders as well as sequencing of the entire foetal genome (Kitzman et al. 2012; Lench et al. 2013). As the technology becomes cheaper, it seems plausible that such detailed prenatal testing will be commonly used (Dondorp et al. 2015).

The test can be used as early as 9–10 weeks of gestation. Unlike invasive diagnostic testing such as amniocentesis, it poses no risk of miscarriage. The accuracy of NIPT is higher than previous forms of prenatal screening for aneuploidy. However, being a screening test, upon abnormal findings, diagnostic testing should be offered (Gregg et al. 2016). The test's features – its non-invasiveness and ability to provide early in pregnancy an abundance of genetic information – are changing the field of prenatal genetics (Dondorp et al. 2015; van Schendel et al. 2014).

1.1   The global debate on public funding for NIPT

It could be argued that there are merits to the user paying for NIPT, at least partially. For instance, it is claimed that charging money for NIPT will promote informed choice, as it will signal to women that the test is optional and will facilitate their deliberation on whether to take it up. However, as Bunnik et al. (2020) argue, evidence for such effect is lacking. Rather, they claim, the fact that the test is paid for out of pocket mainly disadvantages women of lower socioeconomic status, resulting in inequality of access and therefore harming claims to justice and reproductive autonomy.

In its position statement on NIPS, the *American College of Medical Genetics and Genomics* recommended informing "all pregnant women that NIPS is the most sensitive screening option for traditionally screened aneuploidies" (Gregg et al. 2016: 1059). When a high-performance test is offered, but only a certain group of users can afford it, there are ethical implications that should be addressed in policymaking. The inequity applies to both the uptake of the (better) test itself and the accessibility of subsequent publicly funded prenatal services at an earlier gestational age. Women who cannot afford NIPT are denied this better-performing test, and also denied earlier access to related services, such as genetic counselling and pregnancy termination, which has both physical and psychological implications (Vanstone et al. 2014). Implementing NIPT in the national healthcare system with public funding could therefore alleviate concerns about inequality of access.

1.2   Establishing the comparison between Germany in Israel

Past research has shown Israel and Germany to have opposing policies in several relevant fields, such as genetic screening, stem cell research, and preimplantation genetic diagnosis (Hashiloni-Dolev 2007; Raz et al. 2017;

Raz/Schicktanz 2016). In all these cases, Israeli policy is permissive, whereas German policy is more restrictive. Israelis are considered to enthusiastically embrace medical technologies (Prainsack/Firestine 2006), especially those in the field of reproduction. Accordingly, genetic screening programmes are well established, and less subject to social or professional controversies than elsewhere. The limited public debate in Israel is in striking contrast to the thriving social, legal, and ethical debate concerning reproductive genetic technologies in other countries, especially in Germany (Hashiloni-Dolev 2007).

These differences have been attributed to a unique mixture of sociocultural, religious, and political features. Israel's unique stance has been related to its pro-natalism, familism, Jewish heritage, and its views on the beginning of life (Hashiloni-Dolev 2007), its state of conflict with neighbouring countries, and the trauma of the Holocaust leading to an emphasis on survival and abled bodies (Chemke/Steinberg 1989; Prainsack/Firestine 2006). Consequently, ideas that restrict genetic testing and abortion in other countries, mostly disability rights and the rights of the foetus, are less influential (Hashiloni-Dolev 2007; Raz 2005), even among disability rights activists and parents of children with disability who do not oppose testing (Nov-Klaiman/Raz/Hashiloni-Dolev 2019; Raz 2004).

On the other side, German restrictions/caution have been attributed to the view of the foetus as a potential person with at least some individual rights (and requiring protection) (Heinemann/Honnefelder 2002), as well as to the salient presence of disability rights activists in the public discourse (Hashiloni-Dolev/Raz 2010; Raz 2005). A universalistic lesson of the Holocaust on the value of diversity and dignity has propelled criticism of reproductive genetics as a "new eugenics" (Braun 2005; Hashiloni-Dolev/Raz 2010; Raz/Schicktanz 2016). Motherhood itself is also understood differently. Whereas Israeli mothers see themselves as being responsible for preventing suffering and disability in their families (Nov-Klaiman/Raz/Hashiloni-Dolev 2019; Remennick 2006), German mothers are more expected to welcome all children regardless of their condition (Hashiloni-Dolev/Shkedi 2007), although this might be changing with the growing use of prenatal testing (Graumann 2014).

Based on the characteristics emerging from these studies, one might have expected NIPT to be rejected in Germany and adopted in Israel. However, the complex reality is not in line with the initial expectations.

1.3 Mapping out the regulatory framework

We consider three dimensions of the regulatory framework that are crucial for the application of NIPT: the existing provision of prenatal testing; legislation on genetic testing; and abortion laws. Residents of both countries are entitled to services covered by mandatory health insurance. Likewise, an assigned committee approves the inclusion of any technology in the national health insurance scheme. This is the *Health Basket Committee* on the Israeli side and the *Federal Joint Committee* (*Gemeinsamer Bundesausschuss – G-BA*) for Germany.

1.3.1 Prenatal genetic services

Israel

Since 1980 the Israeli *Ministry of Health* has run the "National program for the detection and the prevention of birth defects". This free-of-charge programme offers neonatal screening, prenatal testing, and population carrier screening for reproductive purposes. The prenatal component includes several ultrasound tests for all women, as well as biochemical blood tests that provide, among other information, risk assessments for DS. Women older than 35 or those referred by a medical geneticist due to increased risk are eligible for free amniocentesis (Zlotogora 2014). For every woman who undergoes an invasive test, due to her age or to abnormal findings in previous tests, a chromosomal microarray analysis (CMA) is performed free of charge. CMA, which is currently performed on samples taken in invasive procedures such as amniocentesis, is a high-resolution, whole-genome technique which detects submicroscopic deletions and duplications (Dugoff et al. 2016). In other words, currently, CMA covers a much broader spectrum of conditions than NIPT.

It is noteworthy that, unlike other countries in which a dramatic decrease in invasive testing has been reported since the introduction of NIPT (Hui/ Bianchi 2017), such a trend has not been observed in Israel, according to A. Singer, MD, Head of the *Community Genetics Department* in the *Ministry of Health* (written communications, April 2020).

Germany

In the 1970s, prenatal services became an integral element of the *Motherhood Guidelines (Mutterschafts-Richtlinien)* (Kolleck/Sauter 2019). These binding rules set the prenatal care standards for the healthcare system. They include several basic examinations such as ultrasound for all pregnant women. Additional tests, e.g. invasive diagnostic testing, are subsidised if medically indicated. In a major difference from Israel, further tests like the First-Trimester Screening are not covered according to the guiding principles.

Moreover, unlike in Israel, the combination of invasive testing and CMA has never become routine in Germany and is not covered by mandatory health insurance (Müller-Egloff 2017). Instead, since 2004, the rates of invasive testing have decreased significantly (Kolleck/Sauter 2019). These data reveal a clear trend and priority towards avoiding invasive testing when possible.

1.3.2 Laws on genetic testing

Israel

In Israel, NIPT is subject to the *Genetic Information Law, 2000*, although this law does not explicitly mention prenatal genetic testing, except in relation to testing for kinship. The Israeli law does not explicitly regulate direct-to-consumer genetic testing (DTC-GT) either. This is particularly relevant for NIPT since the test is currently available only privately, with women being able to contact providers directly, without the involvement of a healthcare professional in the public system. DTC-GT, especially in the prenatal context, raises significant ethical and practical concerns, e.g. the quality of the information and counselling that patients receive, potentially affecting the process of informed consent and leading to patients misinterpreting test results (Allyse et al. 2013; Skirton 2015).

It could be inferred that pure DTC-GT is banned, as the law requires informed consent to be obtained, and explanations to be given by an authorised medical figure. However, without explicit clarification, the phrasing leaves room for bypassing the services of public health professionals and using only those provided by the marketing companies, with their inherent bias.

Germany

The German *Genetic Diagnosis Act* (*Gendiagnostikgesetz* 2009) contains a section on prenatal genetic examinations. It is updated when needed by the *Commission on Genetic Testing*, which includes experts as well as several representatives of patient and self-help organisations. The law aims to protect constitutional human dignity and the individual right of informational self-determination, either by protection against discrimination, or by sufficient information giving. This applies to pregnant women but also to the foetuses.

As in Israel, though not explicitly forbidden, pure DTC-GT does not match the required referral by a physician and comprehensive information and counselling. The German legislation emphasises women's right not to perform prenatal testing and not to know the associated findings.

1.3.3 Laws on abortion

The medical conditions that NIPT tests for are currently not treatable. Once one of these conditions has been detected, parents-to-be have two possibilities. They can either prepare themselves and their environment for a child with special needs or terminate the pregnancy. Such terminations are legally possible in both countries, but with several differences in their legislation and regulation.

Israel

Abortions are legal in Israel when performed according to the *Penal Law*, which specifies the circumstances in which a designated committee can authorise a termination request. These include, among other things, foetal handicap, as well as the physical and mental integrity of the woman (*Penal Law* of 1977: *Interruption of Pregnancy*). When legal, abortions are publicly funded.

The Israeli *Central Bureau of Statistics* collects and reports the yearly number of authorised abortions and specifies the numbers approved under each criterion, including those approved due to embryopathies.

Germany

Abortion law is part of the *German Criminal Code* (*Strafgesetzbuch* 1998), but is also regulated by the *Pregnancy Conflict Act* (*Schwangerschaftskonfliktgesetz* 1992), which determines the requirements for counselling. This expresses the constitutional tension between the mother's basic rights on the one hand, and the "unborn life's" dignity and basic right to life and bodily integrity on the other (WD 2017). Following the legislation of 1995, abortion was declared illegal, but is exempt from punishment until week 12 of the pregnancy, and after some obligatory counselling; but it is legal throughout a pregnancy if it results from a crime or endangers the physical or mental health of the mother. Only legal abortions are funded by the health insurance funds. Notably, the vast majority of abortions (96.1per cent in 2019) are officially illegal, but unpunished (Destatis 2020).

The former "embryopathic" (sometimes also called "eugenic") indication was dropped by the legislator in 1995 in order to clarify that a life with or without disability deserves the same protection. However, a child's disability can be interpreted as a threat to the physical or mental health of the mother and thereby serves as an indirect reason for a legal termination (WD 2017). The German abortion statistics do not specify the number of cases in which foetal anomaly was involved.

1.3.4 Findings from the framework comparison

Having reflected on the regulatory background of Israel and Germany, we can reconsider the question of health insurance coverage. The Israeli framework is characterised by more comprehensive provision of prenatal genetic testing, a lower level of regulation and restriction, and no specific friction between NIPT and the abortion law. Thus, it is in principle open towards an inclusion of this technology. The German framework presents significant reservations and conflicts with NIPT on the one hand, but on the other, NIPT fits into the German agenda of avoiding invasive testing (as indeed was the argument of the G-BA).

2.   Discourses on implementation: the stakeholders involved and their positions

The implementation of NIPT involves various stakeholders, including medical professionals, policy bodies, advocacy groups, pregnant women, NIPT producers, and the media. Some of them markedly influence the related public discourse, while others are absent or less notable. In Israel, where there is traditionally less conflict between experts and the public, especially in the field of prenatal care, the process is mainly led by medical professionals and the policy body in charge, i.e. the *Health Basket Committee*. Other voices are hard to find. In contrast, the German discourse has provoked public statements by nearly all stakeholders, vital media reporting, and some related research. Thus, the difference between the discourses begins with the amount and range of easily accessible material. Our analysis focuses on medical professionals, policy bodies, and advocacy organisations.

Israel

NIPT has been marketed in Israel since 2013. The technology was submitted to the *Health Basket Committee* to be considered for public funding, in 2014 and 2019, and was rejected following evaluation in both cases. It is therefore not included in the current basket of health services. Since its introduction, only a few medical societies have addressed NIPT in their opinion papers to different extents. Critical reactions and public statements by advocacy organisations or others are rarely found, with the only statement by a disability advocacy group being supportive.

2.1 Medical associations

The *Israeli Society of Obstetrics and Gynecology*, in an opinion paper (ISOG 2018), refers to NIPT only in their list of tests that pregnant women should be informed of as part of routine follow-up.

Following a previous opinion paper by the *Israeli Society of Medical Genetics* (Michaelson-Cohen et al. 2014), in 2018 this organisation advanced its debate on the recommended use of NIPT. Since NIPT is better than the implemented biochemical screening at detecting the common chromosomal aneuploidies, they recommended using NIPT as a first-tier screening test for trisomies 13, 18 and 21.

It is noteworthy, however, that this society maintains that from a medical point of view, the preferred prenatal test in each pregnancy, including those with a priori low risk, is a diagnostic invasive test coupled with chromosomal microarray analysis (CMA), with its significantly broader scope compared to NIPT.

2.2 Policy body in charge

The *Health Basket Committee* in Israel is composed of representatives of the healthcare system (the *Ministry of Health*, health funds, hospitals), representatives of the *Ministry of Finance*, and representatives of the public (specialists in varied fields of medicine, as well as ethics, economy, social welfare, and others). This diverse composition, according to the *Ministry of Health*, aims to ensure that the decisions made by the committee take social perspectives into account along with the medical ones. In 2019 two scenarios of NIPT implementation were submitted for consideration for the 2020 Health Basket:

either for all pregnancies, or as a second-tier-test for high-risk pregnancies. In January 2020, the committee published its decisions. NIPT was rejected.

2.3 Advocacy organisations and additional stakeholders

In Israel, NIPT has not drawn much public attention or debate and is not discussed in parliament. The *Israeli National Council for Bioethics* has not addressed the issue either.

Moreover, since the introduction of the test into clinical use, no campaign against NIPT has been launched in Israel by disability advocates or by others. In fact, one of the DS advocacy organisations called the *Ministry of Health* as early as 2014 to make sure that NIPT would be affordable for all pregnant women (ATID 2014). They argued that this is important for parental autonomy. To support their claims, they noted that the costs of raising a disabled child, such as one with DS, are far higher than the costs of NIPT. They argued that Israeli society at large and family members alike carry the heavy burdens of supporting and financing these children for their entire lives.

Germany

The introduction of NIPT in Germany was pushed forward in 2012 by *LifeCodexx AG*, a private company that received public funding for the development of NIPT for the German market (Deutscher Bundestag 2015). In 2019, the *G-BA* concluded its assessment by adopting NIPT for trisomies 13, 18 and 21 in the public health insurance under certain conditions. Both the market introduction of NIPT and the involvement of the *G-BA* since 2014 activated numerous stakeholders, public protest, and media reporting (Kolleck/Sauter 2019). Advocates for persons with disabilities even denied the compatibility of NIPT with the German legal framework, but their view did not prevail.

2.4 Medical associations

In sharp contrast to Israel, many German medical organisations engaged in the debate and submitted comments to the *G-BA*, which published them in a collection (G-BA 2019a). This engagement may reflect the tradition of corporatism and self-governance of the German healthcare system, but also the controversial character of NIPT. A broad spectrum of positions was presented, ranging from calls for rejection to unrestricted coverage of NIPT. But most associations come down somewhere in between.

Several major associations welcomed the introduction of NIPT and its evaluation by the G-BA, including the *German Society of Gynecology and Obstetrics* (DGGG 2014), and the *German Society of Human Genetics* (GfH 2012). To them, NIPT – at least for trisomies – is not an ethical slippery slope but an advancement of prenatal testing that avoids the risks of invasive testing and should in principle be available to every woman. Both showed much support for a limited coverage, for women with an increased risk of trisomies (G-BA 2019a).

Other organisations representing prenatal-care specialists emphasised their concerns over the proper implementation of NIPT. They called for clear indications, without which, they warned, extensive and improper use could follow coverage (BVNP 2018; G-BA 2019a).

Others focused more on the possible social and psychological implications of NIPT. For instance, the *German Society of Psychosomatic Gynecology and Obstetrics* (DGPFG 2013) warned against discriminatory effects on people with disabilities, as well as putting greater pressure on women and delegitimising those who decline testing or choose to have a child with disability. Nonetheless, torn between these concerns and the arguments of risk avoidance and equal access, the organisation showed some acceptance of limited coverage, under careful implementation (G-BA 2019a).

2.5 Policy bodies in charge

Even before the market entry of NIPT, the *Commissioner for Matters relating to Persons with Disabilities* tried to prevent this step through a legal opinion stating its incompatibility with several laws (Gärditz 2012). The arguments presented became characteristic of the opposition to NIPT: Without available treatment, the test would be used as a tool for selection, and therefore carries a clear discriminatory message for people with disabilities. For similar reasons, the *Inclusion Council* considers NIPT to violate the *UN Convention on the Rights of Persons with Disabilities* (Staatliche Koordinierungsstelle 2013).

However, this view was not adopted by the *German government* (Deutscher Bundestag 2015) nor by the *German Ethics Council* (Deutscher Ethikrat 2013), which recommended a restricted use of NIPT for women with increased risk of a genetic condition but did not comment on public funding. The council also voiced concerns that the early applicability of NIPT might undermine the restrictions of the abortion laws, and recommended revising them.

Since 2015, a concerned inter-fractional group of parliamentarians has put NIPT on the agenda of the *German Bundestag* (Deutscher Bundestag 2015), and eventually promoted a parliamentary debate. The debate, held on 11 April 2019, presented a spectrum of positions (Deutscher Bundestag 2019; Foth 2021). Many deputies expressed their commitment to the values of dignity, diversity, and the struggle for inclusion of people with disabilities. Nonetheless, NIPT has often been acknowledged as a means to avoid invasive testing that should be equitably accessible to women at a higher risk for trisomies through public coverage.

The German counterpart to the Israeli *Health Basket Committee* is the *G-BA*. Its decision-making body is composed of neutral chairpersons, and representatives of the statutory health insurance funds and healthcare providers. In addition, patient representatives have the right to participate in its discussions.

In its decision of September 2019, the *G-BA* rejected a routinised use of NIPT in the sense of mass screening. Instead, it decided that NIPT could be funded in individual cases for pregnancies with particular risks or suspicious findings. According to the updated *Motherhood Guidelines* coverage is possible when it aims to avoid invasive testing and "is necessary to enable the pregnant woman to address her personal situation regarding the presence of a trisomy under medical supervision" (G-BA 2019b: 3). This is explained by the heavy burden a woman may feel if she might be expecting a child with a trisomy (G-BA 2019c: 4). The request of the patient representatives in the *G-BA* to withhold NIPT until week 12 of pregnancy, while abortions are easily accessible, was rejected.

Although the G-BA explained its decision in an additional statement (G-BA 2019c), it left many commentators unsure about its implications (Rehmann-Sutter/Schües 2020). To finalise the new provisions, however, the G-BA had to "translate" them into an easy-to-understand brochure for insurance fund members, attached to the *Guidelines*. This process required another round of consultations with several stakeholders. According to the brochure's final version, NIPT is covered for a pregnant woman "when other examinations have raised the suspicion of a trisomy, or she, together with her doctor, comes to the conclusion that the test is necessary in her personal situation" (G-BA 2021: 11). In this way, the decision introduces a strongly subjective component and could be widely interpreted in practice.

The regulation came into force in 2022. There was no objection from the legislator, the German Bundestag, although the public debate is not entirely settled.

2.6 Advocacy organisations and additional stakeholders

The discourse on the implementation of NIPT has largely been shaped by civil society involvement and augmented in the media. Some civil society stakeholders that have long been critical of the growth of prenatal genetic testing opposed the market introduction of the test from the outset. However, their opposition has diverse backgrounds (Braun/Könninger 2018).

Some criticism is inspired by Christian values and is often combined with objection to abortion. Thus, several charitable organisations, representatives of the *Roman Catholic Church*, and groups which engage in the protection of (unborn) life opposed the implementation of NIPT (CDL 2012; Zimmermann 2019). The *Protestant Church in Germany*, however, supported limited coverage (EKD 2018).

Another criticism is stressed by some disability advocacy groups and networks with a strong feminist commitment, such as the *Network against Selection by Prenatal Diagnosis* (G-BA 2019a; Netzwerk gegen Selektion durch Pränataldiagnostik/Gen-Ethisches Netzwerk/BioSkop 2014). They believe that NIPT strengthens eugenic practices and the medicalisation and commodification of pregnancies; it undermines the wellbeing and self-determination of pregnant women; and runs counter to the goal of an inclusive society. They claim that prenatal testing should be supported only when it enables a medical treatment. Thus, they also demand a revision of the existing framework of genetic testing, insofar as it can be criticised for similar reasons. From their point of view, NIPT is a major step in an expansive dynamic of genetic testing that is not sufficiently reflected on, discussed, or legitimised by the public or by parliament.

However, the introduction of NIPT received support from other civil organisations, most prominently from *pro familia*, which advocates for sexual and reproductive health and rights. They supported coverage of NIPT for so-called risk pregnancies, stressing the reproductive rights of prospective parents, which should guarantee their access to the means for informed decision-making, but also a right not to know (pro familia Bundesverband 2019).

3. Discussing key themes

So far, we have presented the regulatory and legislative circumstances in which NIPT has been introduced into clinical practice in Germany and Israel, and the discourse of different stakeholders around the use of this technology and its implementation using public funding. While we can learn much from examining the actors involved in medical policymaking, we can equally learn from examining which actors' voices are not heard. Indeed, major differences can be found not only between the regulatory frameworks of Germany and Israel, but also in their discourses about NIPT: their extent, the type of participating actors, and their views.

Several key themes have emerged from the comparison: the balancing of parental autonomy and embryo protection; prevention vs. support; and the extent of public deliberation. In these regards, Germany and Israel approach NIPT from different directions and are concerned with different implications, thus demonstrating the interplay between cultural norms and technology in the shaping of concrete health policies.

On top of parental autonomy, the Israeli framework seems to enhance prevention of disability. This is reflected most prominently in the name of the "National program for the detection and the prevention of birth defects" and the fact that embryopathy is one of the explicit criteria in Israel's abortion law.

However, some changes over recent years might also be interpreted as hints of a growing awareness of disability concerns. Israel ratified the *UN Convention on the Rights of Persons with Disabilities* in 2012. According to Mor (2014), rising disability advocacy had an effect on the Israeli jurisdiction when they barred "wrongful life" lawsuits in 2012. Moreover, with a push from Israeli DS advocacy organisations, Israel's social security organisation changed its policy in 2018 and now gives a "disabled child allowance" to all parents of children with DS at a rate of 100 per cent, at least up to the age of 6. Until 2018, the rate had been determined by an assigned medical committee on a case-by-case basis. This move shifts the "prevention vs. support" balance towards more support. However, both this move and the abolition of "wrongful life" lawsuits, although driven by disability advocacy, do not necessarily reflect a shift toward an agenda of opposing preventive measures in the form of prenatal testing. Indeed, the critical view coming from disability advocacy is absent from the discourse on NIPT. These moves can therefore be seen as another manifestation of the twofold view of disability: the aspiration to prevent it on the one hand, and the sense of duty to support those already born disabled on the other, in line with Raz (2004) and Nov-Klaiman, Raz and Hashiloni-Dolev (2019).

Cost-effectiveness calculations are at the heart of the "prevention vs. support" balance and are a morally sensitive issue (Kibel/Vanstone 2017; Ravitsky 2017). The Israeli case is unique. Even a DS advocacy organisation used the high costs of raising a disabled child, which fall on family members and society at large, as an argument in favour of subsidising NIPT. In Germany, however, even among those who favour public funding of NIPT, reference is not made to the societal costs of supporting affected children. Such economic considerations would be perceived by the German public as implying that a person's value is based on their economic contribution to society, which is a violation of the dignity of individuals with disabilities and would pave the way for discrimination against them. Similarly, an official aim of preventing disability would be perceived as discriminatory, and contradictory to the political agenda of inclusion, which has been pushed forward since Germany's signing of the *UN Convention on the Rights of Persons with Disabilities* in 2007. Indeed, some German proponents of the test use the opposite argument and claim that prospective parents can benefit from the test in terms of preparedness rather than prevention.

The German legislative and regulatory frameworks reflect a stronger emphasis on further groups beyond the women who are the direct consumers of prenatal testing, namely individuals with disabilities (protection against discrimination) and foetuses (their right to live). In Israel, however, foetuses have no legal rights (Hashiloni-Dolev/Weiner 2008), and therefore the implications of genetic testing are not viewed from the angle of their protection. Instead, the focus in Israel is more on the personal implications to the woman (her right to reproductive autonomy). However, the sheer existence of a comprehensive prenatal testing programme with public funding, coupled with the recommendation from professional organisations to test and supported with a permissive abortion law, implies a view that society benefits from prevention as well.

In Israel, NIPT has raised only limited deliberation and hardly any public debate. Engagement in the process is mainly professional and focuses on the test's technical performance. It does not refer to the potentially negative implications of the test, such as the effects on people with disabilities, or connect such large-scale screening of the population with eugenics. Lay people, religious representatives, political parties, or other groups did not spur debate on the test, leaving the process to be led by medical professionals.

It would therefore have been reasonable to expect Israel to adopt the test. However, its rejection is in fact not counter to the known Israeli logic. In the *Health Basket Committee*, NIPT competed with other technologies from diverse fields of medicine over a small and rigid budget. NIPT would thus come at the expense of other, non-related, medical technologies. Moreover, it was proposed to replace or to be integrated within a well-established, publicly funded prenatal screening programme. In other words, the gain from including NIPT in the Israeli *Health Basket* would not be as great as in a country that has not implemented a broad public screening programme, such as Germany. Furthermore, in a country that highlights maximal detection, the inclusion of NIPT with its relatively limited scope would be a step in the wrong direction. As Israeli professionals argue, and as common practice suggests, invasive testing combined with CMA is the goal, rather than NIPT. Therefore, the rejection of NIPT is actually not surprising.

The established screening programme could also explain the lack of public controversy over the test. From a public point of view, NIPT might not be perceived as big news or represent a new approach in principle, but rather a technical improvement to an existing system (Lôwy 2020; van Schendel et al. 2017).

By contrast, the introduction of NIPT into clinical practice and its assessment for public funding has prompted much debate in Germany. This debate involves various actors, including health professionals, religious groups, political parties, disability advocacy groups, and the media, and covers a wide spectrum of views. The opposition to NIPT can be described as a mixed group with some overlapping criticisms and a strong basis in civil society as well as some representation in public institutions and medical professions. Their opposition is twofold. On the substantive level, they consider NIPT a questionable tool in terms of its meaning for women's health, the integrity of pregnancy, the foetus, persons with disabilities, and society in general. The criticism is reinforced by an expected expansion in testing as a result of the decision by the G-BA, and by special features of the German abortion law, which tolerates abortions without a medical indication up to 12 weeks. Since NIPT enables earlier testing, the legal and technical barriers to selective abortion due to foetal anomaly are reduced (Heinrichs/Spranger/Tambornino 2012). On the procedural level, the G-BA is repeatedly criticised for its limited scope of investigation. It is important to recognise that the opposition is not just directed against the addition of NIPT, but is also an attempt to revise significant aspects of prenatal care, including the rules relating to genetic testing, their interplay with abortion, and the governance of the field.

This is one major difference between the countries' discourses on NIPT. While in Israel it is limited to an expert discourse on a specific adjustment in the field of prenatal testing, in Germany it extends to a societal discourse on pivotal rules governing prenatal testing, including matters of abortion. While the Israeli assessment of NIPT is a matter of course within a rarely questioned scheme of prenatal testing and its governance, the German discourse on NIPT questions the pre-existing prenatal care regime and functions as a matter of deep controversy.

The G-BA's decision on the inclusion of NIPT under public health insurance was big news. Non-invasive tests for trisomies are explicitly included within the public services for the first time in certain, somewhat flexible cases, which may reflect a shift by the German policy toward other Western countries' policies, including the Israeli one, which encourage prenatal testing.

The G-BA's explicit goal is not to screen (out) as many pregnancies as possible, but to avoid invasive testing. However, under the rules adopted, it leaves much room for interpretation, as criticised by some medical professionals. They have stated potential problems and predicted high uptake rates, which seems to contradict the initial idea of a restricted inclusion of NIPT and which could generate high costs for the healthcare funds (G-BA 2019a; Scharf et al. 2019). Further German stakeholders feared that this might undermine the aim of protecting women's right not to know and push towards the prevention of disability. Since the G-BA did not comply, it could be argued that the flexible phrasing is deliberate. Such phrasing could serve to reconcile both ends of the spectrum: those who saw Germany lagging behind in the coverage of prenatal testing, and those who oppose the routinisation of testing.

4. Conclusion

Seemingly counterintuitive decisions were reached both in Israel and in Germany. Given the differences between the countries – based on previous studies and in terms of the actors involved and the legal and regulatory background – an opposite scenario, in which NIPT is included in the Israeli *Health Basket* but rejected from the German health insurance scheme, seemed realistic.

Cultural norms have arguably played a crucial role in these societies' attitudes thus far toward reproductive technologies that have led Israel to adopt them eagerly and Germany to lag behind. Returning to the question of whether convergence in policies occurs over time, we conclude that the answer is not straightforward. The two countries seem to move toward one another in some regards, but not in others. Israel moves toward Germany in its growing awareness of disability advocacy in some policymaking. However, in the realm of policy related to reproductive technologies, the influence of disability critique is not apparent and rather maintains Israel's embracing approach. At the same time, Germany is moving closer to Israel in its growing coverage of genetic services, which have so far been lagging behind. By doing so, Germany is moving closer to other European countries as well, e.g. the Netherlands, in which the coverage of prenatal testing, including NIPT, is more comprehensive (Ravitsky et al. 2021). This change in German policy is justified by the wellbeing of pregnant women and is not, as in the Israeli setting, also associated with preventing disability or prioritising large-scale testing. Thus, we could say that the convergence observed remains ambiguous and may even serve to highlight the differences between Germany and Israel. The German adoption of the technology, justified by avoiding the risk of miscarriage and safeguarding women's health, might have unintended consequences. Time will tell how NIPT is implemented and used by women, and what its long-term effects are.

References

Allyse, Megan/Sayres, L./Havard, M./King, J./ Greely, H./Hudgins, L./Taylor, J./ Norton, M./Cho, M./Magnus, D./Ormond, K. (2013): "Best Ethical Practices for Clinicians and Laboratories in the Provision of Noninvasive Prenatal Testing." In: Prenatal Diagnosis 33/7, pp. 656–661.

Allyse, Megan/Minear, Mollie/Berson, Elisa/Sridhar, Shilpa/Rote, Margaret/ Hung, Athony/Chandrasekharan, Subashini (2015): "Non-Invasive Prenatal Testing: A Review of International Implementation and Challenges." In: International Journal of Women's Health 16/7, pp. 113–126.

ATID (2014): "The Israeli Down Syndrome Organization. In Response to the Article 'A New Era in Pregnancy – A Blood Test for the Detection of Down Syndrome'" [In Hebrew]. (www.atid-il.org.il, accessed 10 September 2019, at 4 May 2022, this link is not available anymore).

Braun, Kathrin (2005): "Not Just for Experts: The Public Debate about Reprogenetics in Germany." In: Hastings Center Report 35/3, pp. 42–49.

Braun, Kathrin/Könninger, Sabine (2018): "Realizing Responsibility. Institutional Routines, Critical Intervention, and the 'Big' Questions in the Controversy over Non-Invasive Prenatal Testing in Germany." In: New Genetics and Society 37/3, pp. 248–267.

Bunnik, Eline M./Kater-Kuipers, Adriana/Galjaard, Robert-Jan H./de Beaufort, Inez D. (2020): "Should Pregnant Women Be Charged for Non-Invasive Prenatal Screening? Implications for Reproductive Autonomy and Equal Access." In: Journal of Medical Ethics 46/3, pp. 194–198.

BVNP (2018): "BVNP-Positionspapier 2018 zum Thema 'NIPT als GKV-Leistung' (aktuelles Methodenbewertungsverfahren des G-BA)." Berufsverband Niedergelassener Pränatalmediziner, Bonn, Germany.

CDL (2012): "Inklusion statt Selektion – Kein weiterer Ausbau Pränataler Eugenik." Christdemokraten für das Leben, Münster, Germany. (https://c dl-online.net/pm-inklusion-statt-selektion-kein-weiterer-ausbau-prana taler-eugenik/135), accessed 23 April 2022.

Chemke, Juan/Steinberg, Avraham (1989): "Ethics and Medical Genetics in Israel." In: D.C. Wertz/J.C. Fletcher (eds.), Ethics and Human Genetics: A Cross Cultural Perspective, Berlin: Springer, pp. 271–284.

Destatis (2020): "Gesundheit: Schwangerschaftsabbrüche." Statistisches Bundesamt, Wiesbaden, Germany. (https://www.destatis.de/DE/Themen /Gesellschaft-Umwelt/Gesundheit/Schwangerschaftsabbrueche/_inhalt. html), accessed 23 April 2022.

Deutscher Bundestag (2015): "Vorgeburtliche Blutuntersuchung zur Feststellung des Down-Syndroms. Antwort der Bundesregierung auf die Kleine Anfrage". Drucksache 18/4574.

Deutscher Bundestag (2019): "Tagesordnungspunkt 3: Vereinbarte Debatte: Vorgeburtliche Genetische Bluttests." Plenarprotokoll 19/95, Stenografischer Bericht 95. Sitzung, pp. 11315–11339, 11506–11509, Berlin, Germany.

Deutscher Ethikrat (2013): "The Future of Genetic Diagnosis – from Research to Clinical Practice." Berlin, Germany. (https://www.ethikrat.org/en/publi cations/kategorie/opinions), accessed 24 April 2022.

DGGG (2014): "196. Stellungnahme der DGGG zur Nichtinvasiven Pränataldiagnostik zur Bestimmung des Risikos von fetaler Trisomie 21 mittels molekulargenetischer Tests." Deutsche Gesellschaft für Gynäkologie und Geburtshilfe, Kassel, Germany.

DGPFG (2013): "'Ihr Kinderlein kommet' – Wie gilt das im Jahre 2014?" Deutsche Gesellschaft für psychosomatische Frauenheilkunde und Geburtshilfe, Hamburg/Hanover, Germany.

Dondorp, Wybo/de Wert, Guido/Bombard, Yvonne/Bianchi, Diana/ Bergmann, Carsten/Borry, Pascal/Chitty, Lyn/Fellmann, Florence/ Foranzo, Francesca/Hall, Alison/Henneman, Lidewij/Howard, Heidi/ Lucassen, Anneke/Ormond, Kelly/Peterlin, Borut/Radojkovic, Dragica/ Rogowski, Wolf/Soller, Maria/Tibben, Aad/Tranebjaerg, Lisbeth/val El, Carla/Cornel, Martina (2015): "Non-Invasive Prenatal Testing for Aneuploidy and Beyond: Challenges of Responsible Innovation in Prenatal Screening." In: European Journal of Human Genetics 23/11, pp. 1438–1450.

Dugoff, Lorraine/Norton, Mary E./ Kuller, Jeffrey A. (2016): "The Use of Chromosomal Microarray for Prenatal Diagnosis." In: American Journal of Obstetrics and Gynecology 215/4, pp. B2–B9.

Dupras, Charles/Birko, Stanislav/Affdal, Alija/Haidar, Hazar/Lemoine, Marie-Eve/Ravitsky, Vardit (2020): "Governing the Futures of Non-Invasive Prenatal Testing: An Exploration of Social Acceptability Using the Delphi Method." In: Social Science & Medicine 17, 112930.

EKD (2018): "Nichtinvasive Pränataldiagnostik – ein Evangelischer Beitrag zur ethischen Urteilsbildung und zur politischen Gestaltung." Evangelische Kirche in Deutschland, Hanover, Germany.

Foth, Hannes (2021): "Avoiding 'selection'?–References to history in current German policy debates about non-invasive prenatal testing." In: Bioethics 35/6, pp. 518–527.

Gärditz, Klaus Ferdinand (2012): "Gutachtliche Stellungnahme zur Zulässigkeit des Diagnostikprodukts 'PraenaTest'." Der Beauftragte der Bundesregierung für die Belange behinderter Menschen, Berlin, Germany.

G-BA (2019a): "Anlage zur Zusammenfassenden Dokumentation; Beratungsverfahren Methodenbewertung Mutterschafts-Richtlinien (Mu-RL): Nicht-Invasive Pränataldiagnostik zur Bestimmung des Risikos autosomaler Trisomien 13, 18 und 21 mittels eines molekulargenetischen Tests (NIPT) für die Anwendung bei Schwangerschaften mit besonderen Risiken." Gemeinsamer Bundesausschuss, 19 September 2019.

G-BA (2019b): "Beschluss des Gemeinsamen Bundesausschusses über eine Änderung der Mutterschafts-Richtlinien (Mu-RL): Nicht-invasive Pränataldiagnostik zur Bestimmung des Risikos autosomaler Trisomien 13, 18 und 21 mittels eines molekulargenetischen Tests (NIPT) für die Anwendung bei Schwangerschaften mit besonderen Risiken." Gemeinsamer Bundesausschuss, 19 September 2019.

G-BA (2019c): "Tragende Gründe zum Beschluss des Gemeinsamen Bundesausschusses über eine Änderung der Mutterschafts-Richtlinien (Mu-RL): Nicht-invasive Pränataldiagnostik zur Bestimmung des Risikos autosomaler Trisomien 13, 18 und 21 mittels eines molekulargenetischen Tests (NIPT) für die Anwendung bei Schwangerschaften mit besonderen Risiken." Gemeinsamer Bundesausschuss, 19 September 2019.

G-BA (2021): "Bluttest auf Trisomien. Der nicht invasive Pränataltest (NIPT) auf Trisomie 13, 18 und 21. Eine Versicherteninformation." Gemeinsamer Bundesausschuss, November 2021 (https://www.g-ba.de/downloads/17-9

8-5156/2021-11-09_G-BA_Versicherteninformation_NIPT_Ansichtsexemp lar.pdf), accessed 23 April 2022.

Gendiagnostikgesetz (2009): Gesetz über genetische Untersuchungen bei Menschen, Bundesgesetzblatt Jahrgang 2009 Teil I Nr. 50 (https://dejure .org/BGBl/2009/BGBl._I_S._2529), accessed 26 April 2022.

GfH (2012): "Stellungnahme der Deutschen Gesellschaft für Humangenetik (GfH) zur Analyse fetaler DNA aus dem mütterlichen Blut." Deutsche Gesellschaft für Humangenetik, Munich, Germany.

Graumann, Sigrid (2014): "Die UN-Behindertenrechtskonvention und der Anspruch behinderter Menschen auf gesellschaftliche Anerkennung – Sozialethische Überlegungen zur Praxis der Pränatal- und Präimplanta-tionsdiagnostik." In: G. Duttge/W. Engel/B. Zoll (eds.), "Behinderung" im Dialog zwischen Recht und Humangenetik, Göttingen: Universitätsverlag Göttingen, pp. 71–82.

Gregg, Anthony R./Skotko, Brian G./Benkendorf, Judith L./Monaghan, Kristin G./Bajaj, Komal/Best, Robert G./Klugman, Susan/Watson, Michael S. (2016): "Noninvasive Prenatal Screening for Fetal Aneuploidy, Update: A Position Statement of the American College of Medical Genetics and Ge-nomics." In: Genetics in Medicine 18/10, pp. 1056–1065.

Haidar, Hazar/Dupras, Charles/Ravitsky, Vardit (2016): "Non-Invasive Prenatal Testing: Review of Ethical, Legal and Social Implications." In: Bioéthique Online 5 (https://id.erudit.org/iderudit/1044264ar), accessed 2 May 2022.

Hashiloni-Dolev, Yael (2007): A Life (Un) Worthy of Living: Reproductive Ge-netics in Israel and Germany, Springer Science & Business Media.

Hashiloni-Dolev, Yael/Shkedi, Shiri (2007): "On New Reproductive Technolo-gies and Family Ethics: Pre-Implantation Genetic Diagnosis for Sibling Donor in Israel and Germany." In: Social Science & Medicine 65/10, pp. 2081–2092.

Hashiloni-Dolev, Yael/Weiner, Noga (2008): "New Reproductive Technologies, Genetic Counselling and the Standing of the Fetus: Views from Germany and Israel." In: Sociology of Health & Illness 30/7, pp. 1055–1069.

Hashiloni-Dolev, Yael/Raz, Aviad E. (2010): "Between Social Hypocrisy and So-cial Responsibility: Professional Views of Eugenics, Disability and Repro-Genetics in Germany and Israel." In: New Genetics and Society 29/1, pp. 87–102.

Heinemann, Thoma/Honnefelder, Ludger (2002): "Principles of Ethical Deci-sion Making Regarding Embrionic Stem Cell Research in Germany." In: Bioethics 16/6, pp. 530–43.

Heinrichs, Bert/Spranger, Tade Matthias/Tambornino, Lisa (2012): "Ethische und rechtliche Aspekte der Pränataldiagnostik." In: Medizinrecht 30/10, pp. 625–630.

Heyd, David. (1994): Genethics: Moral Issues in the Creation of People, Berkeley: University of California Press.

Hui, Lisa/Bianchi, Diana W. (2017): "Noninvasive Prenatal DNA Testing: The Vanguard of Genomic Medicine." In: Annual Review of Medicine 68, pp. 459–472.

ISOG (2018): "Monitoring of Low Risk Pregnant Women." Israeli Society of Obstetrics and Gynecology, Opinion Paper No. 6 [In Hebrew].

Kibel, Mia/Vanstone, Meredith (2017): "Reconciling Ethical and Economic Conceptions of Value in Health Policy using the Capabilities Approach: A Qualitative Investigation of Non-Invasive Prenatal Testing." In: Social Science & Medicine 195, pp. 97–104.

Kitzman, Jacob O./Snyder, Matthew W./Ventura, Mario/Lewis, Alexandra P./Qiu, Ruolan/Simmons, Lavone/Gammill, Hilary S./Rubens, Craig E./Santillan, Donna A./Murray, Jeffrey C./Tabor, Holly K./Bamshad, Michael J./Eichler, Evan E./Shendure, Jay (2012): "Noninvasive Whole-Genome Sequencing of a Human Fetus." In: Science Translational Medicine 4/137, pp. 137ra76.

Kolleck, Alma/Sauter, Arnold (2019): "Aktueller Stand und Entwicklungen der Pränataldiagnostik." Büro für Technikfolgen-Abschätzung beim Deutschen Bundestag, Berlin, Germany.

Lemke, Thomas (2005): "From Eugenics to the Government of Genetic Risks." In: Robin Bunton/Alan Peterson (eds.), Genetic Governance: Health, Risk and Ethics in the Biotech Era, London: Routledge, pp. 95–105.

Lench, Nicholas/Barrett, Angela/Fielding, Sarah/McKay, Fiona/Hill, Melissa/Jenkins, Lucy/White, Helen/Chitty, Lyn S.(2013): "The Clinical Implementation of Non-Invasive Prenatal Diagnosis for Single-Gene Disorders: Challenges and Progress Made." In: Prenatal Diagnosis 33/6, pp. 555–562.

Lôwy, Ilana (2020): "Non-Invasive Prenatal Testing: A Diagnostic Innovation Shaped by Commercial Interests and the Regulation Conundrum." In: Social Science & Medicine 113064.

McCoyd, Judith L M. (2010): "Authoritative Knowledge, the Technological Imperative and Women's Responses to Prenatal Diagnostic Technologies." In: Culture, Medicine, and Psychiatry 34/4, pp. 590–614.

Michaelson-Cohen,   Rachel/Gershoni-Baruch,   Ruth/Sharoni,   Reuven/Shochat, Mordechai/Yaron, Yuval/Singer, Amihood (2014): "Israeli Society of Medical Genetics NIPT Committee Opinion 072013: Non-Invasive Prenatal Testing of Cell-Free DNA in Maternal Plasma for Detection of Fetal Aneuploidy." In: Fetal Diagnosis and Therapy 36/3, pp. 242–244.

Mor, Sagit (2014): "The Dialectics of Wrongful Life and Wrongful Birth Claims in Israel: A Disability Critique." In: Studies in Law, Politics, and Society 63, pp. 113–146.

Müller-Egloff, Susanne (2017): "Methoden der Invasiven Pränataldiagnostik." In: Alexander Strauss (ed.), Ultraschallpraxis in Geburtshilfe und Gynäkologie, Berlin: Springer, pp. 441–459.

Netzwerk gegen Selektion durch Pränataldiagnostik/Gen-Ethisches Netzwerk, BioSkop (2014): "Gemeinsame Stellungnahme zur geplanten Erprobungsrichtlinie 'nichtinvasive Pränataldiagnostik zur Bestimmung des Risikos von fetaler Trisomie 21 mittels molekulargenetischer Tests'." Essen, Germany.

Nov-Klaiman, Tamar/Raz, Aviad E./Hashiloni-Dolev, Yael (2019): "Attitudes of Israeli Parents of Children with Down Syndrome toward Non-Invasive Prenatal Screening and the Scope of Prenatal Testing." In: Journal of Genetic Counseling 28/6, pp. 1119–1129.

Penal Law of 1977 (1977): Interruption of Pregnancy, in: Laws of the State of Israel, transl. from the Hebrew, Special volume 5737–1977, Government Printer Jerusalem (https://knesset.gov.il/review/data/eng/law/kns8_pena llaw_eng.pdf), accessed 26 July 2022.

Prainsack, Barbara/Firestine, Ofer (2006): "'Science for Survival': Biotechnology Regulation in Israel." In: Science and Public Policy 33/1, pp. 33–46.

pro familia Bundesverband (2019): "NIPT – nicht-invasiver Pränataltest als Leistung der GKV? Stellungnahme des pro familia Bundesverbands im Rahmen des Stellungnahme-Verfahrens des G-BA." Frankfurt a. M., Germany.

Ravitsky, Vardit (2017): "The Shifting Landscape of Prenatal Testing: Between Reproductive Autonomy and Public Health." In: Hastings Center Report 47, pp. 34–40.

Ravitsky, Vardit/Roy, Marie-Christine/Haidar, Hazar/Henneman, Lidewij/ Marshall/Newson, Ainsley J./Ngan, Olivia M.Y./Nov-Klaiman, Tamar (2021): "The Emergence and Global Spread of Noninvasive Prenatal Testing." In: Annual Review of Genomics and Human Genetics 22, pp. 309–338.

Raz, Aviad (2004): "'Important to Test, Important to Support': Attitudes toward Disability Rights and Prenatal Diagnosis among Leaders of Support

Groups for Genetic Disorders in Israel." In: Social Science & Medicine 59/9, pp. 1857–1866.

Raz, Aviad E. (2005): "Disability Rights, Prenatal Diagnosis and Eugenics: A Cross-Cultural View." In: Journal of Genetic Counseling 14/3, pp. 183–187.

Raz, Aviad E./Schicktanz, Silke (2016): Comparative Empirical Bioethics: Dilemmas of Genetic Testing and Euthanasia in Israel and Germany, Cham: Springer.

Raz, Aviad/Schües, Christina/Wilhelm, Nadja/Rehmann-Sutter, Christoph (2017): "Saving or Subordinating Life? Popular Views in Israel and Germany of Donor Siblings Created through PGD." In: Journal of Medical Humanities 38/2, pp. 191–207.

Raz, Aviad E. (2018): "Reckless or Pioneering? Public Health Genetics Services in Israel." In: Hagai Boas/Yael Hashiloni-Dolev/Nadav Davidovitch/Dani Filc/Shai J. Lavi (eds.), Bioethics in Israel: Socio-Legal, Political and Empirical Analysis, Cambridge: Cambridge University Press, pp. 223–239.

Rehmann-Sutter, Christoph/Schües, Christina (2020): "Die NIPT-Entscheidung des G-BA: Eine ethische Analyse." In: Ethik in der Medizin 32/4, pp. 385–403.

Remennick, Larissa (2006): "The Quest for the Perfect Baby: Why Do Israeli Women Seek Prenatal Genetic Testing?" In: Sociology of Health & Illness 28/1, pp. 21–53.

Scharf, Alexander/Maul, H./Frenzel, J./Doubek K./Kohlschmidt N. (2019): "Postfaktische Zeiten: Einführung von NIPT als Kassenleistung. Eine Vorläufige Bilanz." In: Frauenarzt 12/19, pp. 778–82.

Skirton, Heather (2015): "Direct to Consumer Testing in Reproductive Contexts – Should Health Professionals Be Concerned?" In: Life Sciences, Society and Policy 11, p. 4.

Staatliche Koordinierungsstelle (2013): "Bioethik – Menschen mit Behinderungen – UN-BRK. Positionspapier der Staatlichen Koordinierungsstelle nach Art. 33 UN-BRK." Berlin, Germany.

Strafgesetzbuch (1998): Deutschland Strafgesetzbuch (StGB) neugefasst durch B. v. 13.11.1998 (https://dejure.org/gesetze/StGB), accessed 4 May 2022.

van Schendel, Rachèl /Kleinveld, Johanna H./Dondorp, Wybo J./Pajkrt, Eva/ Timmermans, Danielle R.M./Holtkamp, Kim C.A./Karsten, Margreet/ Vliestra, Anne l./Lachmeijer, Augusta M.A./Henneman, Lidewij (2014): "Attitudes of Pregnant Women and Male Partners towards Non-Invasive Prenatal Testing and Widening the Scope of Prenatal Screening." In: European Journal of Human Genetics 22/12, pp. 1345–1350.

van Schendel, Rachèl/van El, Carla G./Pajkrt, Eva/Henemann, Lidewij/Cornel, Martina C. (2017): "Implementing Non-Invasive Prenatal Testing for Aneuploidy in a National Healthcare System: Global Challenges and National Solutions." In: BMC Health Services Research 17/1, p. 670.

Vanstone, Meredith/King, Carol/de Vrijer, Barbra/Nisker, Jeff (2014): "Non-Invasive Prenatal Testing: Ethics and Policy Considerations." In: Journal of Obstetrics and Gynaecology Canada 36/6, pp. 515–526.

WD (2017): "Schwangerschaftsabbrüche aufgrund einer Behinderung oder vorgeburtlichen Schädigung des Kindes in Deutschland seit 1996." Wissenschaftliche Dienste des Deutschen Bundestags, Berlin, Germany.

Zimmermann, Steffen (2019): "Kirchenvertreter warnen bei Bluttests vor Selektion menschlichen Lebens. Fürst: Der embryonale Mensch besitzt bereits die ganze Würde." (https://www.katholisch.de/artikel/21320-kirchen vertreter-warnen-vor-selektion-menschlichen-lebens), accessed 23 April 2022.

Zlotogora, Joël (2014): "Genetics and Genomic Medicine in Israel." In: Molecular Genetics & Genomic Medicine 2/2, pp. 85–94.

4. PND in Israel: Public Health Services and Uptake in Cultural Context

Aviad Raz

This chapter provides a backdrop for the analysis that follows by taking a broad look at public health genetics services for prenatal diagnosis (PND) in Israel as a network situated within relevant political, cultural and professional contexts, highlighting the social factors that make them possible, indeed desirable, and the dynamics that shape their design and prioritisation.

When PND becomes part of public health, although it is a very personal matter it also follows the logic of control and prevention that is characteristic of public health, which is not necessarily attentive to individual needs and preferences (Stewart et al. 2007; Khoury et al. 2000). Prenatal screening for Down syndrome (DS) provides a striking example of this. Prenatal screening for DS has been viewed for most of its history as a public health problem, with public (sometimes mandated) prenatal screening aimed at reducing DS incidence (Raffle 2001). As Bryant et al. (2008) show, only relatively recently have there been efforts to promote reproductive choice rather than test uptake as the preferred measure of public health DS screening success. While the public health goal is to reduce the prevalence of disease, genetic counselling of the parents of a foetus with DS should ideally be non-directive and conducted in a manner that respects the parents' norms and values. This conundrum of self-determination vs. social pressures is embedded in additional axes of influence, including inequality (of access and funding), healthcare professionals' interests, disability and patient advocacy, family relations and health governance, and so on.

In Israel, the confluence of these factors can be seen in the construction of the "Jewish gene pool" by health professionals as especially prone to inherited disorders (beyond DS), boosting "genetic anxiety" (or "responsibility", depending on one's perspective) and creating a collective sense of risk in which the uptake of PND is exceptionally high – at least among those Israelis who are secular, have a higher income and fewer children, and are of Ashkenazi origin. Furthermore, previous studies of public outlooks on PND in Israel stressed that it is seen by many Israelis as a moral *duty* (Remennick 2006; Raz/Schicktanz 2009a,b). This perception of "collective responsibility" applies not only to doing PND but also to sharing genetic information with relatives. This is also indicated by Israel's Genetic Information Law (2000) which, quite uniquely compared to international regulation, enables healthcare providers to disclose actionable genetic results to family members where consent has not been given for their disclosure (Branum/Wolf 2015).

The chapter begins with an overview of public health services for PND in Israel. Notably, I am not addressing the topic of non-invasive prenatal testing (NIPT) itself as it receives detailed introduction and analysis in other chapters of the book. I am also avoiding the very intriguing topics of in vitro fertilisation (IVF) and prenatal genetic diagnosis (PGD). My focus is on PND that is squarely located as part of the pregnancy and that is furthermore related to genetic testing (therefore omitting the topic of prenatal ultrasound testing, for example). I focus on three contexts that highlight major aspects of the cultural embedding of genetically related PND in Israel: PND and "community genetics", illustrating the unique Israeli social mosaic of ethno-religious communities and their utilisation of PND; PND and the social construction of disability, for example in the context of prenatal screening for DS; and finally, the issue of public/economic pressures concerning PND and the so-called "genetic panel".

PND in Israel: An Overview

The *National Programme for the Detection and Prevention of Birth Defects* was established by the Israeli Ministry of Health (MoH) in 1980. It recommends the following tests, paid for under Israel's universal health insurance: First-trimester screening at 10–13 weeks of pregnancy includes ultrasound to determine nuchal translucency and a blood test for free beta-HCG and PAPP-A; second-trimester tests include maternal serum screening (the "triple test") at 16–18 weeks to identify the probability of DS and neural tube defects for all women. All women older than 35 years are recommended for amniocentesis (paid for by the state). Additional routinely offered prenatal tests include three ultrasound scans. If first- or second-trimester screening tests indicate a chance of more than 1:380 of having a child with DS, neural tube defect, chromosomal abnormality, or a molecularly defined genetic disease, invasive diagnostic tests (chorionic villus sampling or amniocentesis) are offered free of charge. Invasive diagnostic testing is also provided by the state to women with a high chance of an affected foetus as determined in genetic counselling (for example due to family history). The Israeli Law of Abortion (1977) enables pregnancy termination on the basis of foetal abnormalities, with no legal guidelines concerning the severity of the condition or the probability of its expression (Amir/Binyamini 1992a, b). Up to 22 weeks of pregnancy, termination is allowed for relatively mild medical conditions, but after this period a designated committee approval is needed, based on the risk of severe disease and the predicted functional impairment in the foetus (Singer/Sagi-Dain 2020).

The *National Programme for the Detection and Prevention of Birth Defects* also covers adult carrier screening. This screening was originally recommended "pre-conceptionally" but in many cases the test is conducted on prospective parents during pregnancy and thus leads directly to PND. The screening is targeted to couples, usually with the woman tested first and if she is found to be a carrier, her partner is also tested (Zlotogora et al. 2015). The tests are performed either in medical genetic units or in community clinics, and patients with a positive result receive genetic counselling. More extensive prenatal genetic testing can be offered, with coverage shared between the individual and their supplementary health insurance – a point I return to in the section below on public/economic pressures concerning the "genetic panel" in PND. Today, the main diseases included in the national carrier screening programme are Tay-Sachs, CF, fragile X syndrome (FXS), familial dysautonomia and spinal muscular atrophy (SMA). Additional diseases are dynamically added to this panel based on criteria of severity, reliability and prevalence (Singer/Sagi-Dain 2020; Rosner/Rosner/Orr-Urtreger 2009).

PND and "Community Genetics"

The Department of Community Genetics in the Israeli Ministry of Health is responsible for a variety of public health genetics services including prenatal diagnosis. Importantly, the title of the major Israeli public health body overseeing genetics services is the Department of "Community Genetics". This is not a standard title. But what does "community genetics" mean in the Israeli context? This question provides a point of departure for the next section.

Israel has very high fertility rates: 3.1 children per woman on average, with even higher rates in the ultra-orthodox religious Jewish community (6.9), South Bedouins (5.7) and Muslim Arabs (3.37) (Singer/Sagi-Dain 2020). In conjunction with the high tendency for endogamy in various communities (25 per cent among the north Israeli Arab population, see Na'amnih et al. 2015), the result is increased prevalence of specific autosomal recessive genetic disorders in each of these communities. Since the establishment of the national carrier screening programme, its activities have gradually increased, in terms of both additional diseases and varied implementation within different communities. Some of these activities provide an alternative to PND while others lead directly to it. The ultra-orthodox Ashkenazi Jewish (Haredi) community (compromising about 12 per cent of the Israeli population), in which selective abortion is banned by many rabbis, has developed and is operating a special programme ("Dor Yeshorim"), which prevents the marriage of two carriers of recessive genetic diseases (Ekstein/Katzenstein 2001). The Israeli branch of the Haredi carrier screening and matching programme is organisationally and financially supported by the State of Israel and served by Israeli genetics labs (Broide et al. 1993). Among modern-religious Jews in Israel, where marriage is not pre-arranged as in the Haredi community, carrier testing by Dor Yeshorim often leads to PND or PGD (Frumkin et al. 2011). A national carrier screening programme for the prevention of β-thalassemia was implemented in Israel for the Arab-Israeli population and some Jewish communities in which the disease is relatively frequent. Since 2002, targeted carrier screening has also been offered free of charge to other, smaller ethnic communities in which well-established, severe genetic diseases are present at a frequency higher than 1/1000 live births, namely Arab, Druze and Bedouin populations who mostly live in villages and have a high rate of consanguinity. Multiple founder mutations have been documented by Israeli geneticists in these various ethnic populations, often down to the level of specific villages or tribes.

Being secular, having a higher income, fewer children, and being of Ashkenazi origin remain significant factors predicting the uptake of prenatal testing. Out of 377 Jewish Israeli women who were surveyed in hospital maternity departments in 2002 (Sher et al. 2003), 94 per cent of the secular women older than 35 years performed amniocentesis, in contrast to 36 per cent of the religious, and none of the ultra-orthodox (Haredi) women. Indeed, the "35 years" policy has led to a prevailing belief among many Israeli women that age is a sufficient risk factor in and of itself and that women over 35 must have amniocentesis, even with normal triple serum screening results

(Grinshpun-Cohen/Miron-Shatz/Ries-Levavi/Pras 2014; Grinshpun-Cohen/
Miron-Shatz/Berkenstet/Pras 2015). This 94 per cent uptake is often cited as
indicative of the widespread uptake of PND in Israel, but we should remember
that this uptake differs significantly by religiosity and ethnicity. Israel is a
land of contrasts, in this sense as well. On the one hand, a very high number
of non-recommended/elective amniocenteses including CMA are performed
by Israelis who are secular, have a higher income, fewer children, and are of
Ashkenazi origin. On the other hand, Israelis who are very religious and have
a lower income and more children are more likely to reject PND. Most babies
with Down syndrome in Israel are born in religious communities, both Jewish
and Muslim. In religious/traditional Jewish communities, 95 per cent of the
pregnancies diagnosed with Down syndrome are born alive, compared to 25
per cent in largely secular communities (Zlotogora et al. 2007).

Previous studies have indicated that the Arab minority ethnic group, ac-
counting for approximately 25 per cent of Israel's entire population, tends to
underutilise genetic testing, even though the rates of birth defects are considerably higher in the Arab (and especially the Bedouin) population than in the
Israeli Jewish community (Cohen-Kfir et al. 2020). Reasons for this underutil-
isation include religiosity (the Muslim ban on abortion) but also genetic illiteracy and lack of access to services. An ethnographic study of genetic testing
in a Bedouin tribe conducted by the author (Raz 2005a) showed that Bedouin
women were interested in using prenatal tests. They utilised prenatal ultrasound since it could be performed free of charge at local clinics in Bedouin
towns, which many women can often visit on their own. However, in contrast
to the high uptake of ultrasound, the uptake of amniocentesis was very low,
often because the latter required the husband's approval and active participation. Bedouin men objected to prenatal genetic counselling that was critical
of the high rates of consanguinity in the community, which most community
members saw as normative and socially functional. They also objected to amniocentesis for various reasons including religiosity, genetic illiteracy, or cost
(many of the women were younger than 35 so amniocentesis was not automatically covered). Some also perceived genetic counselling as curtailing their autonomy and representing a Jewish conspiracy to limit their reproduction (Raz
2005a; Lewando-Hundt 2001).

PND and the Construction of Disability

The majority of disability activists in Israel support the use of PND and carrier screening to prevent life with disability (Raz 2004). In contrast, in the USA and Europe, and especially in Germany, some in the disability community have voiced strong opposition to PND and carrier screening as sending a discriminatory message that "responsible parenting" means using prenatal tests to terminate an affected foetus (Parens/Asch 2000). Disability scholars around the Western, industrialised world have criticised genetic screening programmes, claiming that: (a) prenatal testing is morally problematic because it expresses negative or discriminatory attitudes about impairments and those who carry them; and (b) prenatal genetic counselling is driven by misinformation because it propagates misconceptions about disability and does not include information on community-based services for children with disabilities and their families as well as on financial assistance programmes and laws protecting the civil rights of persons with disabilities. Perhaps because of such criticism, disability advocacy organisations in the USA and Europe (including Germany) emphasise care and treatment over prevention, lobbying for additional research on treatments and newborn screening, rather than for PND or carrier screening. The latter are framed as individual choices.

Why has no public debate emerged in Israel concerning disability rights and prenatal testing, despite the wide usage of prenatal genetic diagnosis that often leads to selective termination of pregnancy? To answer this question, I conducted interviews with high-ranking officials of support groups "of" and "for" people with genetic conditions and physical disabilities in Israel (Raz 2004; 2005b). Only organisations involved with genetically based disabilities in which a genetic test for the condition was available were contacted. The common attitude that emerged from interviews with most respondents (14/17, 82 per cent) can be described as a two-fold view of disability: support for genetic testing during pregnancy, and support of the disabled person after birth. Support for prenatal diagnosis and selective abortion was also voiced by officials of organisations of disabled people with conditions that are not life-threatening and are characterised by a wide spectrum of clinical symptoms, from severe to mild. Genetic counselling and prenatal diagnosis were seen by these respondents as ways to reduce suffering. While some respondents were aware of the ethical problems inherent in the two-fold view of disability, they still argued for its consistency. On the one hand, for example, selective abortion following prenatal diagnosis of Down syndrome was for encouraged because of the perceived severity of the condition. On the other hand, Israeli DS advocates insisted that DS is labelled a "syndrome" and not a "disease" in the context of supporting those already born with DS.

For many of the above-mentioned respondents, prenatal genetic testing was eugenic and was indeed supported precisely for that reason, since "eugenic" for them meant the improvement of the health of progeny and carried positive rather than negative connotations. The two-fold view of disability – based on the separation of prenatal (preventive testing) and post-natal (supporting disability) – cannot be logically rooted in Orthodox Judaism. The Jewish religion forbids selective abortion. Indeed, Orthodox Jewish women refrain from doing amniocentesis because of this religious restriction. The two-fold view is therefore a secular construction which is furthermore situated in legal, economic and cultural contexts. Rather than having a single, parsimonious cause, it is probably the result of a complex interplay of several inter-connected factors. First, legally speaking, it is enabled by the flexibility of the Israeli Law of Abortion, which does not define the degree of severity of the condition or the probability of its expression (Amir/Binyamini 1992a, 1992b). Second, the preference for preventive genetic testing should be considered against the backdrop of the economic and social hardships of raising a child with congenital disability in Israel. Although Israeli society has adopted a generous restorative approach towards disabled war veterans, this is not so in the case of individuals born with disabling genetic conditions, who – unless covered by other programmes – are provided only a minimum income. As Gal (2001: 239) claims, "despite the overtly inequitable nature of the system of benefits for disabled people in Israel, this issue has not achieved any significant visibility on the public agenda [. . .] The few calls for reforming this system and granting equal rights to all the disabled, regardless of cause of disability, have generally been limited to academic or professional circles." Third, the cultural construction of normality versus disability in Israel should be considered. Congenital disability has been stigmatised in Israeli society as part of the Zionist quest for "Jews with muscles" that will replace diasporic weakness with masculine vigour and militarism (Weiss 2002). Finally, many Israeli healthcare professionals advocate prenatal tests in a directive manner (Wertz 1998).

More is Better? Public/Economic Pressures in PND

In addition to the genetic tests for diseases that are included free of charge in the national carrier screening programme, there are many prenatal genetic tests that users may choose to pay for. About 10 years ago, before advanced DNA new generation sequencing became cost-efficient, Israeli users could choose how many genetic tests (for specific diseases) they wish to add to the so-called "panel" of prenatal genetic testing. Gaucher disease (GD) provides an intriguing example in this context.

In GD, deficiency of the enzyme glucocerebrosidase results in the accumulation of harmful quantities of certain fats, especially within the bone marrow, spleen and liver. Some individuals will develop few or no symptoms while others may have serious complications unless medically treated. Although GD is one of the most prevalent Ashkenazi Jewish genetic diseases, with a carrier frequency of 1 in 15 (Kannai/Chertok 2006), there are strong arguments against providing carrier screening for this disorder. Firstly, the most common GD mutation in Ashkenazi Jews leads to a highly variable but usually mild or symptomless phenotype. In addition, enzyme replacement pills allow patients to lead a near normal life, although treatment is life-long and very expensive. Annual costs can reach USD 400,000 per patient. As Borry et al. (2008) argue, it is ethically questionable to set out systematically to identify carrier couples and offer them prenatal diagnosis and the termination of pregnancy for a condition that will usually not be severe and is treatable. For these reasons, GD was not recommended to be included in the national screening programme by the Israeli Geneticists Association. However, individuals could still pay for it out-of-pocket.

Zuckerman et al. (2007) reported that 10 Israeli genetic centres screened an estimated 28,893 individuals for Gaucher disease between 1995 and 2003, identifying 82 carrier couples at risk for offspring affected by GD type 1. In subsequent pregnancies of these couples, there was a 76 per cent uptake of prenatal diagnosis, leading to a termination of pregnancy for 15 per cent (2 of 13) of the foetuses predicted to be no more than mildly affected and 67 per cent (2 of 3) of the foetuses with predicted moderate disease.

Indeed, when I interviewed the chairperson of The Israeli Association of Patients with Gaucher disease (Raz 2004: 1862), he was (in contrast to his colleagues) very critical of the way GD screening was being conducted at that time in Israel and explained it in terms of economic interests:

Patients and their families should be given the knowledge that enables them to cope with the disease [...]. Genetic counselling for Gaucher should provide, in addition to the genetic results, all the information concerning the medical treatment. Today, genetic counselling does not do that, and the result is unnecessary abortions [...]. It's easy to sell the genetic test to people. If geneticists didn't do Gaucher, they would lose clients. This is purely business.

Prof. Ari Zimran, head of the Gaucher clinic in a major hospital in Jerusalem, commented in this context that:

More than 80 per cent of the foetuses diagnosed with Gaucher will not develop any meaningful clinical symptoms [...]. This screening is performed because of the money involved. Genetic institutes sell services, and the more they sell the better their financial situation is. The Gaucher test is not in the national Basket of Health Services so patients are paying for it, directly to the provider (cited in Traubman 2003).

The case of GD exposes the challenges of leaving PND in the hands of the free market. As Kannai and Chertok suggest in their review of GD screening in Israel (2006: 348): "Prenatal genetic testing for Gaucher may be a business tactic to attract clients". Individuals who are offered a panel of prenatal genetic tests will usually test for all the disorders in the panel. To summarise, screening for GD among Ashkenazi Jews in Israel was included in the providers' panel because it is one of the most prevalent recessive disorders in this community, for which testing is available, and test sensitivity is high. This may have occurred as a kind of "technological imperative", without careful consideration of the benefits and/or harms of this choice; it may have been assumed that screening for more disorders is always desirable – a variation, as Borry et al. (2008) suggest, on the theme of "bigger is better" or "can do, will do". As Zuckerman et al. (2007) suggest: "availability, rather than utility, of a test could be a major determinant of its introduction." In 2008 the Israeli Ministry of Health issued a formal instruction not to include un-recommended tests as part of the panel of genetic tests offered to consumers in genetic labs at Israeli hospitals.

In Lieu of Conclusion

This chapter has examined the design and uptake of public health genetics services for PND in Israel as embedding several cultural scripts (Bowker/ Star 1999). We have looked at different organisational settings and cultural factors involved in PND. The first example was the design of PND for ethnic and religious communities, both as a national strategy underlying the Programme for the Detection and Prevention of Birth Defects within the Department of Community Genetics, and its planned and unintentional adoption by these communities and members. The second context was the justification of PND that leads to selective abortion within the social construction of disability and "genetic responsibility" with the aim of reducing suffering. The third context was about public/economic pressures concerning the genetic panel in PND and carrier testing. These different contexts provide a collage of "Israeli PND", portraying different variations on the theme of self-determination vs. social pressures. Each context illustrates how this theme is further embedded in additional axes of influence, including inequality of access and funding (e.g. the case of PND within ethnic and religious communities, especially the Bedouin community), healthcare professionals' interests (the case of the expanding genetic panel in PND), and disability and patient advocacy (the case of the "two-fold view" of disability by advocates and the public in Israel). All these contexts portrayed something unique to the local ways in which the global technologies of PND are being implemented and used in Israel, adding an important social component to the technological imperative in health care (McCoyd 2010), suggesting that the technological imperative does not work alone. It is already entangled within social, economic and political "imperatives".

While realising the local adaptations of global health technologies is an important feat (and one that the study of NIPT will build on and expand in the later parts of this book), it should be accompanied by a critical look at the "deep structure" of health governance. The local adaptations of health technologies show us how institutional commitments are often reconciled with the more fundamental social and ethical questions and challenges inherent in PND. Targeting ethnic communities for genetic testing, or providing free-of-charge amniocentesis for women over 35, are technical health matters that also have profound normative premises and repercussions. In considering these arrangements we should ask not only how their instrumental rationality can be accounted for but also (to draw on Max Weber's classical distinction), what is the constructive rationality they embody.

This chapter has shown that Israel is both reckless and pioneering – depending on one's perspective (Raz 2019). There has been criticism of Israel for its recklessness and for not looking before leaping, for example in the context of its expanded prenatal panel of genetic tests (Borry et al. 2008). While this criticism is sometimes true, for some countries and in the context of other genetics services, Israel is leading the way. Some scholars have proposed that "Israeli PND" is by and large a product of its biopolitics of reproduction as survival in the face of demographic and militaristic threats (Prainsack 2006; Prainsack/Firestine 2006; Prainsack/Hashiloni-Dolev 2008; Prainsack/Siegal 2006). The analysis presented here usefully complicates this picture by showing how Israeli PND services have been shaped by the ongoing pragmatic concern of public health policymakers with religious and ethnic distinctions within Israeli society. The framing of "genetic risk and responsibility" is being constructed on several levels, not just in the context of the Jewish-Palestinian conflict but also in the context of prevention vs. care. It is by looking at the production of PND services within relevant political, economic and professional contexts that we can discern more fully the upstream factors that make these services possible, and the downstream dynamics that shape their uses and meanings and make them actionable.

References

Amir, Delila/Binyamini, Orly (1992a): "Abortion approval as ritual of symbolic control." In: Clarice Feinman (ed.): The criminalization of a woman's body. Binghampton, New York: Haworth Press, pp. 1–25.

Amir, Delila/Binyamini, Orly (1992b): "The abortion committees: Educating and controlling women." In: Journal of Women and Criminal Justice 3/1, pp. 5–25.

Borry, Pascal/Clarke, Angus/Dierickx, Kris (2008): "Look before you leap: Carrier screening for type 1 Gaucher disease: difficult questions." In: European Journal of Human Genetics 16/2, pp. 139–140 (doi: 10.1038/sj.ejhg.5201960).

Bowker, Geoffrey/Star, Susan (1999): Sorting Things Out, Cambridge: MIT Press.

Branum, Rebecca/Wolf, Susan M. (2015): "International Policies on Sharing Genomic Research Results with Relatives: Approaches to Balancing Privacy with Access." In: Journal of Law, Medicine and Ethics 43/3, pp. 576–593.

Broide, Etty/Zeigler, Marcia./Eckstein Joseph/ Bach, Gideon (1993): "Screening for Carriers of Tay-Sachs Disease in the Ultraorthodox Ashkenazi Jewish Community in Israel." In: American Journal of Medical Genetics 47, pp. 213–215.

Bryant, Louise/Hewison, Jenny/Ahmed, Shenaz (2008): "Conveying information about screening." In: Charles H. Rodeck/Martin J. Whittle: Fetal Medicine: Basic Science and Clinical Practice, Edinburgh: Elsevier, pp. 225–233.

Cohen-Kfir, Nehema/Bentwich, Miriam Ethel/Kent, Andrew et al. (2020): "Challenges to effective and autonomous genetic testing and counseling for ethno-cultural minorities: a qualitative study." In: BMC Medical Ethics 21/98, pp. 1–16.

Ekstein, Josef/Katzenstein, Howard (2001): "The Dor Yeshorim story: Community-based carrier screening for Tay-Sachs disease." In: Advances in Genetics 44, pp. 297–310.

Frumkin, Ayala/Raz, Aviad/Plesser-Duvdevani, Morasha/Lieberman, Sari (2011): "The Most Important Test You'll Ever Take?: Attitudes towards Confidential Carrier Matching and Open Individual Testing among Modern-Religious Jews." In: Social Science & Medicine 73/12, pp. 1741–1747.

Gal, John (2001): "The perils of compensation in social welfare policy: Disability policy in Israel." In: Social Service Review 75/2, pp. 225–246.

Grinshpun-Cohen, Julia/Miron-Shatz, Talya/Berkenstet, Michal et al. (2015): "The limited effect of information on Israeli pregnant women at advanced maternal age who decide to undergo amniocentesis." In: Israel Journal of Health Policy Research 4/23, pp. 1–8 (https://doi.org/10.1186/s13584-015-0 019-6), accessed 26 July 2022.

Grinshpun-Cohen, Julia/Miron-Shatz, Talya/Rhee-Morris, Laila/Briscoe, Barbara/Pras, Elon /Towner, Dena (2014): "A-priori attitudes predict amniocentesis uptake in women of advanced maternal age – a pilot study." In: Journal of Health Communication 20/9, pp. 1107–1113.

Israel Ministry of Health. Screening for foetal Down syndrome (2007) (http://www.health.gov.il/hozer/mr15_2007.pdf) (Hebrew), accessed 09 September 2021.

Israel Ministry of Health. Screening tests for identification of women at risk for carrying a foetus with Down syndrome (2014): http://www.health.gov.il/hozer/mr06_2013.pdf (Hebrew), accessed 09 September 2021.

Israel Ministry of Health, Department of Community Genetics (2007): The Program for prevention of birth defects and genetic diseases in Israel. Summary of 2002–2006. (http://www.health.gov.il/PublicationsFiles/mumim 02_06.pdf (Hebrew)), accessed 09 September 2021.

Kannai, Ruth/Chertok, Ilana R. (2006): "Prenatal panel screening considerations for non-neuronopathic Gaucher disease in the Ashkenazi-Jewish population." In: Israeli Medical Association Journal 8/5, pp. 347–350.

Khoury, Muin J./Burke, Wylie/Thomson, Elizabeth J. (2000): Genetics and Public Health in the 21st Century, Oxford: Oxford University Press.

Lewando-Hundt, Gillian/Shoham-Vardi, Ilana/Beckerelg, Susan E./Belmaker, Ilana/Kassem, Fatma/Jaafar, A. Abu (2001): "Knowledge, Action and Resistance: The Selective Use of Prenatal Screening Among Bedouin Women of the Negev, Israel." In: Social Science & Medicine 52/4, pp. 561–569.

McCoyd, Judith L M. (2010): "Authoritative knowledge, the technological imperative and women's responses to prenatal diagnostic technologies." In: Cult Med Psychiatry. 34(4), pp. 590–614.

Na'amnih, Wasef/Romano-Zelekha, Orly/Kabaha, Ahmed et al. (2015): "Continuous decrease of consanguineous marriages among Arabs in Israel." In: American Journal of Human Biology 27/1, pp. 94–98.

Parens, Erik/Asch, Adrienne (eds.). (2000): Prenatal testing and disability rights. Washington, DC: Georgetown University Press.

Prainsack, Barbara (2006a): "Natural Forces: The Regulation and Discourse of Genomics and Advanced Medical Technologies in Israel." In: Peter Glasner/ Paul Atkinson/Helen Greenslade (eds.), New Genetics, New Social Formations, New York: Routledge, pp. 231–253.

Prainsack, Barbara/Firestine, Ofer (2006): "Science for Survival: Biotechnology Regulation in Israel." In: Science and Public Policy 33/1, pp. 33–46.

Prainsack, Barbara/Siegal, Giel (2006): "The Rise of Genetic Couplehood: A Comparative View of Pre-marital Genetic Screening." In: BioSocieties 1/1, pp. 17–36.

Prainsack, Barbara/Hashiloni-Dolev, Yael (2008): "Faith and Nationhood." In: Paul Atkinson/Peter Glasner/Margaret Lock (eds.), Handbook of Genetics and Society: Mapping the New Genomic Era, London: Routledge, pp. 430–447.

Raffle, Angela E. (2001): "Information about screening: Is it to achieve high uptake or to ensure informed choice?" In: Health Expectations 4/2, pp. 92–98.

Raz, Aviad (2004): "Important to test, important to support: Attitudes toward disability rights and prenatal diagnosis among leaders of support groups for genetic disorders in Israel." In: Social Science & Medicine 59/9, pp. 1857–1866.

Raz, Aviad (2005a): The Gene and the Genie: Tradition, Medicalization, and Genetic Counseling in a Bedouin Community, Durham, NC: Carolina Academic Press.

Raz, Aviad (2005b): "Disability rights, prenatal diagnosis and eugenics: a cross-cultural view." In: Journal of Genetic Counseling 14/3, pp. 183–187 (DOI: 10.1007/s10897-005-0573-0).

Raz, Aviad/Schicktanz, Silke (2009a): Diversity and Uniformity in Genetic Responsibility: Moral Attitudes of Patients, Relatives and Lay People in Germany and Israel, Medicine, Health Care and Philosophy 12(4), pp. 433–442

Raz, Aviad/Schicktanz, Silke (2009b): Lay Perceptions of Genetic Testing in Germany and Israel: The Interplay of National Culture and Individual Experience, New Genetics and Society 28, 4, pp. 401–414.

Raz, Aviad (2018): "Reckless or Pioneering? Public Health Genetics Services in Israel." In: Hagai Boas/Yael Hashiloni-Dolev/Nadav Davidovitch/Dani Filc/ Shai Lavi (eds.), Bioethics and Biopolitics in Israel: Socio-legal, Political, and Empirical Analysis, Cambridge: Cambridge University Press, pp. 223–239.

Remennick, Larissa (2006): "The quest after the perfect baby: Why do Israeli women seek prenatal genetic testing?" In: Sociology of Health and Illness 28/1, pp. 21–53.

Rosner, Guy/Rosner, Serena/Orr-Urtreger, Avi (2009): "Genetic testing in Israel: an overview." In: Annual Review of Genomics and Human Genetics 10/1, pp. 175–192 (Doi: 10.1146/annurev.genom.030308.111406).

Sher, Carron/Romano-Zelekha, Orly/Green, Manfred S./Shohat, Tamy (2003): "Factors affecting performance of prenatal genetic testing by Israeli Jewish women." In: American Journal of Medical Genetics 120A/3, pp. 418–422.

Singer, Amihood/Sagi-Dain, Lena (2020): "Impact of a national genetic carrier-screening program for reproductive purposes." In: Acta Obstetricia et Gynecologica Scandinavica 99/6, pp. 802–808.

Stewart, Alison/Brice, Philippa/Burton, Hilary/Pharao, Paul/Sanderson, Simon/Zimmern, Ron (2007): Genetics, Health Care and Public Policy: An Introduction to Public Health Genetics, Cambridge: Cambridge University Press.

Traubman, T. (2003): Experts warn about unnecessary abortions, but hospitals continue to recommend the test. Haaretz daily newspaper, June 11, 2003 (Hebrew), (https://www.haaretz.co.il/misc/1.887586), accessed 09 September 2021.

Weiss, Meira (2002): The chosen body: The politics of the body in Israeli society, Stanford: Stanford University Press.

Wertz, Dorothy C. (1998): "Eugenics is alive and well: A survey of genetic professionals around the world." In: Science in Context 3/4, pp. 493–510.

Zlotogora, Joël/Haklai, Ziona/Leventhal, Alex (2007): "Utilization of prenatal diagnosis and termination of pregnancies for the prevention of Down syndrome in Israel." In: Israel Medical Association Journal 9/8, pp. 600–602.

Zuckerman, Shachar/Lahad, Amnon/Shmueli, Amir/Zimran, Ari/Peleg, Leah et al. (2007): "Carrier screening for Gaucher disease: lessons for low-penetrance, treatable diseases." In: Journal of the American Medical Association 298/11, pp. 1281–1290.

5. NIPT in Germany
Moral Concerns and Consumer Choice

Kathrin Braun and Sabine Könninger

Policies and practices of prenatal diagnosis (PND) in Germany are characterised by an ambivalence of persistent public concern on the one hand and
increasing routinisation on the other.[1] We will argue in this chapter that this
ambivalence is in fact a pervasive feature of the (West-) German prenatal
diagnosis dispositif (Löwy 2014; 2017).[2]

In German debates on prenatal testing, the legacy of Nazi eugenics and
the concept of "life unworthy of life" have certainly played a role and have given
rise to a certain sensitivity in politics and civil society towards eugenics and
selection practices. Yet whether or how this sensitivity has actually shaped the
ways in which PND is organised, regulated, diffused and performed, is a more
complicated question. This ambivalence, of concern and unease on the one
hand and moves towards normalisation and routinisation on the other, has
also characterised the stance towards non-invasive prenatal testing (NIPT) in

---

1   A note on terminology: The term "prenatal diagnosis" in Germany commonly refers
    to examinations performed on the pregnant woman or the embryo or foetus in utero
    for the purpose of establishing foetal disorders, disease or malformation (Kolleck and
    Sauter 2019: 31; Wolf and Graumann 2016: 14). Conceptually, it forms part of antenatal
    care, but this as a whole is broader and also encompasses medical surveillance and
    review of the woman's health and wellbeing. NIPT refers to a low-threshold procedure
    based on the analysis of cell-free foetal DNA circulating in the woman's blood that
    serves to establish the probability of foetal genetic aberrations. Strictly speaking, NIPT
    and some other procedures are not diagnostic since they actually serve to establish a
    probability, even though a rather precise one. Abnormal findings must still usually be
    confirmed by invasive diagnostics (Kolleck and Sauter 2019: 81).
2   The prenatal diagnosis dispositif, as Ilana Löwy frames it, is the "heterogeneous as-
    semblage of instruments and techniques, professional practices, and institutional and
    legal arrangements that, taken together, made it possible to diagnose fetal anomalies"
    (Löwy 2017: 2).

Germany over the past ten years (Braun and Könninger 2018). Interestingly, in some respects, the German policy approach to NIPT seems to be complementary to that taken in Israel: in Germany, public concern is comparatively strong and vocal but the costs of the test for the most common trisomies 13, 18 and 21 will be covered by the statutory health insurances without setting a specific risk threshold as access criterion. In Israel, in turn, NIPT is not in the national Basket of Health Service and accordingly not part of the universal coverage, but nevertheless partly covered by health funds; however, it has not been a matter of public controversy (Raz et al. 2021). On the contrary, PND is rather seen as a moral duty and more a collective responsibility than a moral concern, as Aviad Raz explains in this volume. In Germany, in contrast, it would be seen as inappropriate to say that NIPT, or any PND, is good because it helps to reduce the prevalence of children with Down syndrome; that would probably cause immediate public outrage. The possibility of using NIPT routinely to screen for Down syndrome is officially refuted. Yet, we will argue, the policy approach that has been taken up to now lacks any effective provisions to prevent exactly this situation.

In this chapter, we explore the controversy around NIPT against the background of previous controversies on abortion and preimplantation genetic diagnosis (PGD).[3] We argue that we see a recurring pattern, which we have termed the "No, but..." pattern. It is characterised on the one hand by a widespread moral unease about reproductive practices that, in effect, involve selective decisions about which children should be born and which should not, and on the other by a political disinclination to take binding decisions to effectively curb them. Since the 1970s, the traditional way of accommodating these countervailing tendencies has been to confirm the morally problematic character of such selective choices *in principle* while nevertheless allowing them under certain circumstances, which – theoretically – are defined as being exceptional and rare (Braun 2016). However, there is no general rule to determine whether such exceptional circumstances are present or not; thus, it becomes a matter of case-by-case decision-making or, as Dominique Memmi (2003) puts is, of delegated biopolitics. In practice, the decision is left to the

---

3   We are mostly drawing on policy document analysis and interviews of experts and policy actors in 2015–2017, supplemented by a review of recent events concerning the issue of reimbursement for NIPT. The empirical research for this article was partly funded by the German Federal Minister for Education and Research, funding number 16I1676.

individual. Thus, the responsibility for the diffusion of reproductive selection practices lies with the individual. Policy actors usually see the need to take fundamental social and ethical implications of such practices into account, but resort to the above-mentioned "No, but…" model to deal with the issue (Braun and Könninger 2018). To understand the structure of this policy pattern better, we will first take a look back at the so-called abortion compromise and the legal regulation of PGD. Subsequently, we will briefly recapitulate the controversy about PND in Germany and then show how the "No, but…" pattern plays out in the case of NIPT.

"No, but…": The Abortion Compromise

In 1976, the German Constitutional Court determined that the liberalisation of abortion law that the German *Bundestag* had passed in 1974 was unconstitutional on the grounds that it violated the state's duty to protect human dignity as enshrined in Art.1 of the German Basic Law. Where human life exists, the Court ruled, it enjoys human dignity (Bundesverfassungsgericht 1975).[4] The development of human life was a continuous process that started with gestation at the latest; it was therefore unconstitutional to suspend the right to life and human dignity for a certain period of life, even if this period was the first trimester of pregnancy. However, the Court also established that under certain conditions, namely a threat to the woman's health (medical indication), birth defects on the part of the child (embryopathic indication), rape (criminal indication), or a general situation of need (social indication), the foetus' rights *could* be balanced against those of the woman. The Court thus established a general norm according to which the foetus' right to life would – normally – outrank the woman's right to self-determination. Simultaneously it established a list of exceptions for which this norm would not apply and the foetus' right to life would *not* outrank the woman's right to self-determination. The "malformed" foetus, as it was termed, thus constituted a case of exception that would suspend its entitlement to life and human dignity. The right to the protection of human dignity and right to life – the logical implication of the ruling – would not apply to foetuses expected to have a "defect"; the legal status of the presumably disabled foetus differed from that of the "normal" one. As a consequence,

---

4   An English translation is available at http://groups.csail.mit.edu/mac/users/rauch/nv
     p/german/german_abortion_decision2.html (accessed 31 August 2021).

the disabled foetus' rights became a matter of case-by-case decision-making. Note that the rationale for allowing abortions under certain circumstances was *not* based on a woman's fundamental right to bodily self-determination, but on a rule-and-exception thinking, a "No-but" figure that seeks to uphold strong normative principles grounded in a universalist deontological ethics but nevertheless allows for decision-making on the question of which children should be born and which not. This type of reasoning would eventually recur both in the legal regulation of pre-implantation diagnosis and in the approach towards NIPT.

Consequently, the *Bundestag* complied with the Court's instructions and passed an abortion law in 1976 that banned abortion *in principle*, but allowed it in cases of a threat to the woman's health, rape, a general situation of need, or "birth defects" of the child.

After German unification, a new law was passed in 1992 that, again, would legalise abortion in the first trimester of pregnancy. Again, the Constitutional Court ruled that it was unconstitutional and prescribed that abortion remain illegal – in principle (Bundesverfassungsgericht 1992). In response, the *Bundestag* passed a new law in 1995 stipulating that first-trimester abortions remain technically illegal, except in cases of rape or a threat to the woman's health, but they are not punishable if the woman has undergone proper counselling (Deutscher Bundestag 1995). In case of a criminological (rape) or a medical indication, abortion is not illegal and not punishable.

This law is still in place today. Thus, technically, it is based on the norm-and-exception or the "No, but..." model, except that the person making the decision is now the individual woman. Up to twelve weeks of gestation, it is she who determines whether she is in a situation of exceptional distress that cannot be averted in any other way than by terminating the pregnancy. The presumably disabled foetus, however, still constitutes a case of exception. The situation has also changed due to another significant change in the law: in 1995, the Parliament also decided to abandon the embryopathic indication in response to pressure from disability rights groups, who argued that it discriminated against people with disabilities (Deutscher Bundestag 1995). From a disability rights perspective, the decision backfired. *De jure* foetal abnormalities no longer constitute a case of exception that justifies an abortion; in practice, however, it is the individual woman who determines that the disabled foetus poses a serious threat to *her* health so that she needs an abortion. Hence, the medical indication has *de facto* substituted the former embryopathic indication (Nationaler Ethikrat 2003: 63). However, since the 22-week time limit for medical abortions was also abandoned, there is as a result *no* time limit on aborting a presumably disabled foetus. Hence, we see a policy that was motivated by moral concerns about selective abortion decisions but in effect individualised them.

"No, but...": The Legal Regulation of Pre-Implantation Genetic Diagnosis

A similar compromise was established for the issue of PGD. After longstanding, controversial public debate that peaked around the years 1999 to 2002 and again in 2010–2011, the *Bundestag* finally passed a law on PGD, the 2011 Pre-implantation Genetic Diagnosis Act (Bundesgesetzblatt 2011).[5] The debate had previously revolved around issues of a new eugenics, the status of the human embryo, the lessons learnt from the Nazi past, the social implications of PGD for women and people with disabilities, versus the desire of couples with an increased probability of having a child with a certain genetically related disease to have a child "of their own" not affected by the disease. The PGD Act inserted a new paragraph into the existing Embryo Protection Act that would allow PGD under certain conditions. The new paragraph stipulates, first, that performing PGD is illegal and can be punished with imprisonment of up to one year. Next, it stipulates that performing PGD is *not* illegal in two exceptional cases: if there is reason to assume that a couple has a "high risk" of having a child with a "serious hereditary disease", or if PGD is performed in order to establish whether the embryo is affected by "serious damage" that with "high probability" will cause a miscarriage or stillbirth. Neither the Act nor the amendments pertaining to it, however, define the terms "serious", "high risk" or "high probability". Instead, it postulates that demands to perform PGD shall be submitted to newly founded ethics committees at state level who then determine in case-by-case decisions whether a risk is "high" and the damage is "serious". In more than 80 per cent of cases, a request is approved (Albrecht and Grüber 2019: 88–89). Thus, the decision does not lie directly with the applicants but, in the vast majority of cases, their individual demands are approved.

At the same time, the Embryo Protection Act continued to ban the use of human embryos for any purpose other than its own preservation (Bundesministerium für Justiz und Verbraucherschutz 1990). PGD means that more em-

---

5   *Gesetz zur Regelung der Präimplantationsdiagnostik (PräimpG)*, hereafter PGD Act.

bryos are generated than will be implanted, so inevitably, some embryos will be discarded because genetic anomalies are detected, and this inscribes a contradiction into the law; it bans the destruction of human embryos in principle but allows it in case of genetic disease or damage.

This tension between moral unease about selective practices and the disinclination to take binding decisions to curb them also comes into play in the controversy about PND and NIPT in Germany, as we will argue below.

The Prenatal Diagnosis Dispositif in Germany

The prenatal diagnosis dispositif, as Ilana Löwy (2014; 2017) terms it, formed in the late 1960s and early 1970s in the context of intersecting developments in society, medicine and law. Formative events were the emergence of amniocentesis and obstetrical ultrasound, the decriminalisation of abortion, the shift in many countries from legislation that would allow involuntary sterilisation on eugenic grounds to a general legalisation of sterilisation on demand, based on individual decision-making, and the framing of Down syndrome as a major strain on public resources. In Germany, amniocentesis was first carried out in 1970. From 1976 onwards, PND was included in the catalogue of antenatal care services (*Mutterschaftsrichtlinien*) and covered by the statutory health insurances (SHI) in cases of so-called pregnancies at risk.[6] The same year, a revision of the Criminal Code allowed for abortion up to 22 weeks of gestation in the case of foetal birth defects, thus opening the way to having an abortion following the result of an amniocentesis. Subsequently, the number of amniocenteses performed increased sharply (Nippert 1999: 63; 2001: 294). In the 1980s and 1990s additional methods of prenatal testing were introduced, such as regular ultrasound examinations in 1979, the "triple test" in 1988, nuchal translucency (NT) measurement in 1996, and in 1999, the first trimester screening test (ETS), which combines NT measurement with analysis of certain markers in the maternal blood to detect trisomies 21, 13 or 18 (Netzwerk gegen Selektion durch Pränataldiagnostik 2002). Today, antenatal care regularly includes three ultrasound examinations, covered by the SHI. If there is an increased probability of

---

6   "Pregnancy at risk" is defined as a pregnancy in which there is reason to anticipate an increased risk to the life and health of the mother or child based on anamnesis or findings obtained (Kolleck and Sauter 2019: 25).

genetic aberration or anomaly, the SHI will also cover an amniocentesis, chorionic villus sampling (CVS), ETS or additional ultrasound examinations. In the absence of increased "risks", ETS is offered as a private service.[7]

Prenatal testing has been a controversial issue in Germany since the 1980s (Achtelik 2015). Criticism and concern are not limited to genetic or invasive testing methods but refer to the purpose of selectively identifying foetuses that are likely to be born with certain impairments or undesired variations from standards of health and normality. In the absence of therapeutic treatment options, critics argue, PND *de facto* operates as a selection technology, serving to decide who should be born and who should not. Criticism comes from pro-life actors, disabilities rights organisations such as the *Bundesvereinigung Lebenshilfe* or the *Aktion Mensch*, and feminists who are in favour of the right to abortion but nevertheless concerned about prenatal selection. One of the most outspoken and longstanding organisations problematising PND, the Network against Selection through Prenatal Diagnosis (*Netzwerk gegen Selektion durch Pränataldiagnostik*), takes a decisively anti-eugenic *and* feminist stance.

The motives of this rather unusual alliance are diverse and overlap only partly. They overlap mainly regarding their concerns about the reinforcement of ableism in society, and otherwise range from anti-abortion attitudes to concerns about an increasing focus on the foetus and its features in prenatal care rather than on the woman and her needs, concerns about social pressures on women to produce healthy and "valuable" children, to a more fundamental, anti-capitalist stance against a lack of solidarity in society and increasing norms of productivity and fitness imposed on individuals, a trend towards further dismantling of the welfare state and shifting responsibility for health, education and wellbeing onto the individual instead.

All these issues have resurfaced in recent discussions on NIPT. In addition, there is increased concern that, due to its low-threshold nature, NIPT might become standard practice in all pregnancies. Furthermore, it is likely to yield significantly more information about the foetus than conventional methods and thereby produce an information overload that cannot possibly be managed by practitioners, genetic counsellors, or pregnant women (de Jong et al. 2010: 275; Schmitz 2016).

---

7   For practices and discussions of prenatal testing in Germany, see Baldus (2006); Waldschmidt (2006); Bundeszentrale für gesundheitliche Aufklärung (2010); Bundesarbeitsgemeinschaft der Freien Wohlfahrtspflege e.V. (2013); Achtelik (2015); Wolff and Graumann (2016).

NIPT: An unsolvable dilemma?

NIPT was introduced in Germany in 2012 and has remained controversial since. At present, it is available to detect trisomies 13, 18 and 21, some sex chromosome aberrations such as Triple-X syndrome and Klinefelter syndrome, some microdeletions such as Cri du chat syndrome, and for foetal sex determination[8] (Kolleck and Sauter 2019: 59; Stumm and Schröer 2018). Data on the uptake of NIPT are hard to obtain since there are no publicly available statistics on the matter. According to LifeCodexx, the most prominent German test provider, 80.000 PraenaTests were performed in 2017, half of them on pregnant women in Germany – equivalent to one in 10.000 pregnancies – and the number of gynaecological clinics performing NIPT increased from 70 in 2013 to over 3.000 in 2018 (Kolleck and Sauter 2019: 145).[9]

Conflicts erupted around market approval, public funding, and most of all around the issue of reimbursement by the SHIs. What sparked these conflicts and what was at stake?

A central issue of contention was the question whether NIPT would lead to further normalisation and routinisation of selective abortions and thereby indirectly to reinforcing negative attitudes in society against people living with disabilities. When LifeCodexx announced the upcoming release of its PraenaTest in 2011, a series of articles in the print media discussed concerns about a trend towards the tentative pregnancy (Katz Rothman 1986), "eugenics from below", and an increasing number of abortions of children with Down syndrome.[10] A legal opinion commissioned by the Federal Government Commissioner for Matters Relating to Persons with Disabilities (Beauftragter der Bun-

---

8   Technically, however, it is illegal in Germany to reveal the sex of the child during the first twelve weeks of gestation.

9   The diffusion of NIPT might further a development that has been occurring for some two decades now: the increased use of early-stage non-invasive testing and a concurrent decline in invasive testing (Kolleck und Sauter 2019: 44). For Bernhard Wieser (2017: 62–63) this indicates that instead of one dramatic testing event, we typically see a testing cascade that starts with low-level, non-invasive tests, such as ultrasound and/or ETS, early in the pregnancy and proceeds to amniocenteses or CVS if the results are anomalous. Some scholars, however, expect that low-threshold NIPT might also lead to more tests and consequently more positive results that need be confirmed through invasive methods (Dondorp et al. 2015).

10   Articles appeared in *Die Zeit, die Tageszeitung* (taz), *Süddeutsche Zeitung, Frankfurter Rundschau, Frankfurter Allgemeine Zeitung, Spiegel online* and several regional papers.

desregierung 2012) argued that prenatal testing for non-treatable conditions such as trisomy 21 was incompatible with the UN Convention on the Rights of Persons with Disabilities. Article 8 of the Convention stipulates that governments have a duty to "combat stereotypes, prejudices and harmful practices relating to persons with disabilities" (UN CRPD Art.8 1(b)). In addition, the opinion held, it was incompatible with the German Genetic Diagnosis Act, which allows prenatal genetic testing for medical purposes only. In the absence of therapeutic treatment options, the opinion argues, testing cannot and does not serve a medical purpose. LifeCodex in return commissioned another legal opinion arguing that the meaning of "medical purpose" should not be restricted to "therapeutic purpose" (Hufen 2013).

Nevertheless, the PraenaTest received approval from the authority in charge, the Regional Council in Freiburg in the state of Baden-Württemberg, who evaluated it in terms of safety and efficacy according to the Medical Devices Law (*Medizinproduktegesetz*), not in terms of ethical or social implications (aerzteblatt.de 2012). In that context, the Premier of Baden-Württemberg at the time, Winfried Kretschmann (Greens), set the tone for the developments to follow by framing NIPT as a matter of individual rather than political responsibility:

> Ultimately, the question is "abortion yes or no". [...] These are very rare cases of a virtually unsolvable dilemmas and moral problems the state cannot solve. This question of conscience [...] has to be left to the woman concerned (dpa 2012).[11]

In the course of this controversy, it became known that LifeCodexx had previously received government funding to develop the test. Critics argued that this funding *was*, after all, a political decision, for which the government was accountable. LifeCodexx had been granted some 300,000 euros from the Federal Ministry for Research and Education for NIPT development (Bahnsen 2011) – a fact that caused considerable outrage, particularly among disability rights organisations (Deutsches Down-Syndrom InfoCenter 2011; KIDS Hamburg 2012; Lebenshilfe 2011; Bündnis zum Welt-Down-Syndrom-Tag 2012; Netzwerk gegen Selektion durch Pränataldiagnostik 2012). Later, in the course of an inquiry by an interfactional group of parliamentarians in the *Bundestag*, it turned out that the government had provided further funding of some 500.000 euros to develop an NIPT for the early detection of trisomy 21. The

---

11   All translations from German to English by the authors.

group of MPs demanded to know precisely how much money the government had allocated to NIPT development and on what grounds. They also asked explicitly what, in the government's view, the medical purpose of the test was (Deutscher Bundestag 2015: 5, 10). The government, however, never really addressed this question. In their response, the government merely conceded that "[m]edical progress constantly poses fundamental ethical questions. This holds particularly true for the possibilities of prenatal and genetic diagnosis" (Deutscher Bundestag 2015: 3).

They did not, however, specify *what* questions these were or in what sense NIPT, in their view, was a case of medical progress. They merely proclaimed *that* fundamental issues existed that should be addressed, but they did not address them. In that sense, the response again exemplifies the ambivalence that characterises the political take on NIPT in Germany in general; a lingering sense of moral unease regarding practices of detecting and aborting disabled foetuses, and at the same time a refusal to renounce these practices.

NIPT: Serving a Medical Purpose?

The question of whether NIPT serves a medical purpose has remained a matter of contention. Critics argue that it does not serve a medical purpose, since currently it cannot open up any therapeutic options for the foetus. An organisation for people living with Down syndrome argued that it would instead reinforce the idea "of allowing socially desirable, well-standardised life only" (Deutsches Down-Syndrom InfoCenter 2011). From this perspective, the government had effectively funded the development of selection technology. Proponents, in contrast, contend that NIPT will reduce the number of invasive tests performed and thus the number of test-induced miscarriages, which in their view counts as a medical purpose – this was also the view of the Federal Government at the time (quoted in Deutscher Bundestag 2015: 4). Therefore, some proponents argue, it should be made available to all pregnant women (e.g. pro familia Baden-Württemberg 2012). This line of reasoning was eventually adopted by the Joint Federal Committee, the G-BA (*Gemeinsamer Bundesausschuss*), the body that decides which medical treatments, pharmaceuticals and medical devices are covered by statutory health insurance in Germany. It establishes a method's or a device's diagnostic and therapeutic usefulness, its cost-effectiveness and its medical necessity. In 2019, the G-BA established that NIPT for trisomies 13, 18 and 21 should be included in the catalogue of services covered by the SHI. This was preceded in 2013 by LifeCodexx applying to the G-BA to include NIPT in the so-called trial procedure so that the test could become an SHI benefit, which was accepted in 2014 (Gemeinsamer Bundesausschuss 2014). The implementation of the decision in 2019, however, was contingent upon the existence of "patient information", which was finally presented to the public in August 2021. Provided that the Federal Minster of Health does not reject the decision from a legal point of view, reimbursement can start in early 2022 (Gemeinsamer Bundesausschuss 2021). We will come back to this point.

In Germany, some 90 per cent of the population are covered by statutory health insurance funds. These are not direct state bodies but self-governing entities in the corporatist tradition. The underlying idea is that the members together form a "community of solidarity" (*Solidargemeinschaft*), the purpose of which is to guarantee that every individual member will receive the medical treatments, services and benefits they need, regardless of income or social status. This is called the solidarity principle. The emphasis, however, is on *medical* treatments and *medically* necessary applications; the community of solidarity is not obliged to provide just any goods or services members need or desire; it is explicitly not committed to reimbursing the cost of lifestyle products. Accordingly, the G-BA is not in charge of assessing these. In practice, some health insurers nevertheless offer reimbursement for NIPT to their members on a good-will basis (Krankenkasseninfo.de, n.d.).

The question of coverage by the SHIs, therefore, has important practical and symbolic implications. Many experts and policy actors we interviewed in our empirical study told us they expected the usage of NIPT to increase dramatically once it was covered. Furthermore, many argued that coverage would send a strong symbolic message to society that detecting foetuses with trisomy 21 or other chromosomal aberrations was a perfectly normal and acceptable thing to do, and therefore supported by the *Solidargemeinschaft*. The decision in favour of reimbursement would be a signal to pregnant woman to use NIPT. In this vein, for instance, the leader of a large self-help organisation for people with learning difficulties told us:

Well, what I consider the main issue is that it may induce an attitude in society that it is a matter of course, that it is completely normal [...] to do the test for Down syndrome, that it completely goes without saying that you don't give birth to a child with Down syndrome. [...] That there is such a test is a signal to people with Down syndrome.

Another interviewee, a pregnancy counsellor, expected that cost coverage would lead not only to routine screening for Down syndrome but moreover to a whole new range of tests to follow:

> However, this is about something else: Do we really want to test our off-spring for all disabilities that can possibly be discovered [...] is this what we want? Since this is what is at stake.

Therefore, we contend, the question of whether or not NIPT serves a medical purpose would fall squarely within the purview of this panel. Yet they never addressed this issue directly, but avoided it.

After LifeCodexx submitted the application to the G-BA in 2013, the committee accepted it and launched an assessment procedure. By doing so, the G-BA implicitly stipulated that NIPT would count as a medical method serving a medical purpose; if it had found it would not serve a medical purpose, the matter would not fall within its remit. The decision met with vocal criticism from disability rights groups, pro-life actors, and feminist and anti-eugenic critics of PND. An alliance of civil society organisations and parliamentarians issued position papers, statements and open letters, voicing concern that providing the test for free would pave the way to routine screening for Down syndrome and other chromosomal or genetic aberrations, and demanding that G-BA take social and ethical aspects of the matter into account.

At the heart of the controversy, which is still ongoing at the time of writing, was and remains the question of medical purpose. Advocates stress NIPT's potential to reduce the number of invasive tests performed and thereby of test-induced miscarriages – implicitly meaning miscarriages of *non-affected* foetuses, while critics deny that the tests can open up any other option than to terminate the pregnancy. One interviewee, a disability rights official, put it like this:

> This test serves exclusively, in my view, the purpose of selection. And when someone says, it is just so that one knows, then one wonders why a health insurance fund is possibly going to spend millions just so that anybody can know anything?

Similarly, an open letter to the G-BA in 2016 by a number of feminist and anti-eugenic civil society organisations objected that the concept of medical necessity in antenatal care had increasingly adopted the meaning of "screening for foetuses with disabilities" (Gen-ethisches Netzwerk e. V. et al. 2016). Critics called for a broader societal debate on NIPT and its social and ethical implications, rather than treating it as a matter of safety and efficacy in a merely technical sense.

The G-BA conceded that NIPT "touched upon fundamental ethical questions that had to be taken into account" (G-BA 2016). Members repeatedly expressed their concern but nevertheless decided against addressing social and ethical issues. The G-BA, in their view, was not the right body to deal with this type of issue; they did not consider themselves responsible for addressing the social and ethical implications of NIPT. The question remained, however: Who else was?

In August 2016, the G-BA decided to clear the way for reimbursement of NIPT for detecting trisomy 13, 18 and 21. The decision was preceded by a surge of position papers, statements, and open letters from civil society organisations and parliamentarians who were concerned that reimbursement would pave the way to routine screening for Down syndrome and other chromosomal or genetic aberrations. Nevertheless, the G-BA commissioned a so-called "patient information"[12] on NIPT for trisomies 13, 18 and 21, which formed the prerequisite for implementing the decision. Patient information is a brief brochure for patients and doctors that informs them about the scope, purpose and possible risks of the treatment or drug in question. Nevertheless, unease about fundamental ethical issues at stake persisted in civil society, in the Parliament, and in the G-BA itself. This became apparent when the chair of the G-BA approached the Health Committee of the *Bundestag* in March 2018 with a letter pointing out that the scope of NIPT would expand in the near future and raise fundamental ethical questions (Beeck et al. 2018). Therefore, he demanded, it was "imperative to launch a parliamentary discussion and consensus-building on the question of whether and to what extent molecular genetic testing procedures can be used in pregnancy" (Hecken, quoted in Fricke 2018: 2). In response to this letter, a group of ten MPs from different political factions issued a position paper in October 2018, also demanding a public and parliamentary debate on the matter (Beeck et al. 2018). Questions to be addressed in such a debate would include:

What could a procedure look like that would serve to assess ethically contested diagnostic and therapeutic procedures in the future? Which body

---

12   The correct translation would be an "information leaflet for the members of the statutory health insurance schemes" (*Versicherteninformation*), but for the sake of briefness, we use the term "patient information".

should deal with these ethical questions, and within which framework? [...] What can we do to counteract prejudices against people living with disabilities, and how can we further improve the participation of disabled people and their families? (Beeck et al. 2018: 2)

The *Bundestag*, in fact, did address the matter and held an "orientational debate" in April 2019. It took two hours and focussed mainly on ethical questions (Deutscher Bundestag 2019), but remained inconclusive; it did not touch upon institutional issues of how to govern NIPT in the future, or produce any decision.

In 2021, following the production of the patient information, a new online campaign was launched by civil society organisations, demanding that prenatal selection through reimbursement for NIPT be stopped. The campaign primarily addressed the *Bundestag*, demanding that they enforce a return of the SHI to its "actual task under §1 SGB V", i.e. the provision that it cover the costs of medically necessary treatment. In addition, the campaigners demanded that the *Bundestag* curb unrealistic promises made by test producers. The test, they insist, cannot guarantee a healthy child, nor can it offer any treatment options for children with disabilities.

In August 2021, a preview of the patient information on NIPT for trisomies 13, 18 and 21, which forms the precondition for implementing the reimbursement policy, was published. Pending its approval by the Federal Minister of Health, the reimbursement policy is scheduled to start in early 2022. From then on, women can be reimbursed for an NIPT for trisomies 13, 18 and 21 – "in well-founded exceptional cases" and after obtaining medical counselling (Gemeinsamer Bundesausschuss 2021). The policy does not define what "well-founded cases" are, but leaves this decision up to the individual woman and her doctor. This scheme, as Christoph Rehmann-Sutter and Christina Schües (2020) argue, differs from that of many other countries in that it does not specify a quantitative risk threshold as an entry requirement for NIPT (or reimbursement) – which is remarkable since the G-BA has stated explicitly and repeatedly that reimbursement should be limited to exceptional cases and not lead to routinisation of NIPT. In effect, however, the policy amounts to NIPT on demand: it is sufficient for the woman to expresses anxieties about possible foetal Down syndrome or trisomy 13 or 18 to have free access to the test.

The related press release from the G-BA again sums up the characteristic combination of moral concerns and an individualisation of decision-making and accountability. Here, the chair of the G-BA again justifies the committee's reimbursement decision: "It is rationally as well as medically right to offer a safe alternative to those pregnant women for whom the knowledge of a trisomy is personally important" (Gemeinsamer Bundesausschuss 2021: 1). Yet at the same time it calls for legislation, shifting the responsibility for NIPT policy to the Parliament:

> If we are serious as a society and consider a clear set of legal rules for dealing with non-invasive prenatal diagnostics to be appropriate, the Parliament must address these ethical and moral questions in light of the ever-evolving innovations (Gemeinsamer Bundesausschuss 2021: 1).

At present it seems highly unlikely that the Parliament is inclined to respond to the demand and enact binding legislation. *De facto*, we can conclude, NIPT in Germany is governed by a combination of consumer choice and public cost coverage: the producer offers tests on the market, the individual woman chooses to take them, and the statutory health insurance covers the cost. This arrangement, we would hold, sets high incentives for private sector companies to develop and market further tests for further conditions; the current policy provides no clear rationale or criteria for confining reimbursement to trisomy 13, 18 and 21.

Conclusion

NIPT is still a matter of controversy in Germany, evoking a sense of moral unease and some outright protest. Nevertheless, the policy approach that has emerged to date effectively results in a combination of individualised decision-making and public reimbursement. It thus shows a pattern that has already characterised the German policy approach towards selective abortion and pre-implantation genetic diagnosis. We have termed it the "No, but..." approach here. It stipulates that selecting which kind of children are desirable and should be born and which not is morally wrong or at least problematic *in principle*, but permissible under certain conditions. Whether these conditions apply or not is then a matter of case-by-case decision making by professionals in consultation with the individual – or, in practice, the other way round. With NIPT the decision is delegated to the individual woman, although she is advised to seek counselling. Thus, we see a tension between a moral unease towards selective practices on the one hand, and a reluctance to impose effective restrictions on the other. In effect, the tension is being resolved through individualised decision-making, loosely coupled with professional consultation.

Early on, NIPT in Germany was defined as a deeply personal matter, akin to abortion. By doing so the responsibility for dealing with it in a morally and socially acceptable manner was shifted onto the individual, away from the level of policy-making. This move, however, also obscured policy decisions that had effectively been taken, namely the decision to support the development of the test through public funding. Moreover, we contend, the decision by the GBA to launch an assessment procedure and open the way to reimbursement, the decision to commission a patient information before the assessment procedure was completed, the decision to reimburse NIPT for trisomies 13, 18 and 21 on demand and without specifying further requirements – these were political decisions as well. In short, the decision to leave decision-making to the individual is a political one. This is all the more important as reimbursing NIPT on demand provides a strong incentive for manufacturers to further promote, diffuse and expand their products. Thus, a politics of individualising NIPT inevitably has social and economic implications that may reinforce a self-propelling dynamic of normalisation and routinisation, whether politically intended or not.

References

Achtelik, Kirsten (2015): Selbstbestimmte Norm: Feminismus, Pränataldiagnostik, Abtreibung, Berlin: Verbrecher Verlag.

aerzteblatt.de (2012): Down-Syndrom-Bluttest formal korrekt: Politik. (https://www.aerzteblatt.de/nachrichten/51092/Down-Syndrom-Bluttest-formal-korrekt), accessed 02 November 2021.

Albrecht, Steffen/Grüber, Katrin (2019): TAB Arbeitsbericht 182: Aktueller Stand und Entwicklungen der Präimplantationsdiagnostik, Berlin: Büro für Technikfolgenabschätzung beim Deutschen Bundestags (TAB).

Bahnsen, Ulrich (2011): "Früher erkennen. Ein neuer Test weist Krankheiten bei ungeborenen Kindern nach – gefahrlos und schon in der 10. Woche. Diese Möglichkeit wird eine neue Debatte erzwingen." In: Die Zeit online, 18 August (https://www.zeit.de/2011/34/MTrisomie?utm_referrer=https%3A%2F%2Fwww.ecosia.org), accessed 22 September 2015.

Baldus, Marion (2006): Von der Diagnose zur Entscheidung: Eine Analyse von Entscheidungsprozessen für das Austragen der Schwangerschaft nach der pränatalen Diagnose Down-Syndrom, Bad Heilbrunn: Julius Klinkhardt.

Beauftragter der Bundesregierung für die Belange behinderter Menschen (2012): Gutachterliche Stellungnahme zur Zulässigkeit des Diagnostikprodukts "PraenaTest", Bonn: Bundesministerium für Arbeit und Soziales.

Beeck, Jens/Henke, Rudolf et al. (2018): "Vorgeburtliche Bluttests – wie weit wollen wir gehen?", 12 October (https://www.netzwerk-praenataldiagnostik.de/praenatal-diagnostik/bilder/180703_Interfraktionelles_Positionspapier_NIPD.pdf), accessed 28 October 2021.

Braun, Kathrin (2016): "From Ethical Exceptionalism to Ethical Exceptions: The Rule and Exception Model and the Changing Meaning of Ethics in German Bioregulation." In: Developing World Bioethics 17/3, pp. 146–156.

Braun, Kathrin/Könninger, Sabine (2018). "Realizing responsibility. Institutional routines, critical intervention, and the 'big' questions in the controversy over non-invasive prenatal testing in Germany." In: New Genetics and Society 37/3, pp. 248–267.

Bundesarbeitsgemeinschaft der Freien Wohlfahrtspflege e.V. (2013): Pränataldiagnostik: Information über Beratung und Hilfen bei Fragen zu vorgeburtlichen Untersuchungen, Cologne: Bundeszentrale für gesundheitliche Aufklärung.

Bundesgesetzblatt (2011): Gesetz zur Regelung der Präimplantationsdiagnostik (Part I, No. 58). (http://www.bundesgerichtshof.de/SharedDocs/Downloads/DE/Bibliothek/Gesetzesmaterialien/17_wp/PID/bgbl.pdf?__blob=publicationFile), accessed 02 November 2021.

Bundesministerium für Justiz und Verbraucherschutz (1990): Gesetz zum Schutz von Embryonen. Embryonenschutzgesetz vom 13. Dezember 1990 (BGBl. I S. 2746), das zuletzt durch Artikel 1 des Gesetzes vom 21. November 2011 (BGBl. I S. 2228) geändert worden ist. (https://www.gesetze-im-internet.de/eschg/BJNR027460990.html), accessed 02 November 2021.

Bundesverfassungsgericht (1975): BVerfGE 39, 1 – Schwangerschaftsabbruch I. (https://www.servat.unibe.ch/dfr/bv039001.html), accessed 02 November 2021.

Bundesverfassungsgericht (1992): BVerfGE 88, 203 – Schwangerschaftsabbruch II. (https://servat.unibe.ch/dfr/bv088203.html), accessed 02 November 2021.

Bundeszentrale für gesundheitliche Aufklärung (2010): Pränataldiagnostik: Ein Handbuch für Fachkräfte aus Medizin und Beratung, Cologne: Bundeszentrale für gesundheitliche Aufklärung.

Bündnis zum Welt-Down-Syndrom-Tag (2012): "Gemeinsame Erklärung zum Welt-Down-Syndrom-Tag" (https://www.ds-infocenter.de/downloads/Gemeinsame_Erklaerung_WDST.pdf), accessed 28 October 2021.

de Jong, Antina/Dondorp, Wybo J./de Die-Smulders, Christine E. M./Frints, Suzanne G. M./de Wert, Guido M. W. R. (2010): "Non-invasive Prenatal Testing: Ethical Issues Explored." In: European Journal of Human Genetics 18, pp. 272–277.

Deutscher Bundestag (1995): "Beschlussempfehlung und Bericht des Ausschusses für Familie, Senioren, Frauen und Jugend (13. Ausschuss)." In: Drucksache 13/1850, pp. 1–28.

Deutscher Bundestag (2015): "Antwort der Bundesregierung auf die Kleine Anfrage der Abgeordneten Hubert Hüppe u.a.: Vorgeburtliche Blutuntersuchung zur Feststellung des Down-Syndroms." In: Drucksache 18/4574, pp. 1–12.

Deutscher Bundestag (2019): "Stenografischer Bericht 95. Sitzung." In: Plenarprotokoll 19/95, pp. 11311–11550.

Deutsches Down-Syndrom InfoCenter (2011): "NIPD – Nicht-Invasiver Bluttest zur Bestimmung von Trisomie 21 richtet sich gegen Menschen mit Down-Syndrom. Stellungnahme zur NIPD," 8 September (https://www.ds-infocenter.de/downloads/Stellungnahmen_zurNIPD.pdf), accessed 28 October 2021.

Dondorp, Wybo/de Wert, Guido/Bombard, Yvonne/Bianchi, Diana W./Bergmann, Carsten/Borry, Pascal/Chitty, Lynn S./Fellmann, Florence/Forzano, Francesca/Hall, Alison/Henneman, Lidewij/Howard, Heidi C./Lucassen, Anneke/Ormond, Kelly/Peterlin, Borut/Radojkovic, Dragica/Rogowski, Wolf/Soller, Maria/Tibben, Aad/Tranebjærg, Lisbeth/van El, Carla G/Cornel, Martina C. (2015): "Non-invasive prenatal testing for aneuploidy and beyond: challenges of responsible innovation in prenatal screening." In: European Journal of Human Genetics 23/11, pp. 1438–1450.

dpa (2012): "Kretschmann sieht Bluttest auf Down-Syndrom kritisch", 23 July (https://www.baden-wuerttemberg.de/de/regierung/ministerpraesident/interviews-reden-und-regierungserklaerungen/interview/pid/kretschmann-sieht-bluttest-auf-down-syndrom-kritisch/), accessed 28 October 2021.

Fricke, Anno (2018): "Welche Rolle sollen pränatale Bluttests künftig spielen?" 14 August (https://www.aerztezeitung.de/Politik/Welche-Rolle-solle n-praenatale-Bluttests-kuenftig-spielen-228146.html), accessed 28 October 2021.

G-BA (2016): "Nicht-invasive Pränataldiagnostik bei Risikoschwangerschaften – G-BA beginnt Verfahren zur Methodenbewertung – Beratungen zur Erprobung ruhend gestellt" Pressemitteilung 32/2016, pp. 1–3.

Gemeinsamer Bundesausschuss (2014): Bekanntmachung: Einleitung von Beratungsverfahren zu Erprobungs-Richtlinien gemäß § 137e SGB V (http s://www.g-ba.de/downloads/39-261-1975/2014-04-17_Bekanntm-Einl-Ber atungsverfahren.pdf), accessed 02 November 2021.

Gemeinsamer Bundesausschuss (2021): "Methodenbewertung: Versicherteninformation zum vorgeburtlichen Bluttest auf Trisomien liegt nun vor." Pressemitteilung Nr. 28 / 2021, pp. 1–4.

Gen-ethisches Netzwerk e. V. et al. (2016): "Offener Brief an den Gemeinsamen Bundesausschuss (G-BA) aus Anlass von Tagesordnungspunkt 8.2.1 der öffentlichen Sitzung des G-BA am 18. August 2016", 12 August (https://www.gen-ethisches-netzwerk.de/files/16_08_12%20Offener %20Brief%20G-BA.pdf), accessed 28 October 2021.

Hufen, Friedhelm (2013): "Zur verfassungsrechtlichen Beurteilung frühzeitiger pränataler Diagnostik dargestellt am Beispiel des Diagnoseprodukts PraenaTest®." Legal opinion commissioned by LifeCodexx AG, Konstanz.

Katz Rothman, Barbara (1986): The Tentative Pregnancy: Prenatal Diagnosis and the Future of Motherhood, New York: Penguin.

KIDS Hamburg (2012): "Pränataldiagnostik und gesellschaftliches Bewusstsein", Hamburg: KIDS Hamburg e. V. Kontakt- und Informationszentrum Down-Syndrom (https://www.kidshamburg.de/wp-content/upload s/2018/10/Praenataldiagnostik.pdf), accessed 06 January 2022.

Kolleck, Alma/Sauter, Arnold (2019): "Aktueller Stand und Entwicklungen der Pränataldiagnostik." Berlin: Büro für Technikfolgenabschätzung beim Deutschen Bundestag (TAB).

Krankenkasseninfo.de (no date): NIPT (Nicht-Invasive Pränataldiagnostik). (h ttps://www.krankenkasseninfo.de/test/nitp), accessed 28 October 2021.

Lebenshilfe (2011): Stellungnahme des "Rates Behinderter Menschen" in der Lebenshilfe zu Fragen der Diagnostik bei Embryonen, Berlin: Bundesvereinigung Lebenshilfe für Menschen mit geistiger Behinderung e.V.

Löwy, Ilana (2014). "Prenatal diagnosis: The irresistible rise of the 'visible fetus'". In: Studies in History and Philosophy of Biological and Biomedical Sciences 47/B, pp. 290–299.

Löwy, Ilana (2017). Imperfect Pregnancies: A History of Birth Defects and Prenatal Diagnosis, Baltimore: Johns Hopkins University Press.

Memmi, Dominique (2003): "Governing through speech: The New State Administration of Bodies." In: Social Research 70/2, pp. 645–658.

Nationaler Ethikrat (2003): Genetic Diagnosis Before and During Pregnancy: Opinion, Berlin: Nationaler Ethikrat.

Netzwerk gegen Selektion durch Pränataldiagnostik (2002): "Pränataldiagnostik in der Schwangerenvorsorge." In: Rundbrief 13/ Sonderheft Rechtsgutachten: Betreuung schwangerer Frauen nach den Mutterschaftsrichtlinien, p. 5.

Netzwerk gegen Selektion durch Pränataldiagnostik (2012): "Stellungnahme des Netzwerks: Neuer Bluttest droht die vorgeburtliche Selektion von Menschen mit Down-Syndrom zu perfektionieren", 21 March (https://www.hebammen-nrw.de/cms/fileadmin/redaktion/Aktuelles/pdf/Anlage_zur_Pressemitteilung_2_.pdf), accessed 28 October 2021.

Nippert, Irmgard (1999): "Entwicklung der pränatalen Diagnostik." In: Genethisches Netzwerk/Gabriele Pichlhofer (eds.), Grenzverschiebungen: Politische und ethische Aspekte der Fortpflanzungsmedizin, Frankfurt: Mabuse, pp. 63–80.

Nippert, Irmgard (2001): "Was kann aus der bisherigen Entwicklung der Pränataldiagnostik für die Entwicklung von Qualitätsstandards für die Einführung neuer Verfahren wie der Präimplantationsdiagnostik gelernt werden?" In: Bundesministerium für Gesundheit (BMG), Fortpflanzungsmedizin in Deutschland. Symposium held by the Bundesministeriums für Gesundheit in collaboration with the Robert Koch-Institut, 24–26 May 2000 in Berlin, Baden-Baden: Nomos, pp. 293–321.

pro familia Baden-Württemberg (2012): "Press Release: Vorgeburtlicher Bluttest auf Trisomie 21 muss erlaubt werden, eine frühzeitige und umfassende Beratung muss sichergestellt sein", 31 July (https://www.profamilia.de/fileadmin/landesverband/lv_baden-wuerttemberg/Pressemitteilung_Bluttest_Juli_2012.pdf), accessed 28 October 2021.

Raz, Aviad/Nov-Klaiman, Tamar/Hashiloni-Dolev, Yael/Foth, Hannes/Schües, Christina/Rehmann-Sutter, Christoph (2021): "Comparing Germany and Israel regarding debates on policy-making at the beginning of life: PGD,

NIPT and their paths of routinization." In: Ethik in der Medizin (https://d oi.org/10.1007/s00481-021-00652-z), pp. 1–16.

Rehmann-Sutter, Christoph/Schües, Christina (2020). "Die NIPT-Entscheidung des G-BA. Eine ethische Analyse [The decision of the German Federal Joint Committee to cover NIPT in mandatory health insurance. An ethical analysis.]" In: Ethik in der Medizin 32/4, pp. 385–403.

Schmitz, Dagmar (2016): "Ethische Herausforderungen der neuen nichtinvasiven Pränataltestung." In: Der Gynäkologe 49, pp. 442–447.

Stumm, Markus/Schröer, Andreas (2018): "Sollen die Indikationen für nichtinvasive Pränataltests erweitert werden?" In: Der Gynäkologe 51/1, pp. 24–31.

Waldschmidt, Anne (2006): "Pränataldiagnostik im gesellschaftlichen Kontext", December 2006 (https://www.imew.de/de/barrierefreie-volltexte-1/volltexte/praenataldiagnostik-im-gesellschaftlichen-kontext), accessed 28 October 2021.

Wieser, Bernhard (2017): How Genes Matter: Genetic Medicine as Subjectivation Practices, Bielefeld: transcript.

Wolff, Janna/Graumann, Sigrid (2016): "Aktueller Stand und Entwicklungen von Pränataldiagnostik." Gutachten im Auftrag des Deutschen Bundestages, vorgelegt dem Büro für Technikfolgen-Abschätzung beim Deutschen Bundestag (TAB). Evangelische Hochschule Rheinland-Westfalen-Lippe.

Commentary – "Yes, but…" vs. "no, but…": Ambivalences towards Prenatal Diagnosis in Israel and Germany

Kathrin Braun, Sabine Könninger, Aviad Raz

The differences between Israel and Germany in terms of policies, practices and attitudes towards prenatal diagnosis and selective abortion are significant. They are deeply embedded in cultural scripts and institutional frameworks, and are remarkably persistent. These differences have often been explained by referring to religion (Judaism vs. Catholicism) and different lessons learnt from the Nazi crimes (the need for self-protection for the Jews vs. the universal protection of human dignity). Yet these broad-brush explanations can easily prevent us from seeing other differences or similarities between them, as well as ambivalences and contradictions *within* each country. Our case studies and our conversations with each other, especially about the development of non-invasive prenatal testing (NIPT), give us a more nuanced picture. Although political and cultural differences remain strong, the comparison of NIPT regulations and debates in Germany and Israel also highlights some similarities and convergence. This convergence is reflected in saying "no, but" to NIPT as a public health service in Germany, and "yes, but" in Israel.

In Germany, NIPT is a controversial issue that raises concerns about the routinisation of selective abortion, eugenic pressures on (prospective) parents to produce fit and healthy offspring, and a hostile societal attitude towards people living with disabilities. Despite protests notably from disability advocacy groups against reimbursement by the statutory health insurance, the relevant authority has decided to reimburse the test for trisomies 13, 18 and 21, theoretically on a case-by-case basis, thus saying "no, but" to NIPT.

In Israel, by contrast, NIPT is largely seen as a means to reduce suffering and strengthen parental reproductive autonomy, and this view is shared by representatives of disability advocacy organisations. There have been no fundamental ethical or political concerns about routinisation of NIPT. Yet while it is widely accepted as a public health instrument, it has not been included in the national Health Basket and is thus not covered, even on a case-by-case basis. This shows that in addition to cultural values and ethical principles, budgetary aspects also play a role in shaping NIPT policy. Thus, Israel in a sense said "yes, but" to NIPT.

Economic factors figure in yet another way. In Israel, NIPT is provided by international companies (under arrangements with the Israeli medical system). In Germany, by contrast, there is a strong local provider, the biopharma company LifeCodexx, which received public funding to developing its NIPT product. It seems that promoting the local economy in this case outweighed moral concerns about the technology.

Thus, we can say pointedly that in Israel, NIPT receives moral support from the government, while in Germany, it receives financial support.

One convergence that can be seen concerns the individualisation of decision-making about selective testing. In Israel, reducing the prevalence of genetically related diseases through the use of prenatal testing is an accepted policy objective, but nevertheless the genetic counselling of prospective parents is ideally non-directive and the ultimate decision is left to them. In Germany, this objective does not exist, at least not in public discourse, even if in the case of the NIPT the reimbursement of costs by the statutory health insurance can be read as de facto encouragement to use the test. Here too, counselling is supposed to be non-directive and the decision is left to the individual. The ultimate decision to perform a selective abortion is even more individualised and liberalised in Germany, since women can have a mid- or late-term selective abortion on the basis of a decision made by the individual woman and her physician, whereas in Israel such requests have to be approved by a committee. Thus, in both countries, any possible proliferation of reproductive selection practices can be interpreted as the result of self-determination, and accountability for it is placed on the individual. Yet leaving the choice up to the individual is a political decision too: a politics of individualising NIPT has social and economic implications. It can place further pressure on women and couples in general, not least through the marketing strategies of companies interested in increasing their sales.

Ideological differences notwithstanding, then, we also see commonalities between the two countries. Both Israel and Germany use the solidarity principle in health care, and in both countries PND and NIPT are quite common practice. In both countries it is also possible to have a selective abortion following prenatal testing, although based on different juridical constructions. In Israel, the reason for an abortion may be given as a disability or genetic disposition of the foetus. In Germany the embryopathic indication has been officially abandoned, but a mid- or late-term abortion can still be legal if the woman argues that continuing the pregnancy would endanger her own physical or psychological health.

Yet we also see internal ambivalences, cleavages and incoherencies in both countries: PND and NIPT are not uniformly welcomed or rejected in either country. In Germany, the dividing line runs along political, ethical and partly religious differences, with ablebodiedness being a relevant category; in Israel it maps along lines of ethnicity, religion and social class.

Both countries have seen an increasing influence of commercial logics and market forces in health care, which have an impact on the use of NIPT. Despite the principle of solidarity in the health care system of both countries, inter-fund competition has led health insurance funds to cover NIPT on a voluntary basis in order to attract and attain members. We conclude that more research is needed to better understand the both enduring differences between the two countries, and the similarities, common trends and tendencies, internal differences and ambivalences. Having direct conversations and exchanging experiences, views and perspectives is certainly a good way to get there.

III. Comparative empirical bioethics of reproductive practices and their social contexts

6. Views on Disability and Prenatal Testing Among Families with Down Syndrome and Disability Activists[1]
A Comparative Analysis of Interviews from Germany and Israel

Tamar Nov-Klaiman, Marina Frisman, Aviad E. Raz, Christoph Rehmann-Sutter

Over the last decade, non-invasive prenatal testing/screening (NIPT/NIPS) has become part of prenatal care in many countries. The technology is based on the presence of cell-free foetal DNA in maternal plasma and can be used early – from 9–10 weeks of gestation – and without the risk of miscarriage associated with invasive prenatal testing such as amniocentesis. However, being a screening test, a positive result requires confirmation by a diagnostic test, usually amniocentesis. Currently NIPT is used primarily to detect chromosomal abnormalities – trisomies 13, 18 and 21, with or without sex chromosome aneuploidies – with highest accuracy in the detection of Down syndrome (DS) resulting from trisomy 21 (Mackie et al. 2017).

Due to its special characteristics, NIPT has heightened the social and bioethical debate that on the one hand argues that prenatal testing supports the autonomy of prospective parents (Chen/Wasserman 2017), and on the other criticises it as a new form of eugenics (Thomas/Rothman 2016). The current controversy is by no means new and has accompanied prenatal testing since its introduction in the 1970s (Löwy 2017; Meskus 2012). The ethical debate about prenatal testing is constantly evolving, thereby providing a dynamic

1   This paper has been previously published in the journal *Social Science & Medicine*, 303 (2022) 115021 (https://doi.org/10.1016/j.socscimed.2022.115021). License: https://driv e.google.com/file/d/1wwEodUZIlgqoskhrwTnHfR5LHvqpZIZP/view?usp=sharing We are grateful for the opportunity to present our study also in the context of this book publication.

standard against which to appraise lay ethical opinions. Various perspectives are brought to the debate, including foetal rights, disability rights, feminist and medical perspectives, and parental autonomy (Bayefsky/Berkman 2022; Löwy 2018; Perrot/Horn 2021; Rehmann-Sutter 2021; Stapleton 2017). Little is known about how the changes in prenatal care are perceived by families who already have a child with one of the conditions for which NIPT tests. DS is especially sensitive in this regard, since it is a condition that is compatible with life. The experience of having a child with DS might influence parents' images of what it means to have such a disability and – as a result – how the practice of prenatal testing, and in particular NIPT, is to be evaluated. This article presents results from a qualitative study in Israel and Germany – two countries with divergent public views on and regulation of genetic testing– based on in-depth interviews with family members of individuals with DS and with disability activists.

Objectives

Since many perceive NIPT to be mainly targeting DS, and because of the test's potential to significantly reduce the birth rates of individuals with DS and to affect society's views of DS, DS organisations and families of individuals with DS are prominent stakeholders in the debates about testing. One example is the "Don't screen us out" campaign, which was launched in the UK in response to the decision to publicly fund NIPT in pregnancies at high risk of trisomy 21, 13 or 18 (Ravitsky 2017). The aim of our study is to explore the views of activists and family members of individuals with DS regarding prenatal testing in general, and NIPT in particular.

Previous studies have shown a spectrum of attitudes toward prenatal testing among parents and siblings of children with DS (Bryant et al. 2005; Inglis et al. 2012). In a study by Kellogg et al. (2014), North American mothers acknowledged the impact NIPT might have, i.e. that it might lead to increased rates of terminating affected pregnancies, reduce the availability of services for persons with DS, and increase social stigma. However, more than half the participants said they would consider using NIPT in future pregnancies. The study by van Schendel et al. (2017) of Dutch parents' views of NIPT showed positive attitudes linked to the test's accuracy and safety. The test was appreciated for reducing false reassurance, reducing unnecessary invasive procedures, and enabling preparation for a child with special needs. Early uptake of the test was seen positively when termination of pregnancy is sought, due to reduced maternal-foetal bonding. However, some feared that this would result in less considered terminations that could eventually lead to regret. Dutch parents also shared expectations of a rise in abortion rates, leading to less acceptance of individuals with DS and fewer resources available to them.

One critique raised repeatedly in these studies concerns inaccurate and imbalanced information about DS provided by medical professionals (Kellogg et al. 2014; van Schendel et al. 2017). Balanced information is necessary to make considerate and responsible decisions – as early as the stage of deciding whether to take the test, and when deciding how to act following anomalous results (Asch/Wasserman 2009; Kellogg et al. 2014; Skotko et al. 2011). As many authors have stressed (an authoritative statement can be found in Nuffield Council on Bioethics 2017), "balanced" means including direct experiences and views of people with DS and their families.

Parents raising a child with DS described both positive and negative experiences (Cuskelly et al. 2008; Farkas et al. 2019). For some, the personal experience strengthened their existing views, further underlining the desire to avoid disability in order to prevent suffering. Others reported a drastic shift away from concern and rejection to acceptance of disability and appreciation of its positive effects on their lives and its contribution to social diversity (Nov-Klaiman et al. 2019).

Comparing German and Israeli interviewees allows us to explore the effects of culture and societal context (Melhuus 2002) on the lived experiences and perceptions of family members of persons with DS, as well as disability activists, regarding disability and prenatal testing. Inter-cultural comparisons, particularly of societies with contrasting regulation, are a strong tool to explore the shared vs. local factors, whether historical, cultural, financial, or religious, affecting usage of genetic services. Moreover, the specific case of an Israeli-German comparison contributes to a perspective that goes beyond the Eurocentrism characterising much of western science (Posholi 2020). Indeed, previous studies have shown substantial differences between Germany and Israel, e.g. the attitudes of laypeople towards genetic testing for late-onset diseases or testing of adults (Raz/Schicktanz 2009a; b). Other work, however, has mainly studied the views of genetic professionals (Hashiloni-Dolev 2007; Hashiloni-Dolev/Raz, 2010; Hashiloni-Dolev/Weiner 2008; Wertz/Fletcher 2004). Both the findings from these works and the legal and regulatory frameworks in these countries indicate that Israel adopts a relatively liberal and supportive approach to genetic testing, whereas Germany is rather restrictive.

The attitudes towards genetic practices in Germany and Israel cannot be considered without acknowledging their historical roots. Advances in genetic technology and the ever-growing testing options that come with it have been related to eugenics, although in different ways, by the general public as well as in the clinical or the bioethical discourse. Hashiloni-Dolev and Raz (2010) found that German genetic counsellors regarded Nazi eugenics as setting moral limits for contemporary practices, and highlighted the value of diversity in society. Interestingly, while the Holocaust is considered a primary defining element in Israeli culture (Zertal 2005), many Israeli genetic counsellors have dismissed the idea that the lessons learnt from Nazi eugenics should guide their current work and have detached their practice from historic atrocities (Hashiloni-Dolev/Raz 2010).

The very event that drove Germany to its restrictive approach is arguably the same event that underlies Israel's contrasting outlook. This culture, still bearing the powerful memory of victimhood in the Holocaust, emphasises survival (Chemke/Steinberg 1989) and prioritizes strong Israelis, thereby leaving little room for disability. Weiss (2004) has suggested that both the Zionist movement, which aspired to the rehabilitation of the Jewish body, and the Jewish religion, which is not tolerant of severe physical and mental disability, are further reasons for the Israeli aspiration to competent and whole bodies. In Germany, the Holocaust is a collective trauma of guilt experienced by descendants of a generation of perpetrators (Bar-On 1989) who must distance current practices of "selective" termination of pregnancies from eugenics (Foth 2021; Rubeis 2018).

The aim of this study is to explore the views of disability activists and family members of individuals with DS. It would be particularly interesting to understand this group of concerned people, since they might have insight into the ambivalence towards testing for DS, or might be offended by DS screening programmes such as NIPT. Expert ethical evaluation offers only one layer for the comparison of cultures. Moral reasoning provided by laypeople, although informal and ambivalent, is the one we 'live by' (Raz/Schicktanz 2009a). We draw on interviews with laypeople belonging to these groups for a descriptive analysis rather than an evaluative one. Previously (Nov-Klaiman et al. 2019), we have studied qualitative interviews with this group in Israel. Now we present a comparative interpretation and evaluation of an Israeli-German sample. In the comparative analysis we focus particularly on how participants made sense of the relation between parental responsibility, views on disability and NIPT/prenatal testing. This analysis will hopefully contribute to a better understanding of the perceptions of those who are particularly concerned with DS in Israel and Germany.

Methodology

As part of a larger project to compare prenatal diagnosis in Israel and Germany that began in 2017, semi-structured interviews were conducted with different stakeholders in both countries, following IRB approval from the research ethics committees at the authors' respective universities. Interviewees included health professionals specialising in obstetrics and gynaecology and/or genetics; women without unusual medical family history; parents or other close family members of children with DS; and disability activists. In total, 42 interviews were conducted in Germany and 52 in Israel. Stark differences in themes between Germany and Israel emerged from the interviews with family members of children with DS and DS organisation representatives, who are the focus of the comparative analysis conducted for this article. Data reported in this work reflect interviews conducted throughout the project. Over this period, two relevant changes in healthcare policies took place. In Germany it was decided in 2019 that NIPT would be covered by public health insurance in individual cases. In Israel, in 2018 parents of children with DS became eligible for a 100 per cent social security disabled child allowance, which until then had been determined on a case-by-case basis.

Participants

The inclusion criteria for interviewees selected for the current study were having a child or a close family member with DS or being a DS organisation representative, i.e. stakeholders with a direct experience of DS who are therefore those arguably most concerned by the possible effects of prenatal testing. The term 'activists' refers to office holders and representative of DS-related organisations and self-help groups. Some respondents were both parents and activists. Israeli participants were Jewish individuals belonging to a spectrum of religiosity – secular, modern Orthodox and ultra-Orthodox – and they varied in their ages and number of children. The recruitment process began by contacting five representatives of Israeli DS organisations – of whom four are also parents of children with DS – who agreed to participate in the study.

These representatives assisted us, through their social networks, in recruiting additional participants. Using the snowballing method, 21 interviews were conducted with Israeli organisation representatives and parents of children with DS. In some cases, the child with DS was born before NIPT was available. Sixteen German participants were recruited via information brochures distributed at obstetric/gynaecological and midwifery practices and pregnancy counselling centres, through online posts and snowball sampling. Twelve of the German interviewees have a family member with DS. Four interviews were conducted with disability activists (one of them parenting a child with DS).

All respondents received a recruitment letter describing the study. They agreed to participate and signed an informed consent form. Interviews in Israel were conducted by the first author (a PhD student in medical sociology with training in qualitative methodology), and in Germany by two medical anthropologists trained in qualitative methodology. There was no professional relationship between the interviewers and the interviewees. Consistency between interviewers was maintained by using the same interview guide and comparing interview analysis in team workshops.

Instrumentation and procedures

The research team used an interview guide, which was structured to probe participants' experiences and views of disability, the impact of having a child with DS on subsequent pregnancies and their management, attitudes toward prenatal testing (with a focus on NIPT), and the consequences of these technologies, for the respondents and for society at large. DS organisation representatives were also asked about their organisation's official position. Some questions explicitly probed moral views, e.g., "Does prenatal testing carry in your opinion any specific message to individuals with DS or other disabilities and their families? If so, what kind of message?", and "What do you think of the decision of some prospective parents to terminate pregnancies diagnosed with DS?". Additional questions considered broader frames of influence, for example "How would you describe the influence of your community in deciding about taking the test?". Data were collected in both countries through semi-structured interviews in the local languages (German in Germany and Hebrew in Israel). Interviews were carried out in person or over the telephone and lasted between 45 and 90 minutes. They were transcribed verbatim and anonymised. Thematically selected quotes were translated from these languages into English and given pseudonyms.

Data analysis

This study pursued a descriptive rather than an evaluative analysis. Classifying statements as ethical was discussed by team members during the thematic analysis. We were looking for references of the respondents to the benefits and harms of prenatal testing and whether they considered them good or bad.

In each country, interview transcripts were coded and analysed thematically, based on the grounded theory approach (Strauss/Corbin 1990). Coding served to identify recurring discursive themes and categories of themes within and across groups of participants (e.g. users and non-users of NIPT, secular and religious, and German and Israeli) (Denzin/Lincoln 1994). Interviews were translated to English to enable their reading by both German and Israeli team members. The research team discussed the first few interview transcripts together, examining the relevance of the themes and agreeing on needed modifications and reclassifications. The first author then continued with the coding, discussing new findings as they appeared and their relationships to the codes in team meetings, where agreements were reached to prevent the potential bias of a single rater. The iterations stopped when all authors agreed on all the themes and no new themes were identified, suggesting that theoretical saturation of the sample was achieved, taking place after analysing about half of the interview transcripts (Corbin/Strauss 2008). Preliminary codes, such as views about disability, and arguments supporting and opposing NIPT, were established following a review of the literature prior to the interviews. Further themes – mainly those related to the social context which is characteristic of each location and associated with decision-making about pregnancy management – were identified from the transcripts. As interview transcripts were read and discussed together by both German and Israeli team members, foci of comparison emanated from this dual juxtaposition of cultural perspectives, exoticising "the familiar" and familiarizing "the exotic"through mutual reflection (Sørensen 2010).

Results

The views of parents and activists are presented together since we did not find differences between these groups. Respondents who are both parents and activists presented comparable views in both their roles. In addition to presenting themes on views about disability (ii) and arguments supporting and opposing NIPT, which were drawn from the preliminary literature review, we focus on the emerging theme of responsibility as (future) parents (i). We also describe three additional themes that were commonly found to form the argumentation for the respondents' views on NIPT: (iii) eugenics, (iv) guilt, and (v) perceptions of how prenatal diagnosis and disability are publicly seen.

*Abbreviations:
IL=Israel; GE=Germany; P=Parent/family member of an individual with DS; A=Activist

(i)   Responsibility as parents

Many Israeli respondents linked testing with parental responsibility, arguing that there is a duty to avoid suffering by preventing disability. This was a recurring theme, as clearly described by Efrat:

> A friend of mine was pregnant around the same time I gave birth to my child and she decided not to have the tests, and I remember that in my view it was "How can you be a friend of mine, see what happened to us and decide not to have the tests?" It was extremely irresponsible in my view. (IL, P, Efrat)

Anna-Lena, a German parent of a child with DS, made a parallel reference to other women who use prenatal screening tests, however in a completely opposite sense:

> I also notice that when I talk to other pregnant women, if they say they are going for a nuchal fold scan, I think, "Why are you really doing this?" I mean, "Would you not want a child if it had something like this? And you know my child!" (GE, P, Anna-Lena)

While Efrat questioned the responsibility of her friend's decision not to test, Anna-Lena questioned other women's decision to test. Both critiques are motivated by their own situation with a disabled child, which in each of their views clearly demands a different decision. While having a child with DS can evidently entail very different experiences for parents, we found that the view in favour of testing was common amongst the Israeli respondents while the view against taking the tests for granted was more common amongst the German respondents. Both women essentially argued: How can you see me and my child with DS and still make the decision you have? In their respective sociocultural contexts, it seemed appropriate to reach opposite conclusions from observing the situation parents of children with DS are faced with. This is a strong recurring signal throughout the interviews.

Within the Israeli secular community, aiming for a healthy child is considered an accepted norm and the expecting parents' right, perhaps even their duty. Using testing and pregnancy termination to avoid disability is therefore clearly articulated and not a taboo. In contrast to the common secular Israeli perception of a duty to test in order to "ensure" healthy children, German parents emphasised their perceived duty to accept the child no matter what. Parents did not see themselves as being entitled to perfect children.

> I don't think you have a right to a healthy child. Well, I don't think you have any right to it. I mean, you get pregnant and I think you simply accept that things won't all go smoothly. (GE, P, Lena)

Holding the view that responsibility during pregnancy is exercised through testing, especially in light of their personal experience, some of our Israeli interviewees expressed their wish to maximise the detection of possible abnormalities in subsequent pregnancies. That is, they would not "settle" for a screening test such as NIPT because it can only detect a limited scope of conditions and can produce false results.

> N: If I were pregnant now, I would have performed chorionic villus sampling at the beginning of the pregnancy.

> I: So NIPT is no longer an option for you?

> N: Of course not. Come on, you don't fall into the same pit twice. It wasn't a minor tumble. It isn't, you know, a tiny scratch on your little finger. (IL, P, Noga; had a False Negative result with NIPT)

In comparison with the Israeli sense of duty to eliminate uncertainties in pregnancy through testing, accepting the uncertain nature of pregnancy was more characteristic of the German respondents. This could be related to a general acceptance that one cannot – and therefore should not – make all efforts to protect oneself from the risks associated with pregnancy and childbearing. The tests are often regarded as providing false reassurance, as explained by Paula:

> Well, it really is outrageous. What kind of security is there during pregnancy that everything will be okay in the end? It just doesn't exist. [...] The tests make us go into things completely naively in the hope that afterwards I'll be safe and know that everything is fine. (GE, P, Paula)

In Germany, "disability and responsibility" were connected too, though in a different way than for the Israeli respondents, due to their alternative interpretations of these concepts. A common German rationale that we found was that testing is a means to detect disability, which responsible parents need so they can prepare themselves and their environment for the child. Some respondents saw this as crucial. An understanding environment of family and friends would provide parents with the support and love they felt they needed in their time of difficulty. Interviewees described, in contrast, the difficulties experienced by other parents who were unable to build on supportive environments.

The preparation enabled by NIPT came in the form of emotional readiness as well as practical arrangements. The following quote from Tanja demonstrates how testing enables emotional preparation – a topic that was repeatedly mentioned by our German respondents:

> So I gave birth and I knew that my child had Down syndrome and I was glad that he was there. I know a lot of other women who didn't know it and had children with Down syndrome [...] and fell into a very deep hole. No, well, all the grieving I did in the decision-making phase, when I was going through prenatal diagnosis. They had to do all that grieving after the birth. (GE, P, Tanja)

Practical preparation included choosing a suitable hospital in which to give birth according to the diagnosed condition or choosing appropriate health insurance. The following quote demonstrates how knowing in advance helps in making the necessary healthcare arrangements for the future child.

> The detailed diagnosis, which we did with both children, is something that for me can perhaps influence the decision about which hospital to give birth in. You can also fix some things before the birth. I mean it also has a curative aspect, so not just a selective one. (GE, P, Beate)

Testing was appreciated by both Israeli and German respondents because it provided knowledge, and not just for practical reasons: it also gave expecting parents peace of mind when the results were normal, or certainty when there was an indication of anomaly in pregnancy. Tirzah from Israel explained why she chose diagnosis by amniocentesis following an ultrasound that suggested DS:

> [Confirmation by amniocentesis] allowed me to prepare. I had the time to think what I wanted to do. I think it was very good for me to know this. It gave me the option to choose and later to remind myself that this was my choice [to give birth to him]. Knowing that it was my choice helped a lot. This feeling that it didn't "fall" on me, but it was my own choice. A choice made with logic and with the will to deal with something different. (IL, P, Tirzah)

Lisa from Germany also described in her words the benefits of knowing. For her, testing was a key to eliminating uncertainties and their associated discomfort and potential shock at birth.

> And then it was somehow so clear to us that we just wanted to know. I mean, I didn't want to go through this whole pregnancy – mhm – [I didn't want to] wander around with such an uncomfortable feeling, is it like this or isn't it, and somehow it was also clear that we didn't want our first greeting of this child when it's born to be perhaps shock or something like that. (GE, P, Lisa)

In addition to these positive effects of NIPT, German respondents also conveyed a great deal of criticism beyond that relating to an erroneous sense of security and control. Similar to a common argument among Israeli ultra-Orthodox respondents, a repeated rationale of the German respondents who criticised the tests was the emotional distress they provoked, and the agony related to the decision-making that followed. Even if the results are correct, the tests are blamed for putting women in situations where they have to make decisions they would rather not. Interviewees like the activist Liselotte emphasised the right not to know.

> The more tests you do, the more decisions you have to make. I mean, the famous right not to know [...]. I mean, the easier it is to carry out a test, the easier it is for you to take the test, and afterwards the woman is left with a decision that she may not have wanted to make. (GE, A, Liselotte)

This message is in line with the following, conveyed by another German activist – Dora – who also argued in favour of reducing testing:

> I would say: have as few tests as possible. Because I believe that you never know what something would be like for you and that the tests are, so to speak, always certain or not certain to some extent, and I think that, a lot in pregnancy is aimed at, I mean it leads to generating more worry than you would have if you didn't do all of that. (GE, A, Dora)

Dora's message is especially interesting when compared with that of Dvora's, an Israeli activist:

> I think life isn't simple and that preventive medicine is the proper medicine. Whatever is preventable, you should prevent. Therefore, do all the possible tests to prevent any problem in the future. (IL, P+A], Dvora)

A different understanding of responsibility is not the only explanation for this contrast, as was shown earlier. It also stems from different perceptions of disability and its effect on disabled people and their families.

(ii) Views about disability

Rather than being a source of suffering, many of our German respondents perceive DS to be a special condition of existence, associated with special needs. DS in itself was not considered a disease. In fact, the manifestations of the syndrome are often disassembled and viewed separately. The structural defects, such as the heart conditions that are common in children with DS, are considered separately, and as something that may be treated by surgery, whereas the untreatable manifestation – the cognitive impairment – is what they consider as DS, but without considering it a devastating trait.

> He's just, he has a disability, but he is HEALTHY, he has no diseases or anything. (GE, P, Anna-Lena)

> What was at the forefront for us wasn't the Down syndrome at all, but the heart defect. Because you don't die of Down's, but you can die of the heart defect. (GE, P, Sabrina)

Beate stressed that families who have children with DS are just as normal and happy as other families:

> I think if you dive into the subject of Down syndrome and trisomy and also get to know people, they are just normal happy families, I mean, they maybe worry a bit more about their health, but otherwise […]. (GE, P, Beate)

However, German respondents did not describe bringing up a child with a disability as carefree. The difficulties associated with raising such children were claimed to be the result of the obstacles that society puts in front of the families. The interviewees spoke more about suffering because of social stigmatisation and a lack of acceptance, and less because of the DS itself. DS was not found to be inherently connected to suffering in Germany as much as it was in Israel.

There is even an emphasis on the positive characteristics of these children in the way some German interviewees describe them. Some interviewees pointed out what a positive impact their children have on other people. Hanna said:

> Life with a child with a disability is so, so enriching. Well, that always sounds such a platitude, but it really is like that. It's something very special because you can think through your own values again and what is practically grafted onto you from outside by this system of having to perform, you can somehow really shake yourself free of it. And there is this saying "Once your reputation is ruined, life gets a lot more relaxed." (GE, P, Hannah)

Among Israeli parents too there were less typical voices echoing German ones, where DS was not seen as inherently disabling and instead the positive aspects of the direct experience of DS were emphasised. Society was seen as the source of these children's difficulties.

> Some people say that these kids are a birth defect. But we say no. They are the light of the house. […] My son taught me a lot. He taught me what is patience, he fine-tuned me, he improved me. […] You need to understand that the child is not retarded, our child is not disabled. The ones that are still disabled and retarded are us, as society that doesn't know how to deal with them. (IL, P+A, Sivan)

A strong emphasis on the positive meanings of disability among Israeli respondents came mostly from the ultra-Orthodox community and carried religious meanings. In those instances, children with DS were described as "higher souls" that were "sent by God" to carefully chosen families.

> I told the kids: "God chose us and gave us this special soul. A pure soul. God chose you to be his siblings and us to be his parents. And that means we will do it in the best possible way, and this is a privilege". And I told them that if their friends say "Oh, poor you, you got a child with Down syndrome" with such pity, then they should know that they were not chosen. We were. It is an honour. (IL, P, Leah)

In interviews from both countries, then, DS was not always seen as an obstacle to a fulfilled life. However, even in Germany, where such ideas were more prevalent, some respondents opposed the clichéd positive view of children with DS. They felt uncomfortable with descriptions such as "sunny children" and claimed that this is not accurate and fair. As Lisa describes it:

> It's such a cliché, I have to say. There are many children who don't fulfil that at all —always being so radiant and so sunny and sweet. There are some children who are quite aggressive. (GE, P, Lisa)

A similar rejection of the portrayal of children with DS as "sweeties" also came from an Israeli head of one of the DS organisations. She advocated a view that rejects seeing them as uniformly cute, and instead discerns their individualities and needs. She called for a society that provides for their needs accordingly:

> Let me tell you a secret: not all Down's children are sweet. They aren't kittens! Each one is an individual. They have talents, needs, dreams and achievements. (IL, P+A, Bosmat)

(iii) Views about eugenics

In line with the widely shared goal of avoiding a life with disability, the idea that prenatal testing will result in a decline in the DS community or even its elimination was not perceived by many of the Israeli respondents as a negative outcome. This was justified by the value of the prevention of suffering, as demonstrated in the following two quotes. One is from an activist in an Israeli DS organisation and the other from a mother of a child with DS:

> A child like this, even with all the advances in science and the available opportunities [...]. Still, a child with DS is a child that brings difficulties into the family that a regular family doesn't have. Not everybody is able to deal with it. [...] Nobody wants a child with disability. If you can somehow prevent it and you know in advance about a disability – if you want you

can have an abortion – I am in favour of that. But I never tell the parents my opinion. Each parent is responsible for their own actions. (IL, A, Ofra)

[As a result of testing] fewer babies with DS will be born and I don't think that's not good. If there is anything I know about in advance, then why [stay pregnant]? But if you don't know, like me, then […] there is nothing you can do. Then you have to cope with what you have. But if you know in advance, then I wouldn't keep it. I say that with real pain, because I gave birth to an adorable child. But not everybody is like him. There are many kids with very difficult problems. I am in touch with parents whose children spend most of the time in hospital […] crying and really suffering. Poor children and poor parents […]. (IL, P, Noa)

Other Israeli respondents, however, opposed the attempt to create a society without DS. Some respondents explained the futility of such attempts because disabilities will always occur for different reasons. Others articulated aspects of the disability critique and described diversity in society as an ideal.

There will always be [people with] special needs. There are so many things that can't be detected genetically. It's not that I think the world will suffer if Down syndrome didn't exist. But this desire to reach perfection, so that everything is according to the norm […]. It doesn't make sense. But also, it will never happen that everybody is the same. That's why I think there is a problem with this desire to reach perfection, not specifically [in connection with] DS. (IL, P, Alona)

In contrast to Israel, explicitly eugenic views were rarely heard in Germany; instead, the fear of selection based on undesired traits was raised multiple times. Several respondents mentioned Nazi history in their interviews. In some cases, this was used to explain older people's views in favour of selection, i.e. arguing this was the result of their upbringing under an ideology that rejected disability. Others mentioned Nazi history to refer to processes that should be avoided. Even the argument of "testing enables preparation" was rejected by some who claimed that it is used simply to cover the true nature and aim of these tests, which is selection. The "slippery slope" argument was sometimes raised, reflecting the fear of an uncontrolled outcome.

I really think that these tests send a message: "It makes sense to avoid having children with trisomy." And I think that it isn't the job of the insurers to fund the selecting out of particular forms of life, and that's what these tests do, or that's what these tests suggest, or that's the consequence of these tests in many cases, and I think what they always argue, that parents want to prepare for what awaits them, in the first place, I don't believe that you can. (GE, A, Dora)

Eugenic ideas are thus openly discussed in interviews from both countries – freely advocated for in Israel, and as a red flag in Germany.

(iv) Feeling guilty

These distinct attitudes are in line with the different kinds of guilt described by our respondents in relation to parenting children with DS, and the uptake of prenatal testing. In Germany, women felt guilty when they encountered abnormality in pregnancy and considered termination. In line with Simandan (2020), who elaborates on the process by which people can come to surprise their own selves, the discrepancy between the acceptance of disability, which they saw as an ideal, and what they actually felt in their situation, made them feel guilty. This demonstrates the impact of the social discourse about inclusion, which may prevent German women from choosing a different path – one of thorough testing and termination.

> So, I surprised even myself, because I'd always thought, "well, I want to live in a colourful world with diversity and where people become happy in their own way and not in one of those things [where you're under pressure to succeed]" and "I don't want to love my child for being in some particular way, but for being at all" and so on. Those were my thoughts before, and I think they also had a basis in my heart, but when I was thrown into this medical-technical [world], I suddenly got to know a completely different side of myself. One that didn't want all this, that wanted more security, more normality. (GE, P, Hannah)

A minority of German parents also expressed guilt over the hardships a child with DS experiences and the associated burden on society as a result of the costs of treatments and care.

> It always plays a role too when I see the costs my son actually generates, through all his health problems. We were constantly at the hospital, he needs a lot of aids and a lot of medication and so on. In some ways I do have a bit of a guilty conscience. (GE, P, Janine)

A parallel type of guilt present in Israel was associated with *not* detecting the condition and thus not sparing the child and the family a life of difficulty, as expressed here by Efrat, who did not have an amniocentesis after what later turned out to be a false negative NIPT:

> Clearly I intensely regretted not having the amniocentesis. And all the time people told me, "You know, it isn't certain that it would have been detected by amniocentesis because it is a case of mosaicism." And each time I felt that people were telling me this even though it wasn't true, just so I wouldn't feel guilty. (IL, P, Efrat)

Another form of guilt was articulated by respondents from both countries and expressed here by Ilanit: realising that testing in subsequent pregnancies sends a negative message to the child with DS whom they already have.

> There is great complexity here. And the issue of the test puts me in that zone. When I come to have the test, what am I actually trying to say as a mother of a child with DS, and who is thankful for having him? Am I saying that in reality I am not thankful? (IL, P, Ilanit)

(v)   Public attitudes about disability and prenatal testing

Despite a clear emphasis in official statements in Germany against routinised selection practices ("Dieser Test ist keine Routineuntersuchung." Gemeinsamer Bundesausschuss 2021: 11), even to the extent of eliminating an "embryopathic" indication in the German abortion law (§ 218 a, 2, German penal law) in 1996, interviewees in Germany described a society that is, in reality, often not receptive to disability. Swaantje said:

> It's absolutely not a free decision at the moment – first of all because of the stigma. A question which I have encountered quite often is: "Why didn't you have an abortion?" (GE, P, Swaantje)

This quote indicates a discrepancy between the ideal, as described in the law, and real life. The official views emphasise a free choice and underline inclusion. In reality, parents report encounters with people that not only demonstrate acceptance of selective practices, but also the expectation of endorsing them.

In the Israeli secular community, respondents described frequent judgmental and negative reactions alongside instances of positive and embracing messages from society. As Alona says:

The biggest difficulty is this look of "How did this happen?" The feeling is that it is something extremely exceptional in our environment and I feel that people pity us. [...] In the current pregnancy I feel pressure from society and from people around us to get tested. People would have really raised an eyebrow had we not tested. [We face] all these questions of "This time you ARE getting amniocentesis, right?" (IL, P, Alona)

Discussion

Our findings portray two different logically coherent triangles of local views about parental responsibility, disability, and prenatal tests in Israel and Germany. Given all the nuances and contradictory evidence that we encountered even within each country sample, this depiction of contrasting logics is an idealisation. It over-emphasises and may exaggerate the contrast. However, it does reveal different *possibilities* for connecting experiences with disability, the power of testing and the concerns about responsibility in two different ways, which seem to form distinct tendencies among Israeli and German respondents. Although the sample is much too small to generalise across a whole population, we can identify some clear indications.

Disability in Israel is perceived by many as a source of suffering that justifies prevention. The role of "responsible" parents is to prevent the suffering of a future child and the rest of the family. This practice of responsibility begins in pregnancy (and even before – in the elaborate pre-conception carrier screening offered to the general population, or premarital carrier matching for the ultra-Orthodox). The availability of the widely implemented pre-conceptional and prenatal testing programmes (Zlotogora 2014), which are funded by the state and recommended by medical professionals, implies that genetic testing is the responsible and expected thing to do before and during pregnancy. This, together with an abortion law that explicitly allows terminations based on embryopathy (*Penal Law Amendment (Interruption of Pregnancy)* 1977), arguably pushes for testing in order to terminate affected pregnancies. This has even been described as a local script of "responsible parenthood" in some studies (Hashiloni-Dolev 2007; Raz/Schicktanz 2009a; Remennick 2006; Rimon-Zarfaty/Raz 2009). This outlook is shared not only by large parts of the population, but also by parents of children with disabilities (see also Raz 2004), including parents of children with DS (Nov-Klaiman et al. 2019), where a two-fold view of disability is prevalent: supporting prenatal testing as a preventive measure while being committed to those already born with disability.

The respondents' views reflect an Israeli environment in which prenatal testing is expected, and pregnancy terminations on the basis of DS are seen as legitimate and, in some cases, even encouraged. No such views were found among the German respondents. According to the German interviewees, to act 'responsibly' primarily means accepting a child with DS and preparing properly. When not rejecting them, they see the tests mostly as a legitimate tool for preparation, rather than sharing the Israeli opinion of them as a legitimate tool for avoiding the birth of a disabled child.

The disability critique in Germany is stronger than in Israel: voices rejecting testing and their implementation in society are clearly audible. In line with the change in the German abortion law so that it no longer includes an "embryopathic" indication, the German public discourse is one that promotes inclusion rather than legitimising selection based on undesired traits. This, coupled with the lingering guilt and aversion related to Nazi history, perhaps explains this different logic. It may be harder for parents of children with DS to express difficult personal experiences which – as in the common Israeli voice – lead them to acknowledge the benefits of prenatal testing through the prevention of suffering.

Social discussions clearly have an impact on personal decision-making. Studies from other countries demonstrate the effect of the social environment on the decision-making process. In Denmark, where the termination rate for pregnancies in which DS is diagnosed is over 95 per cent, parents described the legitimising feedback they received from their social networks as highly valued when choosing to terminate (Lou et al. 2018). Perceived social expectations were found to have an impact in the other direction as well. Parents who decided to continue a pregnancy diagnosed with DS felt vulnerable, knowing that they were choosing a path very rarely taken by others in their society (Lou et al. 2020). This could well underlie decision-making in both Israel and Germany. In Israel prospective parents might find it very hard to decide to have a child with DS, whereas in Germany many find it both hard to decide to have a child with DS and hard to decide not to.

Our findings reflect the previously known contrasting public discourses and cultural differences between Germany and Israel. NIPT – a technology only roughly a decade old – demonstrates the persistence of cultural scripts – values and norms – over time, despite the potential effects of personal experience and global trends such as commercialisation.

This study has limitations. To generalise from the level of personal views to the level of cultural characteristics, we looked for statements that reflect common values and norms within and across the groups of respondents. Our sample, which started with activists and then used snowball technique to recruit further participants, may have created a biased sample and thus missed a broader range of viewpoints. Like all qualitative studies, our study's generalisability is limited by the small sample. Less typical interview statements were discussed by the research team and when deemed meaningful were mentioned as minority views in the findings.

Conclusions

Studying disability activists and parents of children with DS allows us to examine whether the lived experience of those who directly encounter DS changes their perceptions of disability, prenatal testing, and termination of pregnancy. By comparing those groups in two societies that are known to have contrasting views on these matters, we can assess the role society plays in the formation of such views. We might have expected that direct experience of DS would drastically change the views of those involved, thereby making them a unique group within their respective country. However, our findings suggest that in each case society has a strong influence. Many Israeli respondents expressed views that legitimise prenatal testing for pregnancy termination, while the major views amongst German interviewees emphasised prenatal testing primarily as a legitimate tool for preparation or rejected them altogether. This difference arguably reflects the different policies and public debates that broadly characterise these countries.

This study has combined two axes of comparison. The first compares German with Israeli respondents, and the second compares the respondents – disability activists and parents of children with DS – with their wider society. For the first axis, our study provides further evidence of the gulf between Germany and Israel already reported in previous studies (e.g. Hashiloni-Dolev 2007). The passing of time and the emergence of new technologies do not seem to have brought these societies closer to one another. Concerning the second axis, parents of children with DS and disability activists seem to reflect the norms of their socio-cultural environments, thereby emphasising the role society plays in shaping the views of those with direct experience of disability.

Acknowledgement

We are very thankful to all the participants of this study for sharing their insights and experiences. We thank Anika König and Stefan Reinsch for establishing the qualitative study design in Germany and for conducting the interviews there. For suggestions in the process of interpretation we thank Hannes Foth, Yael Hashiloni-Dolev and Christina Schües. This work was supported by Deutsche Forschungsgemeinschaft DFG (funding reference: SCHU 2846/2-1; RE 2951/3-1).

References

Asch, Adrienne/Wasserman, David (2009): "Informed Consent and Prenatal Testing: The Kennedy-Brownback Act." In: American Medical Association Journal of Ethics 11/9, pp. 721–724.

Bar-On, Dan (1989): Legacy of silence: Encounters with children of the Third Reich, Camebridge: Harvard University Press.

Bayefsky, Michelle/Berkman, Benjamin (2022): "Implementing expanded prenatal genetic testing: Should parents have access to any and all fetal genetic information?" In: The American Journal of Bioethics 22/2, pp. 4–22.

Bryant, Louise/Hewison, J. D./Green, Josephine (2005): "Attitudes towards prenatal diagnosis and termination in women who have a sibling with Down's syndrome." In: Journal of Reproductive and Infant Psychology 23, pp. 181–198. (https://doi.org/10.1080/02646830500129214), accessed 18 May 2022.

Chemke, Juan/Steinberg, Avraham (1989): "Ethics and Medical Genetics in Israel." In: Wertz, Dorothy/Fletcher, John (eds.), Ethics and Human Genetics: A Cross Cultural Perspective, Berlin: Springer-Verlag, pp. 271–284.

Chen, Stephanie/Wasserman, David (2017): "A Framework for Unrestricted Prenatal Whole-Genome Sequencing: Respecting and Enhancing the Autonomy of Prospective Parents." In: American Journal of Bioethics 17/1. (https://doi.org/10.1080/15265161.2016.1251632), accessed 18 May 2022.

Corbin, Juliet/Strauss, Anselm (2008): Basics of qualitative research: Techniques and procedures for developing grounded theory (3rd ed.), Thousand Oaks: Sage.

Cuskelly, Monica/Hauser-Cram, Penny/van Riper, Marcia (2008): "Families of children with Down Syndrome: what we know and what we need to know." In: Down Syndrome Research & Practice.

Denzin, Norman K./Lincoln, Yvonna S. (1994): Handbook of qualitative research, Thousand Oaks: Sage.

Farkas, Laura/Cless, Jessica D./Cless, Adam W./Nelson Goff, Briana S./Bodine, Ellen/Edelman, Ashley (2019): "The Ups and Downs of Down Syndrome: A Qualitative Study of Positive and Negative Parenting Experiences." In: Journal of Family Issues 40/4. (https://doi.org/10.1177/0192513X18812192), accessed 18 May 2022.

Foth, Hannes (2021): "Avoiding 'selection'? – References to history in current German policy debates about non-invasive prenatal testing." In: Bioethics 35/6. (https://doi.org/10.1111/bioe.12880), accessed 18 May 2022.

Gemeinsamer Bundesausschuss (2021): Bluttest auf Trisomien. Der nicht invasive Pränataltest (NIPT) auf Trisomie 13, 18 und 21 – Eine Versicherteninformation ist eine Anlage der Mutterschafts-Richtlinien des Gemeinsamen Bundesausschusses (G-BA), pp. 11. (https://www.g-ba.de/downloads/17-98-5156/2021-11-09_G-BA_Versicherteninformation_NIPT_Ansichtsexemplar.pdf), accessed 18 May 2022.

Hashiloni-Dolev, Yael (2007): "A life (un)worthy of living: Reproductive genetics in Israel and Germany." In: Springer Sciences & Business Media 34.

Hashiloni-Dolev, Yael/Raz, Aviad (2010): "Between social hypocrisy and social responsibility: professional views of eugenics, disability and repro-genetics in Germany and Israel." In: New Genetics and Society 29/1, pp. 87–102.

Hashiloni-Dolev, Yael/Weiner, Noga (2008): "New reproductive technologies, genetic counselling and the standing of the fetus: views from Germany and Israel." In: Sociology of Health & Illness 30/7, pp. 1055–1069.

Inglis, Angela/Hippman, Catriona/Austin, Jehannine C. (2012): "Prenatal testing for Down syndrome: The perspectives of parents of individuals with Down syndrome." In: American Journal of Medical Genetics, Part A, 158A, pp. 743–750. (https://doi.org/10.1002/ajmg.a.35238), accessed 18 May 2022.

Kellogg, Gregory/Slattery, Leah/Hudgins, Louanne/Ormond, Kelly (2014): "Attitudes of mothers of children with down syndrome towards noninvasive prenatal testing." In: Journal of Genetic Counseling. (https://doi.org/10.1007/s10897-014-9694-7), accessed 18 May 2022.

Lou, Stina/Carstensen, Kathrine/Petersen, Olav Bjørn/Nielsen, Camilla P./Hvidman, Lone/Lanther, Maja Retpen/Vogel, Ida (2018): "Termination of pregnancy following a prenatal diagnosis of Down syndrome: A qualitative study of the decision-making process of pregnant couples." In: Acta Obstetricia et Gynecologica Scandinavica, 97/10. (https://doi.org/10.1111/aogs.13 386), accessed 18 May 2022.

Lou, Stina/Lanther, Maja Retpen/Hagenstjerne, Natasche/Petersen, Olav Bjørn/Vogel, Ida (2020): "'This is the child we were given': A qualitative study of Danish parents' experiences of a prenatal Down syndrome diagnosis and their decision to continue the pregnancy." In: Sexual and Reproductive Healthcare 23. (https://doi.org/10.1016/j.srhc.2019.100480), accessed 18 May 2022.

Löwy, Ilana (2017): "Imperfect Pregnancies: A History of Birth Defects and Prenatal Diagnosis." In: A History of Birth Defects & Prenatal Diagnosis. (https://doi.org/10.1353/book.55867), accessed 18 May 2022.

Löwy, Ilana (2018): Tangled Diagnoses. Prenatal Testing, Women and Risk, Chicago and London: The University of Chicago Press.

Mackie, Fiona/Hemming, Karla/Allen, Stephanie/Morris, R. Katie/Kilby, Mark (2017): "The accuracy of cell-free fetal DNA-based non-invasive prenatal testing in singleton pregnancies: a systematic review and bivariate meta-analysis." In: BJOG: An International Journal of Obstetrics & Gynaecology, 124/1, pp. 32–46.

Melhuus, Marit (2002): "Issues of relevance: anthropology and the challenges of cross-cultural comparison." In: Anthropology, by comparison, pp. 90–112.

Meskus, Mianna (2012): "Personalized ethics: The emergence and the effects in prenatal testing." In: BioSocieties 7/4. (https://doi.org/10.1057/biosoc.2012.27), accessed 18 May 2022.

Nov-Klaiman, Tamar/Raz, Aviad/Hashiloni-Dolev, Yael (2019): "Attitudes of Israeli parents of children with Down syndrome toward non-invasive prenatal screening and the scope of prenatal testing." In: Journal of Genetic Counseling 28/6, pp. 1119–1129.

Nuffield Council on Bioethics (2017): Non-invasive Prenatal Testing: Ethical Issues, London, UK: Nuffield Council on Bioethics.

Penal Law Amendment (Interruption of Pregnancy) (1977).

Perrot, Adeline/Horn, Ruth (2021): "The ethical landscape(s) of non-invasive prenatal testing in England, France and Germany: findings from a comparative literature review." In: European Journal of Human Genetics. (https://doi.org/10.1038/s41431-021-00970-2), accessed 18 May 2022.

188 Comparative empirical bioethics of reproductive practices and their social contexts

Posholi, Lerato (2020): "Epistemic Decolonization as Overcoming the Hermeneutical Injustice of Eurocentrism." In: Philosophical Papers, 49/2, pp. 279–304.

Ravitsky, Vardit (2017): "The shifting landscape of prenatal testing: between reproductive autonomy and public health." In: Hastings Center Report 47, pp. 34–40.

Raz, Aviad (2004): "'Important to test, important to support'": attitudes toward disability rights and prenatal diagnosis among leaders of support groups for genetic disorders in Israel." In: Social Science & Medicine 59/9, pp. 1857–1866.

Raz, Aviad/Schicktanz, Silke (2009a): Diversity and uniformity in genetic responsibility: moral attitudes of patients, relatives and lay people in Germany and Israel. In: Medicine, Health Care, and Philosophy, 12/4, pp. 433–442. (https://doi.org/10.1007/s11019-009-9215-x), accessed 18 May 2022.

Raz, Aviad/Schicktanz, Silke (2009b): "Lay perceptions of genetic testing in Germany and Israel: the interplay of national culture and individual experience." In: New Genetics and Society 28/4, pp. 401–414.

Rehmann-Sutter, Christoph (2021): "Should prenatal screening be seen as 'selective reproduction'? Four reasons to reframe the ethical debate." In: Journal of Perinatal Medicine 49/8, pp. 953–958.

Remennick, Larissa (2006): "The quest for the perfect baby: why do Israeli women seek prenatal genetic testing?" In: Sociology of Health & Illness 28/1, pp. 21–53.

Rimon-Zarfaty, Nitzan/Raz, Aviad (2009): "Abortion committees as agents of eugenics: medical and public views on selective abortion following mild or likely fetal pathology." In: Kin, Gene, Community: Reproductive Technologies among Jewish Israelis, pp. 202–225.

Rubeis, Giovanni (2018): "Das Konzept der Eugenik in der ethischen Debatte um nicht-invasive Pränataltests (NIPT)." In: Pränatalmedizin: ethische, juristische und gesellschaftliche Aspekte, pp. 100–125.

Simandan, Dragos (2020): "Being surprised and surprising ourselves: a geography of personal and social change." In: Progress in Human Geography 44/1, pp. 99–118.

Skotko, Brian/Levine, Susan/Goldstein, Richard (2011): "Having a son or daughter with Down syndrome: Perspectives from mothers and fathers." In: American Journal of Medical Genetics, Part A, 155A/10, pp. 2335–4237.

Sørensen, Estrid (2010): "Producing Multi-Sited Comparability." In: Thick Comparison: Reviving the Ethnographic Aspiration.

Stapleton, Greg (2017): "Qualifying choice: ethical reflection on the scope of prenatal screening." In: Medicine, Health Care and Philosophy 20/2, pp. 195–205. (https://doi.org/10.1007/s11019-016-9725-2), accessed 18 May 2022.

Strauss, Anselm/Corbin, Juliet (1990): Basics of Qualitative Research. Grounded Theory Procedures and Techniques, Thousand Oaks: Sage.

Thomas, Gareth/Rothman Katz, Barbara (2016): "Keeping the Backdoor to Eugenics Ajar?: Disability and the Future of Prenatal Screening." In: AMA Journal of Ethics, 18/4, pp. 406–415. (https://doi.org/10.1001/journalofethics.2016.18.4.stas1-1604), accessed 18 May 2022.

van Schendel, Rachel/Kater-Kuipers, Adriana/van Vliet-Lachotzki, Elbeth/Dondorp, Wybo/Cornel, Martina/Henneman, Lidewij (2017): "What Do Parents of Children with Down Syndrome Think about Non-Invasive Prenatal Testing (NIPT)?" In: Journal of Genetic Counseling 26, pp. 529–531. (https://doi.org/10.1007/s10897-016-0012-4), accessed 18 May 2022.

Weiss, Meira (2004): The chosen body: The politics of the body in Israeli society, Stanford: University Press.

Wertz, Dorothy/Fletcher, John (2004): Genetics and Ethics in Global Perspective, Alphen aan den Rijn: Kluwer.

Zertal, Iidith (2005): Israel's Holocaust and the Politics of Nationhood. In: Israel's Holocaust and the Politics of Nationhood, Camebridge: University Press. (https://doi.org/10.1017/cbo9780511497537), accessed 18 May 2022.

Zlotogora, Joël (2014): "Genetics and genomic medicine in Israel." In: Mol Genet Genomic Med. 2/2, pp. 85–94. (https://doi.org/10.1002/mgg3.73), accessed 18 May 2022.

A Commentary from Disability Activism in Israel

Rachel Lishansky

I participated in this research because I am a mother of four children and grandmother to twelve grandchildren. My youngest daughter, Nitzan, is a young woman with Down syndrome. I was 36 years old when I became pregnant with Nitzan and so because of my age was not offered any NIPT/NIPS testing. At that time only women over the age of 37 were tested in Israel. Hence, we were completely unprepared physically and emotionally for the arrival into our lives of a baby with Down syndrome.

The name we chose for our daughter, Nitzan, means a flower bud and now 40 years later I can see how appropriate this was for her. Nitzan has been married for almost twenty years to her husband Sagi, who also has Down syndrome. They live together on a kibbutz in a warden assisted hostel with 13 other young people. They go to work every day and enjoy a full range of social and creative activities. Nitzan and Sagi are a loving couple. They care for each other, support each other and they are great together. I often say to people how we all learn from observing their relationship.

As well as being a parent, I am also the head of an organisation in Israel called *Atid*, which means *Future* in Hebrew. In our organisation we encourage preventative medical practice and support the view in Israeli society to test for abnormalities during pregnancy. With today's medical improvements we should be, and in Israel we are, using such methods as widely as possible, including NIPT/NIPS. Testing allows parents to consider their options regarding a pregnancy termination but also provides an invaluable opportunity to be informed and prepared for outcomes should they choose to proceed. I too encourage and support this approach. If a baby is born with Down syndrome (there are approximately 120 each year in Israel), *Atid* strives to do everything to support the whole family and provide the best options for a decent quality of life. This can include home visits, telephone and group support, helping with government agencies, and so much more.

Down syndrome can occur in any pregnancy. The consequences are enormous for the immediate family and their extended network. The impact on parents, siblings and their wider circle is huge. For some parents, the situation is overwhelming and they decide to leave their baby in the care of others; the hospital, foster care and/or adoption. Not everyone can cope with the immense strain of having a child with Down syndrome and families can disintegrate at different stages, causing further ongoing issues. The whole family needs support and encouragement from those around them. I am fortunate enough to have this, but many do not.

Becoming a mother means accepting that your priorities will be different from those you had before. Caring for a Down syndrome child, such as my daughter, requires a huge amount of time and commitment. It took me a few years before I eventually realised that we only have one life and while I would try and do everything to help Nitzan, I also needed to live my own life. I was a working mother and a student. I wanted to encourage Nitzan to be as independent as possible. I wanted her to be responsible so she could live a fulfilled, functioning life as she grew older. Finding the balance between her needs and mine was a constant juggling act, and remains so even today. As a result of publishing two books, plus my long-standing involvement with *Atid* and my active role in the management of Nitzan's and Sagi's hostel life and activities, I am now a recognised name in the field of Down syndrome in Israel. Consequently, over the years I have been approached many times for advice and guidance by couples and families dealing with the issues surrounding a diagnosis or life with a child with Down syndrome.

I am often asked whether if I had known I was carrying a baby with Down syndrome I would have considered terminating the pregnancy. In principle I do support termination of such a pregnancy, but this is not a fair question and I cannot give an objective answer. My daughter is an integral part of our lives, not an abstract, hypothetical situation. To those that ask whether they should terminate their Down syndrome pregnancy, my advice is straightforward. Always consider your opinions and values. If you have support, patience and strength, and you can rise to the challenge, then your life will be certainly interesting, with many successes but also difficult moments and failures. Ultimately each person needs to make their own decision on how to proceed.

Further to this, parents and the wider family not only need to come to terms with their situation but they also need to prepare themselves for the struggles that await them in the wider world. Family, society and many institutions, including education, will all be challenges. They require a strong and well-prepared nuclear family with a "thick skin" to act as a protective wall around them and their child. Even today people and agencies can be ignorant and ill-informed. For the whole family it is a lifelong commitment to ensure that a child with Down syndrome can be supported in the most appropriate and stimulating way. Ideally the state should fund this care, but parents cannot rely on this and need to prepare for when they may no longer be able to be the primary carer for their child.

When I look back on all that we as a family have achieved and gained in our journey with my daughter, I know with all my heart that she and those living with her in her hostel have brought a huge contribution to wider society. What could have been achieved if she and her group had not been affected by Down syndrome is something we will never know. As a society with NIPT/NIPS options and other medical testing we have an opportunity to minimise disability, but just as importantly, we also have a duty to support and care for those who require lifelong help.

A Commentary from Disability Studies in Germany

Swantje Köbsell

The results of the authors' research show a rather distinctive difference between the two countries in the political and the activist discourse on disability
and prenatal diagnosis. Even though the research sample is quite small, it
can be stated that the German discourse on disability, and especially activists'
attitudes, are still very much influenced by "the long shadow of history". Here,
this refers to the eugenic programmes of the National Socialists, which led
to the forced sterilisation of 300.000 disabled and mentally ill persons. Den-
igrated as "ballast existences", "useless eaters" and "life unworthy of life", the
Nazi regime planned and carried out the murder – euphemistically dubbed
"euthanasia" (Greek for "good death") – of about another 300.000 disabled
persons. Research has shown (cf. Friedlander 1995) that the "euthanasia" programme was the first of the Nazi killing programmes that aimed to "purge"
the race of all "spoiling" influences. After the "euthanasia" programme was
discontinued, the staff and the equipment were sent on to the killing camps
to employ their expertise there. These facts have broadly been ignored in the
Holocaust discourse. In Germany, the societal discourse about the crimes
committed against disabled people started only in the early 1980s.

After the Second World War eugenics was largely discredited because of the
National Socialist practices, but re-emerged as a new discipline of human genetics in 1965. The ancestry of this "new" science went unchallenged for a long
time, and its founding fathers who had been active in promoting and teaching
"racial hygiene" (the term in Nazi Germany for eugenics) continued to propagate their ideas about controlling the quality of German offspring, although
now the target was not the health of the *Volkskörper* but the prevention of individual health conditions through genetic counselling. Here the aim was to
identify the precise risk of particular couples to produce disabled children,
and to counsel them to avoid having children of their own when the calculated
risk was deemed too high. Shortly afterwards, prenatal genetic testing became

possible and available. Though officially introduced to support reproductive self-determination, the offer still had the eugenic goal of avoiding the birth of "defective" children. Cost-benefit analysis also played an important role in the process of establishing prenatal testing – how much money could be saved by preventing the birth of disabled children, especially children with Down syndrome, which was relatively easy to detect?

It took a long time for post-war German politics and society to recognise disabled people as victims of Nazi persecution. It was only in 2007, 62 years after the end of the war, that the German parliament declared the Law for the Prevention of Offspring with Hereditary Diseases (*Gesetz zur Verhütung erbkranken Nachwuchses*) of 14 July 1933 to be a Nazi injustice, but the victims of this injustice were not officially recognised as victims of Nazi persecution and are not entitled to any compensation. The central Memorial and Information Point for the Victims of National Socialist "Euthanasia" Killings in Berlin was not opened until 2 September 2014, the last of the four memorials to the victims of the Nazis' racial and extermination policies (Jews, Sinti and Roma, homosexuals, and disabled people) in the German capital.

One of the main achievements of the disability movement and disability studies has been to break the established traditional link of the medical model of disability between disability and suffering through the development of the social model of disability, which was named and formulated first in the United Kingdom. Disability rights movements in other countries, like Germany, developed similar perceptions of disability without calling it a social model. In a medical model disability is perceived as a tragic, individual problem that is equated with suffering, that needs to be cured or must be endured. In this view lack of social participation, education or general access are inevitable consequences of the personal condition. This perception was revolutionised with the advent of social model thinking: here, disability is no longer a personal problem but a social one, and the task for society is to provide conditions that allow people with all kinds of impairments to participate in it equally. In a social model view, disability is not individual suffering, but something that is imposed by society on top of individual impairments (UPIAS 1976) – and can thus be altered. This perception of disability has been reinforced immensely by the UN Convention on the Rights of Persons with Disabilities (CRPD 2006), a major success of the international disability movements. The first article of the CRPD states: "Persons with disabilities include those who have long-term physical, mental, intellectual or sensory impairments which in interaction with various barriers may hinder their full and effective participation in society on an equal basis with others." In Germany, this definition of disability has become the official political stance on disability and can be found in several laws concerning disabled people. On the other hand, scientific and social discourses on prenatal testing in combination with selective abortion, as well as discourses on medically assisted suicide, often argue that these interventions help to avoid individual suffering. This argumentation re-emphasises the link between disability and suffering, thus supporting the medical model of disability.

The German disability movement, as well as German disability studies, which emerged from the movement, has always taken a critical stance towards eugenics. We could even say that it is one of the defining traits of the German disability movement. Every method and technology that may possibly lead to the devaluation of disabled lives is under this scrutiny. A distinctive part of the public and political discourse on prenatal testing and selective abortion is also influenced by the historical experience of Nazi eugenics and in consequence is critical towards the selective potential of new testing technologies. But this is only one side of the coin. On the other we find widespread acceptance for ever finer methods of detecting "defects" in the unborn, mostly in the name of reproductive autonomy and responsible parenthood as well as the prevention of pain and suffering.

Against the backdrop of German history, the disability movement was and still is very vigilant against eugenic practices in any guise – be it prenatal testing, the allocation of medical services according to quality adjusted life years (QALYs), discussions about medically assisted suicide in which "the suffering" of disabled persons is (ab)used, and ethics that divides humankind into persons and non-persons and denies non-persons the right to life, as the Australian ethicist Peter Singer does. The most recent critical debates occurred in the COVID-19 related discussions about triage decisions which were supposed to be "objective" while based on an evaluation system that rated the value lives of people who needed support and assistance in daily life distinctly lower than that of people who lived without this support.

These recent developments have shown that vigilance on the movement's part towards life-denying developments for disabled people is still necessary. We live in times where disabled people paradoxically have more legal rights than ever before, but simultaneously the results of genetic research, discussions about the "just" distribution of healthcare and the discourse on the right to a self-determined death threaten the very existence of disabled people. In public discourse, "inclusion" is the dominant topic, but society's view of disability is still very much informed by ableism, which leads to negative, neo-eugenic attitudes.

References

Friedlander, Henry (1995): The Origins of Nazi Genocide: From Euthanasia to the Final Solution, Chapel Hill, NC: University of North Carolina Press.

Gesetz zur Verhütung erbranken Nachwuchses (14. Juli 1933) (RGBl. I S. 529) accessed 22.5.2022.

Singer, Peter (1999 [1993]): Practical Ethics, Cambridge: Cambridge University Press.

UN (United Nations) (2006): Convention on the Rights of Persons with Disabilities (CRPD), (https://www.un.org/development/desa/disabilities/convention-on-the-rights-of-persons-with-disabilities/convention-on-the-rights-of-persons-with-disabilities-2.html), accessed 18 May 2022.

UPIAS (Union of the Physically Impaired Against Segregation) (1976): Policy Statement, (https://disability-studies.leeds.ac.uk/wp-content/uploads/sites/40/library/UPIAS-UPIAS.pdf), accessed 18 May 2022.

7. Socio-Cultural and Religious Views on Prenatal Diagnosis in Israel and Germany

A transnational conversation between Tsipy Ivry and Hille Haker initiated by Anne Weber and Christina Schües

This conversation between Tsipy Ivry, Chair of Medical and Psychological Anthropology at Haifa University (Israel), and Hille Haker, Endowed Chair of Catholic Moral Theology at Loyola University Chicago (USA), results from an exchange about religious implications and narratives in the context of prenatal diagnosis. Both participants speak from a specific religious background. Their positions are not representative of a whole religious belief system, but reflect their perspective on their own field of research. They shed some light on the different religious values that might organise and inform women's and parents' decision-making during pregnancy, especially with regard to choosing NIPT or other diagnostic procedures. Thus, the following should be read as a starting point – not a finalisation – of the discussion, and hopefully invites further conversations.

On the 18. October 2021, we met online. Afterwards the conversation was transcribed by Isabella Burton-Clark and revised by Anne Weber and Christina Schües.

Christina Schües: With a warm welcome to you, Tsipy Ivry and Hille Haker, we would like to open our conversation, which will be looking at the similarities and difference of the "Meanings and Practices of Prenatal Genetics in Germany and Israel." Since our project is a cooperative, interdisciplinary and transnational study, the idea of conversation is central. Comparing practices of, in this case, prenatal diagnosis in two countries is not straightforward: we can compare laws and regulations because they are mostly nationally defined, but practices of acting and thinking don't stop at border control. Researchers who study reproductive technologies, or the people who are using them, may be influenced by different discourses and traditions, cultures and religious beliefs that are not necessarily nationally formed. Thus, by engaging you in a transnational conversation, it is clear that you will not speak *for* a country.

When you, Tsipy, talk about your research in Israel, you speak as an Israeli woman, researcher, anthropologist, but not in a totalising sense as though "the Israelis do such and such." And the same for Hille: you speak as a German thinker who now lives in Chicago, but obviously you do not stand for Germany. So, in this sense, I think the idea and practice of conversation becomes very important, because it will entangle, combine, and bind together different and similar ways of thinking that emerge, and be inspired by and exhibited in these different countries. A country, or a nation, is certainly not a kind of "bucket" with closed borders. Our conversation today will be cooperative and transnational. But as well as crossing borders, it will also cross disciplines.

Tsipy, you make it very clear that you are not a theologian but an ethnographer who studies religious communities, orthodox communities; so in this sense you are interested in beliefs and how they are enacted. Hille, you are a theologian and an ethicist. You are also working in philosophy, and thus your work goes beyond theology. Both of you are interested in different belief systems and practices, yet you approach your field from different angles, so we'll have a transnational as well as an interdisciplinary conversation. Neither of you is purely a theologian and we, Anne and I, are well aware of this. When we came up with the idea of this conversation it was very clear that we did not want just to talk about principles, or to compare some sayings from the Bible or the Talmud. We are interested in practices and how they are dealt with, and what motivates them. It is our overall idea to open up a space between the two of you, Hille and Tsipy, which allows for a conversation about the different aspects of prenatal testing practices. After these preliminary remarks I now hand over to Anne, who will lead us into this conversational space.

Anne Weber: Thank you Christina, and also from my side a very warm welcome to you, Tsipy and Hille. Hille, you are a theologian as well as a philosopher engaged in social and political ethics, feminist theory and bioethics. For our readers who are not that familiar with religious ideas on birth or life, or the Christian arguments on prenatal testing, I would like to start on a more general ground: From your perspective and in terms of your own research, what moral or religious values appear important to women or parents during pregnancy or when considering prenatal care?

Hille Haker: First of all, thank you very much indeed for giving us the opportunity to engage with each other's work, and with each other in conversation. As a kind of a premise to everything, I would like to state that there are always multiple perspectives when you enter into theological interpretations or conversations, and so I will be introducing my personal approach to theological ethics – in this case Catholic theological ethics. However – and this might already mark a difference to rabbinic ethics – in the Catholic Church there are also so-called authoritative Church teachings. In this regard, theologians are the ones who engage in conversations with these Church teachings as conversation partners. Accordingly, our task as theologians is not only to transmit what we call the *Magisterium* (that is, what the Vatican comes up with) to clergy and lay people, but also to constructively engage with and judge, assess, evaluate – and in my case I must also say dissent from – those teachings. Since many people do not realise this is one of theology's tasks, I would like to emphasise it. We sometimes even say that theology is the place or space where the Church does its thinking. It can be understood polemically, but if you think about it, moral reasoning is also pursued academically and scientifically, and then it's channelled back into the imperatives, or into teachings that can then be implemented and pragmatically practiced in different communities and local churches. That said, it is clear that I do not speak for about 1.3 billion Catholics worldwide, but as a theological ethicist, as a moral theologian and social ethicist, who engages in a conversation on prenatal diagnosis, in this case with the Catholic Church, from my own academic and scholarly perspective, which is informed not only by theology but also by ethical theory and by cultural anthropology, medical anthropology, and most importantly of course by the experiences of women.

Against this background it is not easy to answer your question, because from whose perspective should I respond? Let me tentatively note that there's one common ground upon which we all stand as Catholics – whether we are lay people, engaged in liturgical practices, a woman, a mother, or a theologian, people who are closer to the Vatican's thinking on bioethics or people criticising their approach – and that is the concept of dignity, of human dignity. It's a difficult concept, certainly, but it is important to highlight it. In contrast, American discourse on bioethics is not grounded in human dignity, but rather draws on the concepts of freedom and liberty. Comparing European and US American debates already shows how the grounding of the ethical framework relates to contextual, cultural, historical and also normative facts.

Tsipy Ivry: Hille, maybe my next question appears characteristically anthropological: Could you please give an example of how human dignity matters to women when they approach decisions about prenatal testing, and whether to undergo prenatal testing at all? Or how human dignity informs the decision on what to do with a "suspicious" result, i.e. with an indication? I mean, at each and every point of this imagined route, there are dilemmas where women or parents look for guidance.

Hille Haker: Oh, I absolutely agree. I did not mean to dismiss or discard all these dilemmas, but looked for a common starting point on the understanding of what is considered a moral – or you could also say Catholic – orientation, and at the same time a starting point for women, for families, who are under the pressure of situations in pregnancy that raise moral dilemmas. And the normative frame that Catholic teaching refers to is built on the idea of human dignity. So even if you enter into a situation with a specific set of values, or a culturally, religiously or historically linked prejudgment, in the Catholic context the notion of human dignity gives the overall normative orientation for ethical decision-making processes. As a consequence, and in contrast to other moral pre-judgments – as the premises of one's moral reasoning – such as autonomy or freedom, drawing on human dignity in ethical dilemmas in prenatal testing can mean, for example, that children with a disability are welcomed into the world. On a practical level this translates into giving special attention to children or people with disabilities. For instance, when we meet on Sundays for the Eucharist, there will be children or adults with disabilities, and they seem well respected. Maybe not primarily in a reflexive, concrete sense, but rather in a performative one, such as the way they are seated during Holy Mass. At least in my home parish in Germany, there were a few children with Down syndrome, and among them there was this one boy who wanted to be the Pope when he grew up. So he would come up to the priest in the middle of the Eucharist and play along with the Eucharist. Since people accepted him in his special condition, nobody judged him or stopped him from doing this.

Besides this personal example, it is common in Germany for people to do their best to integrate every person despite their individual abilities and disabilities. Of course, alongside these attempts come paternalist tendencies. I don't want to draw idealistic pictures here, since there is still enough discrimination towards people with disabilities. Nevertheless, coming out of the really dark, dark history of Nazi Germany, with systematic euthanasia and Darwinist ideologies and only a few Christians, like Cardinal Graf von Galen who spoke out publicly against it, this catalysed the emphasis on human dignity, which still motivates us to integrate people with disabilities on a personal as well as an institutional level. So starting with human dignity in this respect might already be very contextual, but regardless of the concrete history of Germany's guilt, its value is upheld and conserved in religious as well as secular contexts. Considering our topic of prenatal diagnosis, it creates problems since dignity and autonomy can collide. However, the Catholic Church safeguards and focuses on human dignity even when women are faced with prenatal dilemmas. Tying human dignity to universal respect and its possible universalisation takes the question "Do people with disabilities have the right to life?" off the table. For a moment at least, we suppose, "Yes, of course"... Does that help as a first explanation, Tsipy?

Tsipy Ivry: Yes, it helps very much. I must confess that I've never lived in a Christian country. My other field of research is in Japan, whose history is also shadowed by a period of eugenics. So I've been always extremely impressed with revelations of acceptance of disability in Christian communities as I find them on the web. When I teach my course "An Introduction to the Anthropology of Reproduction" I sometimes show the students a video of a couple who gave birth to a baby with anencephaly. Even though it is a very difficult condition they accepted the child, and it was amazing to see how they put a cap on the baby's head, how they embraced and sang to the baby. There was a whole way of including this baby into the family and the siblings, and this was extremely impressive and surprising from my perspective because – and I'm not saying it judgmentally in any way, because I really don't feel judgmental towards either of the areas that I'm speaking about – in Israel even the Haredi communities, I feel, are extremely ambivalent towards disability. On the one hand, you hear the narratives about how "these children," are special gifts and they're God-given, and how "this specific child chose me to be his or her mother, and therefore I am suitable to be his or her mother," and you hear how these children pray so beautifully and how they're loving and caring and special and how "we love them," and so on. However, on the other hand, you also hear how difficult it is to raise these children. For instance, one of the women who took part in my empirical research studies and who I'm still in contact with, gave birth to a child with Down syndrome, and one of her relatives called her to give her blessing. So she said to the young mother, "Oh, you're so blessed, and God gave you this special gift," and this woman answered, "What do you mean? Are *you* willing to receive this gift?" So, I always feel there's a lot of ambivalence surrounding children and adults with disabilities, and this ambivalence and tension shows in the Halakha, it shows even in the rabbinic law, you can really sense it, you can really point out the tensions and the ambivalences. In other words, this ambivalent position towards disabilities translates into Jewish law and into Orthodox Jewish communities. I'm wondering whether there's any diversity that you can find, about the status of or attitudes towards people with disabilities, whether there's any diversity to do with the actual conditions of care for children and adults with disabilities: the setting, the framework, economic resources for care? I can give a very distant example: in the early 2000s, when I did my fieldwork in Japan, the doctors and the women used to tell me the people with Down syndrome in Japan have higher IQ or intelligence rating compared to other countries. They explained this with reference to the quality of nurturing and educational facilities for people with disabilities in Japan. Later on, when I continued to do fieldwork, I found complexities and ambivalences within these statements. Nevertheless, it made me wonder whether the discourse about people with a disability being welcomed into a community or not has something to do with the actual economic and technical setting.

Hille Haker: Thank you! That is quite difficult to say. First of all, I have to tell you the narrative used by the Haredi women or communities is new to me. Saying a child with disabilities is a special gift from God seems to me a rather secondary thought, meaning it occurs after these children are born in order to counter possible hardships. Secondly, at least in the German context, and that's slightly different from the US, many of the healthcare and caring institutions are actually run by either the Catholic Church or the Protestant Church as a substitute for the state. That means they're mostly financed by the government or by the state. So it is not just a parish or a religious community but actually a nationwide institutional setting, which supports interaction, education and care for people with disabilities. Although this might sound promising at first glance, it is ambivalent at a second, because for decades after the war, children with disabilities would, at least for day-care, be taken out of their families and sent to these special institutions. This way they are part of society but at the same time hidden away from the public: the children with disabilities would be picked up by school buses in the morning, would be then cared for in these institutions, and would be brought back to their homes in the evening. For sure, for the individual family this system makes a difference economically or socially, and takes away at least a little bit of the burden. The flipside, however, is that we didn't see many children with disabilities in everyday life. So, relating these findings to the questions on prenatal diagnosis, I am just trying to understand: how did this system influence the perception of prenatal genetic diagnosis when it was introduced into the broader public in the 1970s? How would families who had a known trait of a condition or a disability or disease, react to and evaluate being channelled into human genetics? When I started working on prenatal diagnosis in more depth, and alongside the introduction of blood tests and probability testing in the 1990, the situation changed even further, since it appeared that the possibility of giving birth to a child with disabilities was still there, but the idea was to prevent it and "help" at least the women who had a greater risk due to their age. All of a sudden it was not only families with a particular family history that were included in the programs, but any woman above the age of 35. The advanced technologies worked at the medical level but also matched social developments, certainly in Germany but also other countries, of having children later in life. The development is much more complex than sketched out here, but needless to say all women, Catholic women included, were facing a new attitude towards children with disabilities.

Christina Schües: I'd like to ask a question of clarification concerning two themes that you introduced earlier. You, Hille, referred to the idea of a pre-judgment. On the one hand, you introduced the idea of dignity as a very important normative focus for the German discourse. On the other hand, you brought up – and quite rightfully – the atrocities of Nazi Germany. Furthermore, Tsipy, you were telling us about Japan's history and its quite ambivalent rhetoric of accepting children with disabilities. With regard to the source of pre-judgment, in what sense do Israel's history of the Shoah and Germany's Nazi history matter, and in what sense are they entangled with the religious discourse?

Hille Haker: I would really say that history matters in both cases. Both are mediated by religious thought, so my understanding of the history in Israel is that there's a very strong emphasis on natalism, on giving birth – not just as a moral pre-judgment. This is, in my understanding, on the one hand linked to the specific historical or even political situation of the 20th century, i.e. the state of Israel urging Jewish citizens to increase the overall population. On the other hand, it is mediated by basic Jewish thought and its very pronatal or pro-life narratives. Tsipy, am I following on from your thoughts and insight?

Tsipy Ivry: I never know, as an anthropologist, how to categorise Jewish thought, whether it's pronatalist or eugenic. In a broad sense, there are eugenic aspects. I wouldn't call them that, but in anthropology we have etic and emic perspectives; so from an outside perspective, there are dimensions of

Jewish thought that might in certain circumstances be addressed as eugenics. When writing about Jewish religious communities, I always make a point of emphasising the diversity in the texts that are considered canonical in the Halakhic tradition, in how prayers are led, and in many other aspects. However, very broadly speaking, I would agree that Jewish thought implicitly and explicitly focuses on pronatalism, meaning to be fruitful and multiply. That said, what really counts, what really works, within Jewish communities, is not the "be fruitful and multiply" – it's less about being fruitful and multiplying. The underlying thought – at least if we think about religiously observant communities – is rather about raising devoted – and that means *religiously* devoted – Jewish families. In other words, the Halakhic discourse, and Halakhic discussions on the feat of reproducing Jews, go much deeper than the mere obligation to be fruitful and multiply. So, on the one hand, especially after the Holocaust, it is definitely pronatalist. On the other hand, there is also a dimension to it that is more pragmatic and in a sense practical, since it addresses questions about – and I'm cautious about the terminology – how we make families that really can work, can function. Looking from a broad perspective, I think that's one of the main questions. In this regard, rabbinical thinking is about how large families can fulfil their obligations, as family and as religious devotees. So yes, it is about procreation, but not at any price. Jewish thought and the concept of pronatalism, I would sum up, address the question of how to create viable families.

Hille Haker: That would actually resonate very much with what I know from bioethics discussions with Jewish scholars. Certainly, generalisation in this context is impossible, but considering your explanation, the religious narrative is not just about being pro-life, it is also about being pro-health and pro-flourishing. This might even hint at why Israel embraced prenatal diagnosis on an institutional level as well as the social level. At least, it seems that the whole social setting, in this temporal context, coincided with a wave of technological development that also concerned health. Against this backdrop I might even say that, comparing the situation in Germany, in Israel prenatal diagnosis was embraced, not just because of the technologies (and kind of a fetishisation of technology), but also because the ethos of being pro-life always included attention to and concern for flourishing – and I use the term "flourishing" deliberately because it resonates so much with this wider understanding of the family and how it should function.

As an aside, you also mentioned something that has always impressed me as a Catholic Christian: rabbinic moral deliberation. It is a really interesting model of practical reasoning. As I tried to emphasise at the beginning, theology and theological tradition, either Catholic or Protestant, the Christian tradition, also knows discourse and deliberation on practical and ethical topics. However, it has changed over the centuries, and especially in the Catholic tradition it became rather abstract reasoning with a top-down morality. What I would like to stress here is another aspect: even though Christian ethical deliberation was similar to rabbinic reasoning for many centuries, it was always tied to what we call *the confessions*. So practical reasoning actually happened during confessional conversation and thus was tied to the priest's judgment. They had the challenging task of finding out how to deal with a particular sin, or guilt. In what we call *penitentials* you can trace the attempt to find coherent judgments and redemption, giving many practical examples. Basically, that is how Catholic moral theology, developed over the centuries. That gives quite a good idea of how much historical settings – not only the big history but also the history of moral reasoning – matter, for our tentative comparison, too. Would you say that this captures some of your findings and thoughts? Can you relate to practical reasoning in the rabbinic context that is decision-oriented, i.e. proactive and prospective rather than retrospective, or is it both?

Tsipy Ivry: I think that rabbinic reasoning is again based on principles that protect and guide viable families. So how it approaches punishment, or more precisely, how the rabbinic reasoning approaches the notion of sin and how to work with confessions, is always related to the goal of the functioning family. So for example, in post-diagnostic abortion, if a rabbi rules that a post-diagnostic abortion is permissible, and he knows that the woman, the couple, are going to feel extremely guilty and they're not going to get rid of the guilt afterwards, his mission is to find a way to enable them to go on with their lives in a good way. He knows that it's not that simple and they're going to suffer quite a lot after a post-diagnostic abortion, but his vision, his mission, is how to make this family work, function, how to make them viable families. I think this is the moral reasoning that leads the way for rabbis.

Hille Haker: I see. I would like to move one step further since from my perspective in the Catholic Church it is really exactly the opposite! If you, as a woman, have an abortion, you excommunicate yourself performatively, i.e. with your act. That is the moral reasoning. For now, without idealising these Catholic moral practices or systems at all, this moral causality of a specific deed and ex-communication as a direct consequence matters in our discussion of reactions to prenatal diagnosis. When it was introduced, it already stood on the shoulders of previous teaching and a decision that really "rocked" Catholics throughout the world: the internal Catholic discussion on the prohibition of so-called artificial birth control in the late 1960s.

Holding couples and families accountable for their actions on the one hand, and having almost no Catholic family complying with that teaching on the other, showed a disconnect between the moral teaching, top-down teaching, and the everyday moral challenges or judgments of Christians. So in the pews or in the confession boxes you could note a complete moral disconnection that touched the obsession with sin and guilt to a point where every moral ruling became toxic. So, adding another perspective to our thoughts on the religious implications of the attitude towards prenatal diagnosis in the Christian context, it has to be said that in addition to the pronatalism narrative in Judaism, in Christian ethics it is already situated in a very guilt-driven and sin-driven context. I know that from my Catholic mother, for example, who actually gave birth to eight children during the late '50s and then '60s, that when the birth control pill was introduced in Germany Catholic women lived with conflict: "Are we allowed to use birth control or not, and do we then have to go to confession about it, or how does this really work?" But over the '70s, '80s, '90s, couples and families started to step away from this conflict and made up their own mind about what to do. Sociological studies show that the big rift between the Church's teaching and what families actually did was not because of different understandings of flourishing families, but resulted from a concern about personal wellbeing. So, with respect to prenatal diagnosis now, how do the two groundings, the moral grounding of dignity and the experienced disconnect between the couples and families and the Church teaching, and their priests, how did that play out? I don't have the anthropological data for that; however, I would say that prenatal diagnosis is not only very broadly established in women's healthcare in Germany, but is also now accepted. There are still discussions going on at the margins, but these concern the different techniques, or how far we should go. It is not about whether to consider prenatal diagnosis or not. For Catholic women, Catholic families, I would say that the disconnect has become even deeper because of the sexual abuse scandal in the Church and the complete disintegration of its moral authority from any moral dilemmas or moral practical reasoning. The Church's teaching, and especially the moral authority of priests or clergy, is almost completely lost, resulting in only marginal use of confession. So the whole centuries-old system of how the Catholic people did their moral reasoning and are held accountable within their communities has dramatically changed in my generation, up to a point where it has now almost collapsed. The attitude towards prenatal diagnosis, at least in Germany, is not all about reactions to the Nazi history but in my view at least, really show layer upon layer the changes within Catholic communities, the Catholic Church and their authority. The complex ramifications caused by these changes leave the women and families as moral pioneers. In the Catholic or even the German context there is no moral labour, as you show in one of your articles – there is no moral labour that the women or the families can do with their priests.

Tsipy Ivry: That was really illuminating and clarifying. I've been writing for a while now about the negotiation, the moral labour that goes on between the women or couple and the rabbis. This is part of a struggle: it's a strategic struggle over their authority. Listening to you, Hille, I was wondering, how does the division between religion and state play out in Germany? What's the status of religion within the secular German state? Because in Israel this is a huge issue: here there is freedom *of* religion but very little freedom *within* religion. In other words, if you're Jewish, then you're bound to the Jewish authorities, who are given authority by the state. Against this background, the invitation rabbis extend to couples or women for consultation, to do the moral labour together and share the burden, has more than one side. Surely, and in accordance with my observations, a huge part of it is based on genuine compassion that the rabbis feel towards women and couples. Part of my fieldwork has been on an organisation of rabbis that mediates reproductive medicine, with the mission of supporting the couples in being fruitful and multiplying in a viable way. Part of their support also includes the offer of counselling on prenatal diagnosis, because this is part of reproductive medicine and couples deal with it. At the same time, another dimension of this support is that rabbis are very much aware of the dangers to their own authority. By offering such consultations they're trying to make their authority relevant, they're trying to make religion relevant to the couples. I would argue that part of this invitation to consult the rabbis is about preserving their own authority. Doing this they draw from a huge "Jewish library," from texts collected and systematised over at least 3000 years. So there's enough of tradition of discussion and dispute among rabbis to supply the substrate, if you like, for all kinds of rulings, all kinds of precedents. I was really dazzled by the virtuosity of these rabbis, how they negotiated different layers of the canon, of Jewish literature, the Mishna and the Gemara, thereby preserving and making their own authority relevant in a state –within which their political presence and participation is established, on the one hand; and on the other, where there is increasing tension around state-sanctioned religious restriction in public areas. Although religion is secured within the state's apparatus, there's a lot of resistance to it from non-religious Jews. Moreover, the variety of religious and heretical unities challenge rabbinic authorities as well. Consequently, in a way, rabbinic authority is under negotiation: it has to prove itself all the time, it has to prove its relevance – this is in a way part of the invitation to mediate very difficult ethical decisions, reproductive decisions; it is part of a larger story about rabbinic authority being negotiated, being challenged all the time. This setting can become paradoxical: there was a woman I met during fieldwork, who approached her rabbi and said "I reached the decision to terminate a child with Down syndrome," and it was really important to the rabbi to give her a ruling, a rabbinic ruling, so that she wouldn't feel that her own decision is autonomous but is supported by rabbinic ruling.

Besides this question about the configuration of religious authority in the state, I was also wondering about mechanisms or rituals to deal with abortions, for instance, after a positive diagnosis. Confession is also a central practice in Judaism, and there are many different meanings and reasons for applying rituals. In Japan, for instance, there are rituals for aborted foetuses that have been practiced for hundreds of years. The *Mizuko kuyō*, for example, is a ritual to ask for forgiveness from the unborn foetus. Women who wish to do this buy a little piece of land in the backyard of a Buddhist monastery, and put a little figure of Jizo-sama, who is the god of the children, on the ground and let the priest perform a ritual for them. The deity is supposed to ensure that the children can cross the river from life to death, and through this ritual leads them from one side to the other. The purpose of the ritual is partly to console the spirit of the fallen foetus, the unborn foetus. But it also works for the women, since they visit this backyard of the Buddhist monastery again and again, asking for forgiveness from the foetus. Even though we are not talking about Japan, for me it is an illuminating example of a ritual mechanism to deal with guilt. So I'm asking myself, how do religious Christian Catholics deal with guilt? Do they have any mechanism, religious mechanism, to deal with it?

Hille Haker: Thank you so much, Tsipy, for your questions and examples! So far, we have shared some thoughts about the background assumptions, i.e. our moral and social contexts, when entering into this kind of conversation about prenatal diagnosis. From my perspective, and allied to what Christina and Anne have already emphasised, it is of the utmost importance to find a common ground for understanding by introducing our different cultures and histories. Reflecting on and explaining these general premises is a good starting point for what we have implicitly done next, entering into a conversation about decision-making processes, and about who has the authority to say what or to deliberate, and to co-deliberate. I want to come back to that in a minute, but what seems to me very important to discuss with you is the perspective of the women and families. So whatever decision has been made, how do people, how do families, how do women cope with the decision they have made? Because we started the conversation about the care work of families who have to be able, or have to be *enabled*, to care for a child, for a prospective adult, with disabilities. This and the institutional setting most certainly influence how you decide and also deal with a decision you have made. I would like to focus a little bit more on the individual decision-making process.

As I mentioned at the beginning, in Germany there is this institutionalised system for care. Taking into account what you have explained about counselling and also your question about how religion and the state relate, I would say there is also an institutionalised system for counselling. In other words, family counselling in whatever matters is supported and in part run by the Protestant and the Catholic Churches, subsidised again by the state, so that this system of counselling is partly secular and partly religious. Consequently, if you need counselling on questions of pregnancy, birth control and so on, as an individual you can choose which form you turn to – religious or secular. Now, even though numbers of Christian devotees in Germany are going down, and there is also religious pluralism regarding the growing Muslim population, the situation, the social and cultural base for decisions, especially in the context of reproduction, is still very much informed by secularised Christianity. However, people don't go to churches or priests to get help with existential problems. They turn to family counselling centres and institutions such as Caritas or Diakonie, which are based on Christian principles and ethos, but are largely run by lay people such as social workers, psychologists and so on. So, given the context of decision making before or during pregnancy, I would say people mostly turn to them not for an authoritative statement, but for help in discernment. I would say, in distinction to what you say about the groundedness of the moral authority of the rabbis and addressing the fact that Catholic priests have lost much of their moral authority, in Germany social workers and psychological counsellors working in the Christian institutions help couples or families when they experience conflicts during pregnancy. In this regard, the option of getting a prenatal diagnosis and dealing with potential conflicts remains much more of a task for the individual conscience. Alongside what I said about human dignity as the main moral orientation, for me at this point freedom and autonomy enter the discussion. So, taking your examples of the rabbis who take the decisions and consequences upon themselves, almost like scapegoats, I really wonder if that would be possible in Germany or even the USA. I think, at least in the Catholic context, it would not: First of all, because there would not be any wiggle room in the decision about abortion, and second, because there is no longer any authority. To me, that again is not only a result of secularisation or a more secularised culture, but is caused by the moral toxicity surrounding the whole issue of reproduction. That said, however, for some time German secular law – perhaps due to the remaining power of the bishops, and the bishops' conferences – obliged women who decide to terminate a pregnancy to have – in addition to medical expertise – mandatory counselling before any abortion. I would say if one tracks that down historically, it has a lot to do with the societal power, the political power of the Christian churches and the fact that other parts of German secular law, such as education, are a so-called *res mixta*. However, even though such counselling was mandatory it was at the same time non-directive. As a legal matter, and after post-unification reform of the German abortion law in the 1990s, termination is still against the law – taking into account the coherence of the German Constitution. It is illegal but the woman – or medical professionals, for that matter – will not be penalised – at least not as long as the mandatory counselling has been received. No matter how critical I am towards the Church teaching's idea of sexual morality, I must say I am a fan of mandatory counselling because I do believe it really does good, giving a chance potentially to introduce unknown options or different perspectives to women or couples for their individual situations. Many social workers would, however, disagree. The surprising part is that, even though this mandatory counselling enables Christian principles to show their existential dimensions, the Vatican under John Paul II eventually intervened in the German Church and prohibited all the institutions who were counselling couples in so-called pregnancy conflicts. The result is that they can still offer counsel but they cannot sign the form that you need to terminate the pregnancy. This of course also concerns prenatal diagnosis, and once again leaves the woman potentially alone with her moral labour. Even though some clerics, and even the bishop of Limburg, resisted the order from Rome and upheld the counselling institutions for a while, they faced penalties. Although this particular bishop helped to set up a foundation for counselling in questions of prenatal diagnosis, it was really scandalous that the Vatican mostly suppressed such bottom-up efforts. One single not-for-profit organisation called *Donum Vitae* has survived all these years through donations, and against the Church's ruling. So, with these examples, I want to tell you that I don't know the end of the story yet, for Germany. However, over the last few decades, you can see a deep rift between the official teaching and what is needed on the ground, a rift between the Church's self-understanding and the ongoing secularisation of German culture. There is also a lot of, I would say, religion-internal mourning about this situation going on in Germany, also about the lack of Catholic priests due to, in my view, the obtuse political decision not to ordain women. There are many factors that go beyond our conversation here, but with respect to decision-making, I would say it is now much more personalised, individualised, and channelled into the medical system. Accordingly, the doctors or medical counsellors now play a greater role in the decision-making process, and the individual conscience decision has much more weight than at least what you say about some of these communities in Israel. Even if that is the case, with respect to what you asked about the coping mechanisms, the accountability, the responsibility, the guilt, the forgiveness, the reconciliation – I think that with decreasing religious commitment here, too, women are very much thrown back upon their own means and resources. Since the termination of pregnancy in general has been taboo or even stigmatised for decades in Germany, such individual coping sometimes results in tremendous psychological problems. There are always waves of public feminist reckoning with this situation, but when it comes to coping with terminations of pregnancies after prenatal diagnosis, there still seems to be a great taboo. Trying to address this situation, some hospitals, for example a clinic in Mainz, have introduced a practice for anyone who has a stillbirth, a late miscarriage, or a termination. They are supported by a non-profit organisation, and will accompany couples during this time and give them a so-called *Moses Körbchen*, a Moses Basket, in which they put a candle and other things that this support group has prepared in the background, and they encourage the couples maybe to put a letter to their child into the basket. I was so intrigued by your story about the river, it's the journey the child has to make, accompanying the child and the women or couples with this little gesture, accompanying the families in this really tragic situation. In this context the whole question of morality is taken out, the "morality of guilt," the morality of "is that allowed or not?" is completely taken out of the

214 Comparative empirical bioethics of reproductive practices and their social contexts

story here because they deliberately do not ask how a child died. I find that an exceptional practice, and I wished that such practices would be encouraged further. At the same time and as a Christian, a part of me is grieving, because there were religious rituals once, helping people to cope with loss and with guilt, too, bringing it back to the community and not leaving individuals alone with their experiences. Even with the Moses Basket, the coping remains very individualised – partly because abortion is so stigmatised. Even the Church is not against prenatal diagnosis in particular; it rejects abortion after prenatal diagnosis. Consequently, as a Christian woman you know that you are excommunicating yourself from the most important community, the community with God, and that's far more than a social exclusion, it is a spiritual exclusion. This setting makes you really shy away from even daring to speak, so you have to close it off, close it away, in your own conscience, which makes it a very difficult situation for the individual. So doctrinally and ethically really, I totally disagree with my Church regarding its practices and attitudes. I find its teachings and judgments at this point against life and against human dignity, un-Christian even. That is why I said at the beginning, theology and moral theology need to be more in conversation with the doctrinal level and with these authoritative judgements.

Tsipy Ivry: Hille, what you described mirrors the setting in Israel: The notions of exclusion and inclusion are key here, too. In the very beginning you emphasized how important it is to make everyone welcome regardless of his or her abilities or disabilities. Women find themselves in a position where they must judge which child is allowed into the human community.

It seems to me that in any society prenatal testing raises questions about the inclusion or exclusion of "new" members. In a circular motion it also raises questions of inclusion or exclusion of "old" members, i.e. the parents, particularly the pregnant woman. At these points, the dynamics of inclusion and exclusion tend to turn paradoxically. For instance, a woman – who for any reason finds herself in a position that is non-inclusive toward a foetus with a disability – will exclude herself performatively from the community with God. In other words, her inability to include becomes a reason for exclusion either in the sense of self-exclusion or explicitly as communal and social exclusion.

Christina Schües: What both of you have just outlined is touching and inspiring at the same time! Tsipy, may I refer to what you mentioned on the basis of our empirical experience during the interviews in Israel? When women are faced with the decision to use invasive testing (e.g. amniocentesis) some would say, "No, I don't want to use this because it may harm the foetus or the pregnancy." With NIPT this reason to say "no" is no longer valid. If women do not want to know the genetic disposition of the foetus, how can they then justify saying "no" to testing? In Germany, they may turn to religious belief, or explain in a very secular way that they don't want to know the future or details about the child/foetus and they want to take "what comes." In Israel, it seems that women can certainly refer to religious belief. However, a non-religious, i.e. secular, not wanting to know and saying "no" to testing seems rather irrational and irresponsible. Thus, do you think that PND has become a practice as a matter of course that considers saying "no" is "only reasonably" possible for religious women? Is religious belief the only socially acceptable reason to say "no"?

And if so, what does this tell us about the relation between religion and high-tech reproductive medicine? On the one hand, religion seems tied up with a demedicalisation in which the course of pregnancy is God's will, and on the other it is tied up with high-tech medicalisation when it comes to a willingness to actually use reproductive biomedicine; and all of these evaluations seem to depend on the ruling of the rabbis, their narratives, and the means allowed to create viable families. Thus, behind my question I'm wondering about the religious narratives at work and the value of life, especially the value of the foetus's life more concretely, which is hotly debated in German discourses of medical ethics.

Tsipy Ivry: I do think that in Israel, a kind of "acceptable no" to testing is easier for religious women. However, my findings show that doctors as well as people who identify as non-religious tend to feel anger toward religious women who refuse testing or even part of the testing. As for "secular" women, one more or less "acceptable" reason to say "no" is infertility. If the child was conceived after long and painful fertility treatments, it might be acceptable in Israel for the woman to say that this is a "precious pregnancy" [herayon yakar: yakar also means "expensive"] and therefore she wants to give birth in any case. Such reasoning is rare!

Another way to think about your question is to rethink the term "secular." In Israel there are several New Age communities that do not fall into the category of institutional religion but practice a myriad styles of spirituality. Among them are anthroposophic communities, as well as communities in which New Age spirituality is practiced eclectically. In such communities there is a generally resistant attitude toward biomedical interventions. Typically, women there opt for minimal prenatal care, minimal testing, homebirth, home schooling, veganism. So these people are non-religious, but are highly likely to say no to NIPT. There is a range of explanations that these women might give for refusing NIPT; maybe the metanarrative is the wish to connect with or get closer to "nature." Israeli doctors are often as intolerant of New Age women's rationales as they are of religious women's rationales.

And to your further question about the relation between religion and reproductive technologies, that is, the question of how it is that, on the one hand, women are saying they would not get an abortion for religious reasons, and on the other, Jewish orthodoxy has such an important role in Israel reproductive technologies? I have actually been writing about this question from several perspectives. I think the important thing to keep in mind is that the Jewish orthodox idea is that technology is provided by God, and that it can be "koshered" – it can be adapted to rabbinic law on the condition that rabbis are allowed into the technological and medical arena.

Anne Weber: Please allow me to add some thoughts and questions on what we have talked about so far. Concerning Tsipy's question about Christian coping rituals and what you mentioned, Hille, about the practice of the "Moses Basket": As far as I know and have experienced working as a counsellor in a small hospital in Paderborn, such practices have become quite common. Here it is called "Sternenkinder," and although it may not be a religious ritual in a liturgical sense, in my diocese it is supported by the archbishop. The idea is very similar to what you have described: accompanying people who are living through crisis instead of judging them, accepting the existential trauma of such experiences, and helping to create a context in which they can find a way of coping. Despite all the criticism of the Church's teachings, especially in the area of sexual morality and reproduction – which I definitely share with you, Hille – I find this at least a positive, i.e. more humane and compassionate development. Still, the question is how such counselling in individual, singular cases plays out, and what criteria and religious narratives could be implemented in order to avoid arbitrariness.

Hille Haker: Absolutely. The central question is, how do you accompany people, how do you counsel people in the prenatal context? I would say that what happens in the hospital and even in the counselling institutions is often very different from the normative framework of the Church's teaching. I work a lot with hospital chaplains and midwives who accompany women during labour and also afterwards, in the process of late abortions. In such practical contexts, far away from their desks, the hospital chaplains, the ministers, be they priests or not, see that they need to accompany the women and not judge them. But there is a lot of room between Earth and Heaven, so even a simple task such as accompanying depends a lot on the attitude of the person in charge. However, in general and aside from the question of quality, I consider the counselling as well as the coping to be a moral practice. And if it is not based on toxic narratives, instead of a guilt-driven practice it can become one of solidarity, a compassionate practice.

Anne Weber: Yes. Taking your thoughts on the task of theology to claim a discourse with the Church's teachings, especially on existential topics, this work is still ahead of us, isn't it? The guilt-driven traditions and practices, in my understanding, originate from a very specific but also very dominant line of religious interpretation of existential contexts. It will be essential to look for other interpretative frameworks in the Christian tradition, which don't just challenge the very influential Augustinian ideas on procreation and reproduction, for example, but also make minority perspectives visible in theological discussions. So, jumping ahead of Christina's questions about the religious narratives of life's value, what theologians need to do is to broaden their horizon, i.e. remember the unheard voices of tradition, give room to and use other frames of interpretation. So even if there is a dominant narrative of life, family or sexuality in Church teachings, to me as a Christian and a feminist it is key – especially in the context of reproductive medicine – to show other lines of religious or Christian concepts and bring them into the discussion as well.

Hille Haker: Yes, absolutely. Before we go to the question of the value of life, let me emphasise that in my own work, I always try to counter this tradition of a very conservative, very normative kind of reasoning, and really expand on the tradition of the ethics of good life. So, for example, I reflect on modal verbs in moral argumentations, since they already structure the way we reason. Having said this, the normative question of what I *must* not do, or what I may do, is very much linked to the question of what I *can* do, where the limits of my capabilities are what I want, or if I even know what I want, or whether I'm already torn in my intentions, in my ends. Consequently, with this approach you enter a space of existential ethics and an existentialist ethics where freedom does not equate to autonomy, but needs to be seen as an effort. To me, this is also very important for the discussion on prenatal diagnosis and its potential consequences, since the women and couples are always already in relation to others, their social heritage, educations, experiences, capabilities. So although from what we have discussed it appears that women are fully accountable and thus sometimes tremble at the responsibility for their decisions, you always have to take into account that they are responding to a situation in the way they *can* as the person they are. I work a lot with two basic concepts, namely recognition and responsibility. The mutual recognition that happens as a *verb* means not just valuing an unspecific someone but engaging in acts of recognising her as the person she is and can be. Recognition is thus an interactive kind of endeavour that you strive for. For sure, you often fail, and not only in reciprocal symmetric relations; but the responsibility we have is to think deeply about how we respond – not to an abstract entity but to a specific person and her capabilities, the realisation of her freedom. There are many follow-up questions that we cannot discuss here. Going back to what you said, Anne, about finding alternative narratives and interpretative frames, what I wanted to show is that in this concept the questions of guilt or sin cannot be answered as monocausally as Church teachings and traditions suggest. I think that in redoing Catholic moral theology, this becomes a very important endeavour, of course, once again facing the question of grounding the values of moral reasoning.

Just let me quickly try to respond to Christina's question about the value of life, the value of the foetus. This discussion of moral status without any context is very prone to misunderstandings. First of all, let me express how much I appreciate that we didn't begin our conversation with the question: "What is the status of the embryo?" This question takes us too far away from the fact that it follows on from a situation of dilemma. Tsipy showed in a very detailed way that the decision-making process begins at the point of asking the question whether or not to make use of prenatal diagnosis, whether or not to utilise reproductive technology. In this regard, the status question is part of a broader bioethical discussion that also includes questions on dealing with information and the right not to know, on shared decision making, on concepts of health, counselling, authority, on enhancement, gene editing and other topics we have mentioned. So I believe that the status of the foetus, or the value of life in that respect, is really only one factor, and in the concrete decision making perhaps ultimately not even the decisive one. However, it is not a minor issue. Referring to my perspective and what I said at the beginning about dignity, the question of the value of the foetus comes with other questions such as: "What does it say about myself if I cannot welcome a particular child into my life? Can I live with myself as someone who does not welcome a particular child?" I don't want to fall into the trap of both liberal bioethics and Catholic moral theology, that both narrow the questions down to one single issue. Tsipy, I am sure you have some different insight and perspectives to add to our discussion.

Tsipy Ivry: Yes, Hille, I feel the same towards the status question. However, I will try to respond to it, because even though in the context of decision making it might only be one factor among others, I do think for the theoretical discussion it's an important question since it influences other factors, or at least how they are evaluated. Let me try to address it in a comparative way. What I find very interesting is that – regardless of whether the formal status of the embryo or the foetus is considered to be fully-fledged life or partly life, or on the verge of becoming a person, or having subjectivity or not having subjectivity – there is a really strong emotional and moral, ethical reaction that women experience when they find themselves faced with a decision about the kind of prenatal diagnostic technology to choose. Sometimes this reaction comes after an indication or a diagnosis, sometimes it comes after a post-diagnostic decision, and sometimes even after a post-diagnostic termination. So regardless of the formal status of the embryo or the foetus, in my work with women, whether religious or not, I found the process of decision making to be very ethically troubling for all of them. The gap between what is formally considered the right thing to do and what the woman feels is actually very difficult. It appears sometimes to be even more painful when women have not received a religious ruling. In Israel, non-religious women are led to think the termination of a foetus with a disability is the right, responsible thing to do, since having it will disable the mother, the family. However, after the decision to abort, the women are left alone with it, causing them terrible ethical turbulence. So despite societal acceptance of terminating pregnancies with an indication [of anomaly] based on the thought of creating viable families, for the individual woman it is emotionally and psychologically very troubling, to a point where they may remain in this decision-aftershock for years. This is a setting I found repeatedly regardless of the discussion of moral status in the media, among policymakers and healthcare professionals, midwives, or disability rights advocates. This is something that I find important to keep in mind and think about. Now, if I go back to the question of the value of life, of the foetus, you can draw on rabbinic texts. I'm neither a Talmud scholar nor a Mishnah scholar, but in the course of my fieldwork I try to engage with this literature when it emerges in the reasoning mechanisms of interlocutors. In preparation to this conversation I collected a number of Mishnaic and Talmudic verses and tried to grasp this literature's logic, and to come into dialogue with it. So from a broad analysis of rabbinic texts, I would say that as a first rule of thumb they reveal a clear preference for the mother's life and safety. There are really harsh texts in Jewish or rabbinic literature, for example, if a woman is to be executed according to rabbinic law and she's pregnant, her death sentence may be executed immediately, i.e. nobody is going to wait for her to give birth. However, this is less a decision against the unborn child, but in favour of the mother's mental integrity – she shouldn't be tortured by having to wait for her execution. Another very graphic Mishnah example in Oholot says that if a woman is giving birth and the baby that is being born seriously endangers the woman's life by shoulder dystocia, then the baby should be cut apart inside the womb and taken out limb by limb. This sounds very cruel, but it is nonetheless part of the Mishnah. Diagnosing the texts and the literary tradition in general, the implication of the mother's life being prioritised over that of the foetus becomes quite evident. The reasoning behind it goes back to the Halakhic understanding that the embryo is, up until 40 days, considered part of the woman's body. Despite these religious rulings and texts, Haredi women won't even consider an abortion, and even emphasise their religious integrity and community by saying, "We never do abortions for Down syndrome." However, receiving a positive diagnosis of Down syndrome causes them tremendous stress, asking themselves how they are supposed to live with this child. Even though the community will most likely support its upbringing and care, the women fear that having a child with a disability might harm the chances of other siblings finding a "quality" marriage partner. So again you see an ambivalence. On the one hand, the devout Haredi woman would tell you that the ultimate righteous thing to do is to accept each and every choice that God makes, because God is the only one who makes choices. So they would argue: "We might not be able to understand why this is good, but it is definitely good because God chose this child to be born through me and it is good because God's choices are good, by definition." Thus, even consulting a rabbi would mean either doubting God's good choices or being too weak to accept them. On the other hand, the factual reality of this diagnosis was extremely troubling to some of the women. Anticipating such worry and anxiety, many Haredi women choose not to engage in prenatal diagnosis in order to avoid being placed in a position of overwhelming distress. If you look more closely, in the background of this reasoning there appears an informal hierarchy among Haredi women, and if you want to compete in this hierarchical ladder of righteousness, then you shouldn't engage in prenatal testing, because this may testify one's lack of faith in God's choices. Agreeing with this, however, will make the question of coping even more urgent. So, despite any religious ideas and narratives that the mother's wellbeing is clearly prioritised over the status of the unborn child, the dilemma remains, even for ultrareligious women. Another thing I wanted to mention is that the rabbis who say they will take the responsibility upon themselves are actually also outsourcing this responsibility even further. The whole system of consultation consists of outsourcing and shouldering decisions among doctors and other rabbis, it is communal among decisors, among rabbinic and medical scholars. So a rabbi who gives the impression of shouldering the responsibility for a prenatal or a reproductive decision, is acting performatively for the couple. Of course, in the end I don't know whether or not the rabbi feels responsible himself, if he is able to sleep at night. What I want to point out is that to make such a decision, a rabbi needs a network of decisors to be able to share the moral burden.

Hille Haker: May I just expand your thoughts a little bit further from a Christian perspective, Tsipy? I believe that there will always be attempts to respond to the question, "What is the value of life?" Sometimes even posing this question seems naïve, since it is as if we could just put it on a scale like an organ, weigh it, and compare it to other issues. The effort and the attempt to find objective and quantifiable criteria will always be there, since it is a question that concerns all of humanity and the way we live with one another. What seems important to me is that the religious traditions bring a kind of a cautionary tale to the table, since their narratives always point to God's authority: "Be careful. The only one who knows the weight of the issues is God. You don't have the means to weigh them when it comes to life." I think the Jewish and the Christian traditions both caution that it is not up to us to translate values into quantifiable, objective measures. Values need to be accepted, and even though there might be many values that can be translated, for some it is not for us to say. I think the difference between the Jewish tradition and the Christian tradition is that the rabbinic tradition at least acknowledges that having said that, life is life, and life comes with conflicts. That is why there is a long tradition of practical reasoning dealing with life's conflicts. Accordingly, the rabbis would ultimately also refer to God's authority, but faced with these conflicts in practical, everyday life decisions, they, we, do the best we can. To me this explains the sharing of the burden, the consultation among the rabbis. From what you have explained as well, the rabbi actually hides behind the authority, and the whole setting remains paternalistic with respect to the women. In the Christian tradition, the Catholic tradition especially, there's a certain denial of these dilemmas. Philosophically, you can pinpoint this denial to someone like Kant, who always shied away from acknowledging dilemmas, fearing to lose the consistency of a system and thereby its normative integrity. Something similar happened in the scholastic tradition of Catholic theology: the idea that there must be a solution to everything and every question. So when it comes to the value of life, and a conflict between the value of the mother's life and the value of the foetus's life, the Catholic tradition retains the idea of a solution to all dilemmas but comes to the opposite conclusion, i.e. sides with the foetus rather than with the mother. Originally, up until the 19th century the theological discussion of the process of humanisation also referred to the 40th day as the time of ensoulment. Since it was a different time for a boy and a girl, it was called "successive ensoulment." However, by the end of the 19th century and due to the scientific insecurities, ensoulment in the Catholic tradition was set at the point of conception. That takes away any wiggle room here, whether with respect to embryo research or abortion. Consequently, what you end up with in this line of reasoning is a denial of any moral dilemmas on a practical level. You might be able to acknowledge that people, women especially, experience conflicts, but on a theoretical level there is actually no dilemma, since the morally right decision, of course, is to side with the foetus in any given situation. The right to life, as humane and important as it may be, leads ultimately to an attitude towards the mother that demands that whatever she may feel, she must suck it up and accept the situation. Needless to say, this is very absolutist reasoning, but ironically it takes away the moral conflicts with respect to decision-making. I disagree with that reasoning, as you might have seen, because I absolutely resonate with what you say about the women especially, but also the families, being almost wiped out of this story. Speaking from more of an American perspective for a second, in reality both absolutist pro-lifers and absolutist pro-choicers show a denial of conflict that blows away the individual hardship, the weight of the decision-making and the subsequent coping. All that you have said shows me that the bioethical discussion about determining the value of life is this always ongoing effort of putting a life on a scale and then weighing it up against other circumstances; but not only is the metaphor not innocent, the process of trying to determine the value in that way is not innocent either. To tell you the truth, I would like to shy away as long as possible from that metaphor of "weighing." Although I totally agree that the question of welcoming a child or not welcoming a child into your life is the real question, it does not have so much to do with the scales or the weighing. It is a question of who you want to be, how welcoming you can be, and where your limits of welcoming someone else into your life are, and whether or not you can live with acknowledging the limitations of your life, whether or not you can find help and can accept help, to welcome a child into your life.

Tsipy Ivry: So we are talking here about a social scale, the social framing of the decision. I am convinced that the ethical principles and values are always framed and instantiated by cultural, political and social conceptions. To understand them and how they interact is as important to me as the discussion on "the value of life" – difficult as it may be. Having said that, these frames become key to answering the question of what is understood to be an ethically proper process of decision making, or what makes a decision-making process ethically appropriate. Asking "How does one make decisions?" has social as well as individual implications. For our context and with regard to what religious authorities – whether priests or rabbis – find it reasonable for women and families to endure; so questions of suffering, the interpretation, the narrative or the value of suffering, become important. For example, there is no agreement among rabbis about the "status" of suffering (the parents' and the child's suffering): what is suffering and what role does it play within decision making about whether to welcome – if I use the idiom that Hille uses – or not to welcome a child? Neither is there clear consensus on who should be considered when thinking about suffering, avoiding or accepting it – the woman, the child, the family, the community? The consequence of this lack of clarification is a culture of disagreement, that in a contradictory way makes possible a huge diversity of decisions. This corresponds to what I presume to be of utmost importance from a rabbinic perspective when being consulted: that rabbinic knowledge has been negotiated while the decision, the ethical deliberation was being done. As I mentioned before, rabbis are interested in preserving their authority and making it relevant, but another element in this dynamic is to safeguard the integrity of people's life. Thinking of my Haredi informants and their partners and families, another risk within the context of possible reproductive decisions is that if a couple or a woman makes a decision without consulting a rabbi, she potentially dissociates herself from the framework of rabbinic decision making, resulting at some stage in disconnection from the community. Such disconnection is going to be so troubling, and ethically so confusing for her, that the rabbis are not only trying to protect themselves and their authority, but also trying to protect the people by keeping them within the framework of religious and rabbinic decision making. Making rabbinic traditions relevant for the people helps to keep the people intact, because the wholeness of these couples, these families, these communities, depends on their continued connection with a whole apparatus that is spiritual and legal and communal.

Hille Haker: You have shown remarkably the rabbinic logic of protecting the community. It is striking to me how the reasoning is almost the opposite in Catholic Christianity: the protection of the purity of the community and institution by excluding people who have deliberately acquired guilt. So that is the big thing and, in my view, exemplifies the Augustinian legacy in Christian thinking: if you don't know what you are doing, then it is just a sinful thought or act and you can regret it, but if you continue to live in sin, whether it is with respect to birth control or something else, then it becomes an issue of guilt. With respect to abortion, you can know ahead of time that it is wrong and if you still continue to do it, you live in sin. So in order to protect the institution, the community, the purity of morality, you have to be excluded, partly or once and for all. To me that seems almost the opposite intention to what you say is the motivation of the rabbis. Practically speaking, I believe that many priests actually do *not* agree with that exclusion and do not act upon the official teachings, but they try to include and support couples and women in conflict. However, until the official "ruling" is undone and a new conceptualisation of sexual moral theology in this area is found, implemented and acknowledged, it is always up to individual priests to depart from these exclusionist practices, and open solidarity with "sinners" will in the long run also lead to exclusion for them. We see such exclusions from community and Eucharist, i.e. community with God, in several areas in the Catholic Church. Again in the US, President Joe Biden cannot receive Communion because, ideologically, he is pro-choice and that means he holds the opinion that the law of the land, namely abortion, is there for a reason. If conservative Christian wings exclude the US President, you can imagine how they treat a woman who comes out as having made the decision – and that to me is where the ethical violence within the Catholic system begins. It causes a problem, not only practically speaking but also theoretically and certainly theologically, too.

Tsipy Ivry: May I ask a final question? If Catholic contemporary authorities would like to "reform" their discourse and authoritative statements, is there enough substance in the tradition from which to reinterpret or revive traditions to create a more inclusive atmosphere for women and families?

Hille Haker: Absolutely, but I think the very first step is simply to acknowledge what you said in the beginning, that we are dealing with moral dilemmas, or even moral tragedies. Because then, in the practical reasoning the virtue of prudence becomes the central virtue. Even in the scholastic tradition, reading Thomas Aquinas, the virtue of prudence entails tools of practical reasoning that are much more in line with a rabbinic tradition. For example, prudence entails attentiveness to circumstances, the imagination, the remembrance of similar cases, the attention to possible consequences, a certain strategic thinking. In the Thomistic tradition these are called the middle principles, and acknowledging that we're dealing with moral tragedy would allow us to give the virtue of prudence and practical reasoning greater weight in relation to the other principles, or even the other virtues. There is a potential to harmonise the theological tradition with this kind of virtue reasoning, embracing the sources of theological, ethical reasoning, which are scripture, tradition, reason and experience – that is my "solution," and I've been promoting it for years now. Perhaps for Church teaching it is still too uncomfortable to acknowledge moral dilemmas and acknowledge that they are tragedies, that often there is no good solution, if any at all. To bring forth such acknowledgment it is necessary to get away from depicting the ethical questions abstractly and find a more descriptive approach. That is why I think it is so utterly important to have anthropological, ethnographical research like yours, where you can see the ideologies and narratives in the background influencing the decisors, co-creating the dilemma structure. On the one hand, the obligation to welcome every child into your life as God's gift, and then on the other, two sentences down, the existential anxiety of not being able to cope with this gift. Ignoring these background narratives means ignoring the distress, the burden, the despair a woman may experience throughout prenatal diagnosis, trying her best to create a viable family. Legitimising the dilemma by saying that anxiety and suffering are also part of God's gift remains on the confessional or ideological level; it is not experiential, it appears cynical and with a certain cruelty in the judgment – at least, it may well entail ethical violence. So I think only if you go through that door of acknowledging the moral dilemmas *as* dilemmas, will you be able to enter into a conversation, a moral deliberation process, which takes the people with you, and lets them live as the person they are.

Christina Schües: We have come a long way – and we have opened a path for further research and further conversations. Thank you both for the inspiring, deep, and most insightful conversation!

Anne Weber: Even though we will end our conversation at this point, we hope this is not the end but the beginning of an interdisciplinary, interreligious, and transcultural exchange, helping to support a way of moral reasoning that is sensitive to life's challenges and conflicts. Thank you both for sharing your work and insights with us.

8. What Does Prenatal Testing Mean for Women Who Have Tested?

Christoph Rehmann-Sutter, Tamar Nov-Klaiman, Yael Hashiloni-Dolev, Anika König, Stefan Reinsch and Aviad Raz

Women who use prenatal tests have varied reasons for doing so. It is therefore important to learn from women who have used tests, the reasons why, and for what purposes they have tested. Reasons and corresponding aims of testing constitute what we can call the "meaning" of testing for those who have tested.

One aim of those who test is to be able to decide whether to discontinue (or not) the pregnancy. But we can also ask: why should it be desirable to decide about continuing the pregnancy? What does continuing or terminating a pregnancy mean for those who make that decision in their particular situation? Testing and the information it generates are in some way tools for achieving a desirable outcome. It is therefore not enough to state the obvious: that prenatal tests are tools to find out the likelihood that the child about to be born has a genetic disorder, since this leaves open questions about meanings. Why should this be a good thing to know during pregnancy? One reason could be the perception that a disabled child will suffer and/or cause suffering to the family, for example.

Expecting or knowing a result only in technical terms therefore does not reveal the reasonings of women or couples. The reasons why women take a test are personal and as such do not belong directly to the scientific realm. They give the test a particular significance within the dynamic life context of those who decide. In this chapter we use interviews with women and couples who chose to test for a chromosomal or genetic disorder to better understand what these meanings are, in the lifeworld of those using them, using a comparative analysis of a selection of interviews from Israel and Germany. We will try to identify patterns of meaning-making, and see whether there are significant differences between our Israeli and German interviews. We also discuss the findings in the context of the current bioethical literature on prenatal testing and screening, where two interrelated framings are predominant: that prenatal tests enable women to make "informed decisions", and that prenatal tests are key parts of a practice of "selective reproduction", for which information is meaningful.

Germany and Israel differ in their regulation of the field, the scope of prenatal testing they offer under public funding, and the recommendations of professional associations of obstetrics and gynaecology (OB/GYN) and genetics (see chapter 3 in this volume for details). Israel has a widely implemented prenatal testing scheme, which is publicly funded. However, it does not include NIPT (non-invasive prenatal testing, a test based on analysis of cell-free DNA in maternal blood). Since 2022 Germany has had regulation enabling NIPT to be covered by health insurance, but only if the woman is in a conflict by the lack of knowledge and the risk of psychological harm due to the uncertainty (Rehmann-Sutter/Schües 2020). At the time of the interviews (2017–2019), NIPT had to be paid for privately but its availability was widely known and its uptake common practice. The overall uptake rate of NIPT in Germany has been estimated by Gadsbøll et al. (2020) based on best clinical guesses as < 25 per cent of all pregnant women. In Israel, where the first- and second-trimester screening tests are publicly funded for all women, and where amniocentesis coupled with chromosomal microarray analysis (CMA) is often funded, uptake rates of NIPT were relatively low: in 2019 it was about 4.4 per cent of live births.[1]

Below, the analysis focuses on the meanings attributed to varied types of testing – be they invasive, such as amniocentesis (whether or not coupled with CMA, also known as the "genetic chip"), or non-invasive, such as NIPT and the first-/second-trimester screenings.

---

1   Ami Singer, MD, Head of the Community Genetics Department in the Ministry of Health of Israel, personal communication.

Methodology of this analysis

> A word is dead, when it is said
> Some say —
> I say it just begins to live
> That day
> Emily Dickinson[2]

Analysing the interviews a few years after they had been conducted and transcribed was a special experience for us when writing this chapter. It brought the words of the interviewees back to life in a new way. In the context of analytical questions that we have since generated, selected passages of the interviews made new sense. While speaking, our interviewees could not have been aware of the exact questions that we now had while interpreting the transcripts. Prompted by questions from the interviewer, they essentially told us their stories of testing as part of their life. They explained how testing was important and how it was problematic for them in their particular situation.

In an important sense of the term, interpreting the interviews as we do in this chapter has to do with a "double hermeneutics", as frequently emphasised in interpretative phenomenological analysis (IPA). The analytical process of interviews can be described as a dual interpretation process, because first the participants made meaning of their world, and then second the researcher tried to decode that meaning to make their own sense of the participants' meaning-making (Smith/Osborn 2008). In the first step, the participants' interpretation, there are even more layers involved. Tests are offered to women and couples in the context of meaningful packages that already contain interpretations of what it means to be a responsible parent. Women and couples are well aware of social expectations that restrict the freedom of choice they are constantly assured that they supposedly have. And on the side of the interpreters there are multiple interpretative layers too. We first read the interviews in a narrative fashion, in order to understand "the story" of these women. Then we reread the interviews and asked what the interviewee particularly wanted to get across while telling their story to the interviewer, who they already knew was doing "a study" on prenatal testing. And what we have tried to do in writing this chapter was to set a certain reflective distance between us and the

---

2   Dated 1862; no. 278. In: R.W. Franklin (ed.) (1989): The Poems of Emily Dickinson, Cambridge, MA: Belknap.

interviewees' full stories, in order to become more attentive to the meanings they attached to the tests. We were looking for typical meaning patterns that show up in the interview dialogues.

Before we say more about what these "typical meaning patterns" can be, we briefly want to explain the procedure of how interviewees were selected, how the interviews were conducted, and how cases were selected for this analysis. The interviews belong to the empirical part of the German-Israeli comparative interdisciplinary study of prenatal testing, which combined social sciences, philosophy and ethics. It was essentially a qualitative interview study in both countries. Before starting to recruit interviewees, ethical approval for the research was obtained from the ethics committees of the University of Lübeck and Ben-Gurion University of the Negev at Be'er Sheva in 2017. The recruiting process differed in each country due to the different contexts of the respective healthcare systems. We invited women who had either taken NIPT or other tests, or declined them. As part of the broader project, we also interviewed healthcare professionals in obstetrics/gynaecology and genetics, policymakers and activists. The interviews with these stakeholders were however not included in the analysis in this chapter. To recruit women in Germany we used a flyer that was distributed through OB/GYN and midwifery practices and pregnancy counselling centres, through online posts, and snowballing. Women who were interested in being interviewed then contacted us. In Israel, recruitment was done through online posts, relevant organizations (e.g., Down syndrome organizations), the authors' social network and snowballing. All participants gave written informed consent for the inclusion of their interview material in this study, and participants were fully anonymised.

An interview guide was initially developed, revised and extended after the first interviews had been transcribed and analysed. The first questions always focused on the women's individual biographies and the histories of and emotions concerning their pregnancies. We then asked how they had learned about prenatal testing and their attitudes toward it, their experience of professional counselling, and their decision-making process regarding the tests. We were also interested in the role of other people and/or sources of information in this process. Subsequently, we asked whether – and if yes, how – the tests changed their experience of pregnancy. Further questions asked their opinions on the financing of the test: whether it should be covered by health insurance or paid for privately. We also asked about their retrospective evaluation of the test, in particular whether they would do things differently or the same if they became pregnant again. To gain a normative insight, we asked what they thought about women whose choices about testing or acting upon test results were different. We added specific questions for women whose test results had been positive. We asked how they experienced learning about the positive result, whether they had chosen further invasive confirmatory tests, and whether they had terminated the pregnancy. The interview also focused on the experiences of people with disability, and on their attitude towards life with a disabled child and views on terminating pregnancy.

In Germany, in addition to interviews with professionals of various kinds, we conducted 36 interviews with women and couples who had or had declined NIPT. In six of them, we interviewed both partners together, while in one interview only the partner participated. In 14 of our interviews there was a chromosomal disorder in the (extended) family (more details in Reinsch/König/Rehmann-Sutter 2021). In Israel, in addition to interviews with professionals and activists and with women who declined testing, we interviewed 30 women who had varied types of prenatal tests: first-/second-trimester screens, NIPT, amniocentesis with or without CMA. This number does not include women who had no tests or "only" had ultrasound tests (which in our sample was ultra-orthodox women). Six of the interviewees are mothers of children with Down syndrome.

All respondents received a recruitment letter describing the study and including a disclosure statement. German interviews were conducted in German, face-to-face and in a few cases by telephone. In Israel, interviews were conducted in Hebrew over the phone or via Skype. Israeli interviews were all conducted by Tamar Nov-Klaiman. German interviews were conducted by Anika König or Stefan Reinsch. The guideline-based interviews lasted from 45 to 150 minutes, and in most cases more than an hour. Interviews were audio-recorded, fully transcribed verbatim and pseudonymised following transcription.

For this special analysis we used the 19 German and 30 Israeli interviews with women who *had actually taken* a prenatal genetic test. These women had either received a positive result, and after confirmation by amniocentesis had decided to terminate their pregnancy, or to continue it and have the baby with special needs; or they had received a negative result.

Those sections in the transcripts that contained statements about the meaning of prenatal tests (reasons for testing, aims of testing and related topics) were highlighted and interpreted, considering each interview and its narrative individually. Iterative comparison and abstraction was used to compile a table of distinct, typical meaning patterns. This process was done first for each country separately. The categories were then discussed in joint sessions, and meaning patterns adapted by further abstraction to include similar patterns identified in the table of the other country. The result of this process was a joint table of ultimately seven different but interrelated meaning patterns. Many patterns appeared in both German and Israeli interviews, but some were seen more in one country and less in the other.

The procedure was similar to a Weberian ideal-type analysis, which has been formally described by Uta Gerhardt (1994) for qualitative research in particular, and more generally for sociology by Richard Swedberg (2017). In general, the ambition of an ideal-type in sociological theory is to understand and explain a certain cultural phenomenon, i.e. a particular social action that is the focus of our attention. Decisions about prenatal testing can be considered social actions in many important respects. They affect other people beyond the one who makes the decision about testing, and they are also organised actions since they are only possible within social arrangements and using cultural scripts. More explicitly, prenatal testing therefore belongs to what we may call the *pre-partum sociality* of the pregnant woman and couple.[3] While technically looking for features of the foetus, prenatal testing as a social action derives its reasons and aims from within the social relations among the family and in society. It therefore needs to be explained within the social relationships between people.

When we look at the meanings of the prenatal tests, and the reasons and aims that led women to have such tests, we focus on the women's rationales in a specific historical and social context. This could be done very specifically and on a case-by-case basis for each individual. But it is also interesting to see whether we can find some typical patterns in the sense of ideal types. In order to clarify what this notion implies and what ideal types can do (and not do) in theory we now briefly look at this discussion with reference to Weber. As both Gerhardt (1994) and Swedberg (2017) note, Max Weber's work does not give a single authoritative and unequivocal definition of the concept of "ideal type" in his project of *interpretive sociology*. The most comprehensive statement is in his 1904 essay on objectivity. With his idea of ideal types he wanted to explain a specific historical formation (such as "the spirit of capitalism"). Weber strove for

---

3   It is related but not identical to Stefan Hirschauer's concept of "prenatal sociality", i.e. the sociality of the unborn, which is socialisation of the unborn during pregnancy (Hirschauer et al. 2014).

conceptual clarity about a historical formation by means of a synthesis of individual components that he selected in their sharpest, most consistent form. By conceptual clarity he seems to have meant a rational understanding of the meaning of a phenomenon. In chapter 1 of *Wirtschaft und Gesellschaft* there is a second version of the ideal type theory that can be applied to social actions. In Swedberg's reconstruction, this refers to what a hypothetical (or ideal) and typical rational actor can do under certain circumstances. This is a first point to keep in mind: an ideal type explanation assumes, sometimes counterfactually, that the actor is acting rationally, i.e. according to a coherent reasoning. The two criteria Weber then gives for ideal types seem to be (i) that they must be adequate on the level of meaning for what they are intending to explain in reality ("Sinnadäquanz"); and (ii) that they heighten or concentrate the meaning in order to reach a clearer understanding ("gesteigerte Eindeutigkeit"; Weber 2014, Part I, chapter 1, § 1, section 11). This is a second point to keep in mind: claims about ideal types must meet certain criteria. The first is: "What is involved in adequacy on the level of meaning is that the meaning and the action have to fit each other, a bit like the hand in the glove" (Swedberg 2017: 187). This relates to the double hermeneutics, which we have mentioned above: the researchers' interpretation must fit the meanings that actors communicated in the interviews. The heightening or concentration of meaning under the assumption of ideal actors who act rationally and have complete information relates to the explanatory force of an ideal type pattern. We will therefore present ideal meaning patterns with the aim of *adequately representing the meaning* of what women explained and at the same time *heightening and concentrating* this meaning, in order to make it more graspable.

Findings

a) German and Israeli interviews

The major difference we found in the interviews is that Israeli women were more likely to seek to maximise detection by testing, even at the cost of risk due to the invasiveness of the procedure, and even in the absence of a medical indication. For example, a notable proportion of Israeli women who were offered NIPT (but no German women in our sample) declined, not because they refused tests in general or because of the costs, but because they wanted to have more comprehensive genetic tests than NIPT, such as amniocentesis combined with chromosomal microarray analysis (CMA). This was also found in a sub-set of our previous interviewees, i.e. parents of children with Down syndrome (Nov-Klaiman et al. 2019, 2022). This difference can be explained in part by the stronger desire of interviewed Israeli women to find out as much as possible about their future children. For a close analysis of the meanings of prenatal testing for women who had the tests, we decided to ignore the particular test chosen, i.e. the meanings given to testing by women who had either performed NIPT or alternative tests, whether invasive (mostly in Israel) or non-invasive, e.g. first-/second-trimester screens.

In this situation it would not make sense to focus exclusively on the features of NIPT that make it unique from the points of view of both providers and women using it. The focus of our analysis shifted from NIPT to multiple variants of (genetic) prenatal tests. Compared to other methods, NIPT is a clinically risk-free testing procedure. In several interviews women said that they would not have had amniocentesis because of the risk it poses to the continuation of the pregnancy. This however appeared among the reasons why they preferred NIPT over other means of prenatal testing, or why they did not go any further with a diagnostic invasive test, even after a positive result. We wanted to know how women and couples understood the meaning of their *act* of testing in the context of a practice that is more extended in time, social distribution and space.

The meanings of testing cannot be sharply distinguished from the reasons that made women decide to have it. These reasons include the physician's recommendation, the expectations of the family, or the perception that a woman had an elevated risk due to her age (> 35). Reasons give one answer to the question of why they tested. But the question has another level of meaning as well: in addition to reasons for consenting to a procedure of prenatal testing, the women and couples referred to what these tests meant in their life situations. The meaning they are referring to is the *intention* of their act of testing: *What did they do it for?* This is an equally central focus of this chapter.

This question is distinct from the medical description of the tests (in terms of probabilities, reliability, or the medical significance of a diagnosis such as trisomy 21), and also distinct from technical descriptions of the tests (in terms of cell-free foetal DNA fragments sequenced), and from the regulatory description of the tests (in terms of permissibility of an abortion under national law, or of claiming reimbursement from health insurance funds). The women often had ideas about what the testing meant to them in their personal situation. But not all of them had; some, especially women in Israel, also said that they had the tests just because they are offered and performed as part of medical routine in pregnancy management, and they wanted to do things, as one interviewee put it, "by the book", without giving it much thought. But for those who attached a certain meaning to the test, it was for instance to help prepare themselves for a child with special needs, or to evaluate whether their medical, emotional, social, financial etc. resources would allow them to cope with it. Alternatively, testing was important to allow the termination of a pregnancy if abnormalities were detected, because in their view and personal situation, disability should be avoided. These descriptions of personal meanings of prenatal testing were extremely diverse. They included references to the life situation of the woman or couple in their family and in their country, their previous family history etc. In analysing the interviews and using the "ideal type" approach (explained above), we have been attentive to typical *patterns of meanings* used in these highly personal and diverse explanations.

b) Patterns found

In the interviews we find multiple and very different subjective descriptions used by the actors to describe this kind of action, "performing prenatal tests". As we have said, in Germany they mostly referred to NIPT whereas in Israel, except for the first-/second-trimester screening tests with their high uptake rates, more extensive tests such as amniocentesis coupled with CMA are commonly preferred over NIPT. These subjective descriptions are embedded in personal narratives and therefore refer to what was personally relevant for the women and couples in their particular situations. These descriptions are heterogeneous, each guided by their special circumstances and previous experiences, their idiosyncratic views on family, pregnancy and disability. So there are probably no two identical descriptions from different people about what it means to do a prenatal test. Similarities and overlaps can nevertheless be found. We started by looking for patterns and then, by dropping more of the particular details, for typical patterns.

To explain this procedure, let us look at an example. Shimrat is an Israeli woman who at the time of the interview had two children after having terminated her first pregnancy following a diagnosis of Down syndrome, which was suspected at the second trimester screen and confirmed by amniocentesis. She said:

I'm the one who would need to raise her and I'm not willing to do it – not to myself and not to her. I mean, why? I see no reason why. I didn't hesitate. I don't have a partner. I'm a single mum. But even if I had a partner I wouldn't have kept this pregnancy.

I think, to begin with, all these tests exist for prevention. I see no reason to bring a child into the world when you know in advance that something is wrong. It's not, you know, a missing finger or something like that, which you can live with. It isn't a congenital problem that can be fixed. It's something irreversible. It means condemning her to life that isn't ... Not as far as I'm concerned.

In the second pregnancy I was so impatient to have [NIPT] already and get the results and finally breathe. I felt like I couldn't breathe, and I had to breathe.

She explains her situation as a single mother but then quickly goes on to state that this was not the reason why she terminated her pregnancy after receiving confirmation of Down syndrome. But what was it then? There are two main layers of interpretation within her statement. One is about the termination of the first pregnancy, the other about her willingness to have NIPT in her second. On the first level she refers to her understanding of the condition called Down syndrome. In her view, trisomy 21 means that there is more than just missing something, a condition you can live with ("a missing finger"). It will be, as she explains, "something wrong" with the child that cannot "be fixed", and this is something "irreversible". The explanation culminates in a sentence, which however is not spoken to its end: "It means condemning her to life that isn't ..." At the left-out end of the phrase she avoids saying what she means about what that life would be for her child. What did she want to say? Or did she use the fragmentary sentence, the unspoken word, on purpose, in order to hint at what cannot be said? The unspoken word(s) must fit the beginning of the sentence: It means "condemning her". From her beginning with *condemning* we hear that she is speaking about a particular life that in her view is highly undesirable. Otherwise she could not have used a word as strong as "condemn".

She was looking back on a difficult decision she had taken quite a while ago in her first pregnancy. She *had* terminated. Now, using the story of her first pregnancy, she explains why in the following pregnancy she *rushed* to get NIPT. She was desperate ("like I couldn't breathe") and needed to ensure the same scenario would not reoccur. Looking more abstractly at the motives of both actions – termination of pregnancy and testing – we can see they are closely linked. She saw the testing as a preventive tool, allowing both the child and herself to avoid a life that is deeply undesirable ("willing [...] not to myself and not to her").

What is so undesirable as a life that one can say that being condemned to having it? This is something that most generally we call suffering. We therefore decided to use this more abstract term, "suffering" (a term explicitly used by some respondents) to define this meaning pattern: to perform prenatal tests *in order to avoid suffering*. The term suffering covers many concrete visions and fears, some of which may have been in this interviewee's mind. Other people might have different images of what lives or conditions could lead to suffering. But there is one important distinction clearly indicated in this interview statement: the suffering of the child and the suffering of the mother, and perhaps more generally of the family. Based on this consideration we therefore emphasised the two dimensions of this category: testing in order to avoid suffering: not to inflict this suffering on a child, and/or not to inflict suffering on the family and oneself.

After following such an interpretative procedure with all included interviews, we compared the provisional versions of the categories and combined similar interviews into one more general category. Tentatively, we concluded with seven nuanced though interrelated and partially overlapping intentional patterns found in our sample (Table 1):

Table 1: Typical meaning patterns of prenatal testing

1) To test in order *to gain knowledge*,
   which is in itself an empowerment.

2) To test in order *to be prepared*
   for the birth of a child with special needs. This can relate to external aspects: preparation of family and friends, health insurance, housing etc., or to an internal attitude: to get ready to welcome the child, to do the work of grief etc.

3) To test in order to *reduce uncertainty* and to increase certainty.
   This provides reassurance for those who believe the pregnancy is developing well, or confirms or disproves the fears of those who have them.

4) To test in order *to find out and to decide*
   whether one has the resources and capabilities to have this child, thus whether the pregnancy should be continued.

5) To test in order *to avoid suffering*
by avoiding a condition that would inflict harm on the child, and that would also mean suffering for the family and oneself.

6) To test in order to *satisfy the social environment*
which can be the partner, the parents, or wider family and social milieu.

7) To test in order to *fulfil the physician's recommendation*,
which can arise from a wish to do everything by the book, or just out of trust in the doctor.

We shall now explain and illustrate all these meaning patterns and provide supporting quotes from both Israel and Germany.[4]

(1)   To test in order to gain knowledge

Tests can be done for the purpose of gaining the knowledge they promise to provide. Knowledge of course has a function: for instance, it should increase certainty or reduce uncertainty and fear. Knowledge can also have a value in itself. It can be an empowerment. It then also empowers people for the task of making the decisions that need making. The rationale is that knowing is always better than ignorance and that knowledge in a way also provides a means of controlling something over the course of events.

For example, Sarah (IL) said:

[When I receive medical information] it lowers my anxiety, and it empowers me. It gives me the power to make choices. And power in general. In my view, knowledge is power.

She had an amniocentesis with CMA, which she understood to be the most reliable, precise and broad test that there is. Due to her age it was publicly funded in Israel.

---

4   Some of the categories developed in this chapter resonate with descriptions published from the German interviews (Reinsch/König/Rehmann-Sutter 2021).

(2) To test in order to be prepared

Tests can be done in order to be prepared for the birth of a child with disability. This can relate to external aspects, such as preparation of family and friends, finding better health insurance, preparing the home. Or it can relate to an internal attitude: getting ready to welcome the child, to do the work of grief by letting go of former expectations etc.

Lisa (GE) is in a same-sex marriage. Both she and her wife had a child from the same sperm donor who was present in the family as the father (however not legally) and cared for the two children each week. When she was pregnant with her son, an ultrasound found an unusually short femur and white spots in the heart. She then had NIPT, not to terminate but to be better prepared:

> The test was a huge gift. I mean, for us, that at the moment when Noah was born, it meant we could just be very happy about this baby. And, um, this mourning process, which there just is, saying goodbye to something that you kind of imagine, whether you want it or not, that runs alongside it, you just don't have it on your radar.

The preparation that she meant was mainly an internal process that included letting go of certain expectations and, as she called it, "mourning" it. Other women said that preparation included external things such as choosing good health insurance for the child.

Ronit (IL) was also sure that she would not terminate:

> But I wanted the test for my own sake, to know and prepare for the situation. Be prepared for what is coming.

This pattern was found in several interviews in both Germany and Israel among people who, for whatever reasons, were sure that they would not choose to terminate but wanted to know in advance what to expect. In Israel, these descriptions came from religious women.

(3) To test in order to reduce uncertainty and to increase certainty

Some people may have tests to be reassured that the pregnancy is developing well, or in order to confirm or disprove fears if they have them. They either want to be sure of what awaits for the child and themselves, or that the feared disabilities will not be present.

Sandra (GE), who had two girls in her late 30s, used NIPT because it felt better to know for sure that all was fine:

> Right, because it really was this, this reassurance we were hoping for, that was definitely there.

The test fulfilled the function of confirming her and her partner's hope that all was well. Corinna (GE) said that, in addition to many other considerations, the test was done to confirm the feeling or belief that everything with the baby would be fine:

> But we were still somehow very sure, well, it's just more of a confirmation for us that there's nothing there, I mean, that there's actually no problem.

Anna-Lena (GE) explained the testing in terms of the reassurance that they hoped it would give them, not necessarily in order to hear that there would be no problem with the child, but to know what awaited them. She said:

> Because we were so tortured by uncertainty, because first I thought, "OK, I'll, um, [...] we'll just ignore it." I didn't want to do it anyway. [...]
> My husband just wanted to be sure, I think, or just know what it was all about, because [...]. I think he could handle it better.

Their plan was to continue the pregnancy in any case.

(4) To test in order to become capable of deciding

This motive, too, is related to the knowledge that a testing procedure can deliver and the power it can provide. But knowledge and the power it gives are not sought for their own sake, but because they open an opportunity to gain the necessary information that makes it possible to see whether this pregnancy should be continued, and whether one has the resources and capabilities to have this child. The levels of disability associated different possible genetic conditions differ enormously, and people may want to know more concretely what they would be dealing with, in order to find out whether they can in fact do it. This then has implications for their decision to continue the pregnancy or not.

After experiencing a spontaneous miscarriage in her first pregnancy, Nurit (IL) received abnormal findings in an ultrasound test in her second pregnancy. She was offered chorionic villus sampling (CVS) – an invasive diagnostic test – and decided to have it, before determining whether to terminate the pregnancy. Following a diagnosis of Down syndrome, she terminated the pregnancy. She explained why she had testing in the second pregnancy:

> It was important for me to know what it was, for the future as well. I had already had one pregnancy that failed, and I thought there might be a connection. I wanted to know, to have all the information. It's also a big decision to make – having an abortion. I wanted to be 100 per cent sure that there was a problem, a defect, when we chose to terminate this life.

The decision she was facing was difficult, and in order to make the decision about "this life" she needed maximum information about the existence of a defect.

Gali (IL), whose physician informed the couple of NIPT, explained her attitude toward prenatal testing:

> To reach an informed decision we want to know what there is. If there is something that can be treated – then treat it. And if it's something more dramatic – then I don't reject the option of having an abortion.

Corinna (GE) was looking for information from the test in order to consider whether she would have enough strength to care for this child.

> If it turned out to be trisomy 13 or 18, emm, we said, then we just wouldn't *have the confidence* for it at the moment.

(5) To test in order to avoid suffering

Testing can be primarily motivated by the intention of preventing suffering. This can mean doing something to avoid a condition that would inflict harm on the child, and it can also mean to avoid suffering for the family and oneself. As our respondents explained, the parents and siblings can suffer because of the physical suffering of the disabled child, but also from the energy and time dedicated to him or her, at the expense of other family members and by exhausting them. The aim of avoiding suffering is close to the aim of avoiding disability but distinct from it, since disability per se does not necessarily entail suffering, and also because the conditions that fall under the rubric of impairment are so different. It is not the disability that is avoided but the severe burden that it may mean for the child, the future mother and the family.

Dorothee (GE) was very concerned about the burden a disabled child would be for the relatives, and also for their second child. She anticipated a time after she and her husband would no longer be there:

> If my husband and I are no longer there, or something happens, then [...] well, [...] then who would take care of, well, the responsibility lies with our second child, I would think.

Her caring attitude towards the child in this hypothetical situation meant she did not want this to happen, and therefore she decided to test.

When asked whether financial and social aspects of life with disability were among her considerations about prenatal testing, Orit (IL) explained:

> Aspects concerning the child. If a child is born with a syndrome – the issue of which manifestations the syndrome has. Aspects regarding the family. If a child is born with a syndrome and you know about it in advance – you put your family in a situation that you have a child who's going to consume much more energy from you than your other child, who also needs your time and energy. So you hurt them from all directions. This is the consideration mainly. [...] These children suffer. Their families suffer, the other children at home suffer. With all the love and the fact that they are sweet children, they still consume familial energy from their siblings.

Anna (GE) wanted to prevent the severe burden that a disabled child can be for the family and the suffering it can mean. Her aunt was mentally impaired. Her grandmother had to care for her until her death at 95, when the aunt was 75. She said that the experience of this shaped her decision to have a prenatal test at the age of 37:

> And I knew that if I had a child, and especially now so late in life, I couldn't have a handicapped child, because I realise that perhaps I'm already too old [laughs], and because I saw how my grandmother lived, at 95, with this disabled child – my aunt is now 75 – until she died, and I don't believe I'd have had the strength. So it was a very clear, stark decision, simply pro or contra child.

The decision "pro or contra child", as she phrases it, is behind her taking a test. The motivation for testing is to avoid a situation in her future life that she feared she would not have the strength to bear, a child that would overburden her.

Here are a few more examples from our Israeli sample. Stav (IL), who had NIPT, explained:

> I think disability should be avoided in order to spare the family from suffering, and the child itself. The child, meaning that society would be cruel to him or her.

Ella (IL) had NIPT following abnormal findings in an ultrasound scan. NIPT detected trisomy 18, after which she terminated the pregnancy. She said:

> If there are things I can know in advance and prevent to avoid suffering for myself, for my husband, for my children, of a child with a severe syndrome... Look, people always say that [it should be done] to prevent suffering of the child. The truth is that when there is a severe syndrome, the child is usually so cognitively impaired and so handicapped that they're not able to be aware of their situation and their suffering. That's why I refer more to the horror that the family has to go through.

Hadas (IL) had amniocentesis in her first pregnancy without any medical indication. She had one in her second pregnancy too, due to her age. She explained:

> Certain disabilities are accompanied by a lot of suffering and pain, so this is a very difficult life. For both the child and the family. For the siblings too if there are any.

(6) To test in order to satisfy the social environment

Tests can also be done to meet expectations of others. It could be the partner who wants a test to be done, it could be the parents or the wider family that builds the social environment. In principle, expectations of the wider society would fall into this category of meanings as well, for instance if one is trying to behave in a manner that would be seen as socially responsible. This is a way to comply with community norms or to enact cultural scripts. In the interviews with those respondents who said that they tested in order to satisfy the social environment, however, we found more references to relevant close others or to the family.

Shani (IL) referred to general social expectations in explaining her choice to have amniocentesis plus CMA:

In the end, what won the debate was the idea that you don't want an anomalous child. Anomalous by definition, right? Because all children are exceptional in their own way.

"You don't want" refers to what she assumes to be a generally shared opinion in her society. But Hagit (IL) did it for the sake of her mother, who said she should:

My mum was mostly the one putting on the pressure. She's the one who eventually funded my NIPT, which isn't publicly funded. I told her I wasn't planning to have it, so she said she would pay and I should have it. Actually, this is why I did. I wouldn't have had it if she weren't pushing.

For Sandra (GE), the decisions behind whether to test or not and which tests to take were difficult. She and her partner quarrelled a lot over it. He absolutely wanted her to have the test in order to be fully secure that nothing was wrong. The fight continued over the interpretation of the test, since NIPT only provided probabilities, not a clear yes or no. She described her partner as pretty much "paranoid" about all this but, in order to move forward in the relationship, she agreed to have the test done, among other things because of potential reproaches from her partner if she refused:

In the end, I'd be to blame if something was overlooked.

Danit (IL) also told us that her partner desperately wanted her to test. With NIPT, she no longer had any reasons to be scared about testing (as in her previous pregnancies):

This alternative appeared, of a private blood test instead of amniocentesis. My husband held my hand and told me: "I beg you, do this test. You don't know what disability can do to the family. Please listen. No matter how much we pay. Better to have the test and know than not test at all."

In her partner's considerations we find the concerns that disability means suffering to the family. She saw her own pregnancy as problematic due to her advanced age, and saw that her partner was very stressed because of this:

I had NIPT and it was considered something that would relax my husband and the environment that my geriatric pregnancy at the age of 35 would be all right. This was my state of mind. I didn't even eagerly anticipate the results. I knew I was doing it for others.

(7)   To test in order to fulfil the physician's recommendation

Tests in a highly regulated healthcare environment can be chosen out of a wish to do everything right, according to recommendations, to do everything by the book, or just out of trust in the doctor who recommends it.

Sivan (IL) trusted her physician when he recommended she have invasive testing in her situation of being of a more advanced age (over 40):

> He said that in amniocentesis and the added genetic chip most conditions that are tested, or at least a lot of them, are age related. Meaning, at this age there is an advantage for amniocentesis combined with the chip. That's it. At that very moment the decision was made.

Gali (IL) explained that she wanted to do everything right, according to the doctor's recommendation:

> I did everything by the book. Whatever my ObGyn told me. [...] When I'm told to do something, I do it. [...]
> And then the doctor came [and told us about the test] and we said, "actually we have nothing to lose here. More information. No risk. Let's do it." Without thinking too much about it. Without truly understanding what it means. And we did it.

A few observations

In Israel, women seemed to take the performance of tests for granted. This could be partially explained by the fact that a wider selection of tests has been implemented in the national healthcare system for a longer time, supported by professional guidelines and practice that recommend their use. It is therefore much more routinised than in Germany.

When Israeli women think about testing, it seems to be more common than in Germany to take for granted that abnormal results will lead to termination of pregnancy, although such instances were also found in the German sample. This could be explained by different interpretations of disability in each culture. In Israel disability is more often directly connected with suffering.

Meaning patterns 1 (pursuit of knowledge), 6 (satisfaction of social environment) and 7 (fulfilment of physician's recommendation) were found mostly in the Israeli sample. This observation should however be read with caution. Given the small size of our samples in both countries, however, the evidence it provides can only be anecdotal. It cannot warrant any conclusions for either country beyond indicating a certain tendency that would need to be confirmed by more extensive studies.

More often than in Israel, women in Germany saw the decision to test and the decision to terminate or continue the pregnancy as separate decisions. Most women saw them as being not only independent but also different in content. Even Laura (GE), who chose abortion after a confirmed diagnosis of trisomy 21, insisted that they did not make the decision to terminate beforehand, but as a second and most difficult step only after the amniocentesis. This is seen less often in the Israeli sample. In a minority of cases, Israeli women test in order to know (which is separate from the decision to terminate), i.e. even when they know from the outset that they would not terminate. For some Israeli women, however, testing was also separate in a different sense, i.e. in the sense that testing is done automatically, "by the book". Then, if an abnormality is detected, the decision to terminate is a separate one. But it seems that Israeli women often say: "What is testing for if not to prevent?" – meaning they couple the decision to test with the decision to terminate.

As we expected, women rarely gave a medical description of the tests, even if they said it was a test for certain conditions such as trisomies 21, 13 or 18. But what they were focusing on was the expected lived reality of these conditions. Their predominant concern was the personal existential meaning of testing, which involved themselves as the mother. It was not just their own image of the lived reality of disability that was important to their decision-making rationales, but also the image that society or their family (in their view) addressed to them. An important factor was how they expected the family and society to include and support children with special needs, and how their children would be looked at.

Some women used several different intentional patterns to describe their actions in the same interview. This indicates that the patterns, which we suggest to be ideal types of rationales of testing as a social action, are mutually exclusive only on a theoretical level. In reality, people can combine different patterns in their thinking and in their explanatory discourses, representing different facets of a complex deliberation. Some women however concentrated on one core formulation of the meaning, for which they sometimes used varied wordings.

In some interviews we find patterns from which women wanted to distance themselves. One topic that occurred frequently, mainly in interviews with German participants, was concern about developments in society that they saw happening or that they feared would happen in future, which our interviewees saw as problematic if they became dominant in society. For instance, Hanna said that she feared it was becoming more and more "normal" in society to use prenatal tests to check genetic makeup ("um die genetische Ausstattung zu checken"), which would mean society was becoming increasingly ableist ("behindertenfeindliche Gesellschaft"), one in which women would avoid giving birth to children whom society would not welcome ("gesellschaftlich nicht gewünscht"). We have not included these idioms in our list of the typical meaning patterns, since they were not presented as belonging to participants' own actions; and if these idioms have been used in relation to their own actions, then as a negative contrast.

Discussion

We have focused on women's strategies of sense-making about testing during pregnancy. What did the tests mean to them? Which words did they use when they talked about the tests? How did they frame their decision-making about the test when they explained it in the interview? The question of the nature of the ethical challenge confronting them is closely connected with the meaning pattern they associated with the action of testing. Another related question is how they positioned prenatal testing in the context of their lives and in the society in which they live. This question, as understood by parents (or future parents), also depends on the meaning pattern of how they see testing as a social action.

Our findings give insights into the hermeneutics of testing from the point of view of those who decide about the test and make sense of both the test and its results. That such a hermeneutics of testing from the point of view of women who take the tests is related to but distinct from those rationales provided by geneticists and gynaecologists has long been established, by the classic qualitative interview studies of Rothman (1986), and more recent studies by Gregg (1995), Rapp (1999) and Meskus (2012). In order to understand prenatal diagnosis as a cultural phenomenon it is crucial to consider the women's rationales and their perception of the new kinds of conflicts presented by their supposed genetic responsibility as well.

One of the reasons why we were interested in analysing the interviews under the lens of personal meaning patterns was that in recent bioethical literature there is an increasingly predominant view prenatal tests serve the woman or couple either as a tool for decision-making of (we could call this the "autonomy rationale", however demanding this may be in order to enable women to make not just choices but meaningful choices; de Jong / de Wert 2015); or as a legitimate tool to avoid the birth of children with certain conditions, i.e. an instrument in a practice of what has been called "selective reproduction" (Wilkinson 2010; Tarkian 2020). The autonomy rationale found some resonance in our meaning patterns 1 (pursuit of knowledge) and 4 (capability to decide). However, only a few of the women and couples we spoke to used a variant of the autonomy rationale to explain the meaning of their testing. The selective reproduction rationale has been given a scholarly definition by Wilkinson as choosing to have one possible child over another, since "one possible future child is, in some way, more desirable than the alternatives" (Wilkinson 2010: 2). This idiom was rarely explicitly used by women or couples to explain their action in our sample.

However, we did find occasional examples. For instance, Sivan (IL), who was pregnant at the time of the interview, explained that the meanings of raising a disabled child were in the background when deciding about the tests. She said that raising a disabled child is a very difficult and complicated thing. She would therefore prefer to terminate and try again, even at the risk of not succeeding in becoming pregnant.

> We'd rather try again. I mean, have an abortion and try again, even if it's late and even if I'm already 41 or 42. We'd rather try again than be with such a child for life. Try again, even if we might not succeed.

This can be considered a rather explicit expression of "one possible future child is, in some way, more desirable than the alternatives". Similar idioms appeared in a negative way to characterise reasonings people *feared* are becoming predominant in society. The rationale that perhaps comes closest to it is no. 5 (preventing suffering). One may see here an implicit wish to – generally speaking – choose a more desirable child. The desire to prevent suffering is concrete and can be rooted in a caring attitude. This is not the same as parents explaining their action as a choice made from the point of view of "preferences" as to which child should be born instead of another. But from a purely logical point of view, choosing to terminate a diagnosed pregnancy (or testing with the intention of terminating if abnormality is detected) is indeed the manifestation of a preference – that one future child is (for whatever reason) better than an alternative. The meaning therefore remains ambiguous.

We understand Wilkinson's suggestion to operate on the abstract level of a discussion about the permissibility of certain kinds of reproductive behaviour, such as prenatal testing and conditional termination of the pregnancy. On formal grounds he subsumed prenatal testing within a general category of actions that are said to be practices of selective reproduction. He did so regardless of the actual intentions of women and couples who use prenatal diagnosis.[5] On the basis of our study we should be cautious about accepting such a general categorisation, since it would not do justice to the way women and couples who actually *bear* genetic responsibility in making decisions in their families described their views and decisions.[6] If bioethics should relate to the moral considerations of those who actually are making the decisions about prenatal diagnosis, i.e. the pregnant women and their partners, "personalised ethics" as Meskus (2012) has called it cannot rely on vague or formal assumptions about the "general meaning" of prenatal diagnosis as a social action, which is far distant from the actual thoughts and concerns of those making the decisions.

Further studies are needed to develop a more comprehensive and nuanced picture. One crucial limitation of our study is that we asked women after the fact. Explanations of reasons and corresponding aims can be different, depending on the time they are given. Before having a test, people decide to do the test for particular reasons, which might be remembered retrospectively and reported in terms of their actual situation *after* knowing the result of the test, after having made a decision about termination, or after the child is born.

Contributions of authors

Christoph Rehmann-Sutter: Study design, analysis and interpretation, draft, revision; *Tamar Nov-Klaiman:* Field work (IL), analysis and interpretation, revision; *Yael Hashiloni-Dolev:* Study design; revision of chapter text; *Aviad Raz:* Study design, revision of chapter text; *Anika König:* Field work (GE), revision of chapter text; *Stefan Reinsch:* Field work (GE), revision of chapter text.

We thank Marina Frisman and Vera von Kopylow for thematising transcripts and for supporting us in the interview analysis. We are grateful to Monica Buckland and Jackie Leach Scully for an English revision of the manuscript.

---

5   See the critical discussion of this strategy by Rehmann-Sutter (2021, 2022).
6   Cf. chapter 2 in this volume.

References

de Jong, Antina/de Wert, Guido M. W. R. (2015): "Prenatal Screening: An Ethical Agenda for the Near Future." In: Bioethics 29/1, pp. 46–55.

Gadsbøll, Kasper/Petersen, Olav B./Gatinois, Vincent/Strange, Heather/Jacobsson, Bo/Wapner, Ronald/Vermeesch, Joris R./Vogel, Ida (2020): "The NIPT-map Study Group. Current use of noninvasive prenatal testing in Europe, Australia and the USA: A graphical presentation." In: Acta Obstetrica et Gynecologica Scandinavica 99/6, pp. 722– 730 (https://doi.or g/10.1111/aogs.13841), accessed 26 July 2022.

Gerhardt, Uta (1994): "The use of Weberian ideal-type methodology in qualitative data interpretation." In: Bulletin of Sociological Methodology 45, pp. 74–126.

Gregg, Robin (1995): Pregnancy in a High-Tech Age: Paradoxes of Choice, New York: New York University Press.

Hirschauer, Stefan/Heimerl, Birgit/Hoffmann, Anika/Hofmann, Peter (2014): Soziologie der Schwangerschaft. Explorationen pränataler Sozialität, Oldenburg: DeGruyter.

Meskus, Mianna (2012): "Personalized ethics: The emergence and the effects in prenatal testing." In: BioSocieties 7/4, pp. 373–392.

Nov-Klaiman, Tamar/Raz, Aviad E./Hashiloni-Dolev, Yael (2019): "Attitudes of Israeli parents of children with Down syndrome toward non-invasive prenatal screening and the scope of prenatal testing." In: Journal of Genetic Counseling 28/6, pp. 1119–1129.

Nov-Klaiman, Tamar/Frisman, Marina/Raz, Aviad E./Rehmann-Sutter, Christoph (2022): "Views on disability and prenatal testing among families with Down syndrome and disability activists: A comparative analysis of interviews from Germany and Israel." In: Social Science & Medicine 303, pp. 115021.

Rapp, Rayna (1999): Testing Women, Testing the Fetus: The Social Impact of Amniocentesis in America, New York: Routledge.

Rehmann-Sutter, Christoph/Schües, Christina (2020): "Die NIPT-Entscheidung des G-BA: Eine ethische Analyse." In: Ethik in der Medizin 32, pp. 385–403.

Rehmann-Sutter, Christoph (2021): "Should prenatal screening be seen as 'selective reproduction'? Four reasons to reframe the ethical debate." In: Journal of Perinatal Medicine 49/8, pp. 953–958 (https://doi.org/10.1515/jpm-2 021-0239), accessed 26 July 2022.

Rehmann-Sutter, Christoph (2022): "'Selektive' Fortpflanzung durch pränatale Diagnostik?" In: Ethik in der Medizin 34, pp. 7–26 (https://doi.org/10.1007/s00481-021-00658-7), accessed 26 July 2022.

Reinsch, Stefan/König, Anika/Rehmann-Sutter, Christoph (2020): "Decision-making about non-invasive prenatal testing: Women's moral reasoning in the absence of a risk of miscarriage in Germany." In: New Genetics and Society 40/2, pp. 199–215.

Rothman, Barbara Katz (1986): The Tentative Pregnancy. Prenatal Diagnosis and the Future of Motherhood, New York: Viking.

Smith, Jonathan A./Osborn, Mike (2008): "Interpretative phenomenological analysis." In: Jonathan A. Smith (ed.), Qualitative psychology: A practical guide to research methods, London: Sage pp. 53–80.

Swedberg, Richard (2017): "How to use Max Weber's ideal type in sociological analysis." In: Journal of Classical Sociology 18/3, pp. 181–196.

Tarkian, Tatjana (2020): "Die Auswahl zukünftiger Kinder." In: Zeitschrift für Ethik und Moralphilosophie 3, pp. 109–125.

Weber, Max (2014 [1992]): Wirtschaft und Gesellschaft. Max Weber Gesamtausgabe Abt. 1, Bd. 23, Tübingen: Mohr.

Wilkinson, Stephen (2010): Choosing Tomorrow's Children: The Ethics of Selective Reproduction, Oxford: Oxford University Press.

9. "Something is Not Quite Right" – Two Cinematic Narratives about Decision-Making after Prenatal Diagnosis

Christoph Rehmann-Sutter, Christina Schües

The choice of the two films we discuss in this chapter – both released in 2016 – was first motivated by the striking similarity of their titles: *Week 23* and *24 Wochen* (24 weeks). Both refer to the number of weeks of pregnancy, which in both films was linked to a controversial and difficult experience because of prenatal diagnosis and the resulting prognosis. Both films show the moral complexity of the experience, including moral stress, ambivalence towards "medical knowledge", and familial tensions over the outcome and prospect of bringing a "disabled child" into the world. However, the two films differ from each other in many other important respects. *Week 23* is a documentary produced by Ohad Milstein in Israel, shot in Israel and Switzerland and addressing international viewers, while *24 Wochen* is fiction, a drama directed by Anne Zohra Berrached, produced in Germany and addressing a German-speaking audience.

The two films end in opposite ways. In her 23rd week of pregnancy Rahel, the protagonist of the Israeli film *Week 23*, who is carrying twins, learns that one of the foetuses has died in utero. She then has to decide what to do about the surviving foetus – and against the recommendation of her physicians, decides against abortion. As we learn at the end of the film, the child goes on to be born and can be seen toddling around. In the other film, the number 24 refers to the timepoint of a rather tragic late abortion of a foetus with Down syndrome and a severe heart defect. The unborn foetus lives for 24 weeks, and the film ends with an induced stillbirth. Wanting to break a taboo, the protagonist Astrid is going public with her decision to abort.

If we look below the surface and the storyline of the films, any comparison between these two narratives is not straightforward. They do not show similar situations of prenatal diagnosis, or illustrate how it is understood and handled differently in Israel and Germany. Both films intend to raise questions about the medicalisation of pregnancy and the roles of decision-makers. However, the Israeli film is organised around a biographical narrative of an event that actually happened in the film director's own family. Rachel is his partner; the child is their real child, and the story contains the rather unlikely and unforeseeable plots and twists that often characterise real-life stories. Although a constructed narrative, the other film is a story that could perhaps happen similarly to many couples. It aims to show the moral complexity of the practice of prenatal diagnosis as it is commonly experienced in Germany, and contains many realistic elements, even to the point of including real physicians and real psychologists who play themselves (Berrached 2016). The entertaining yet improbable element of the fictional film is that the character Astrid is a well-known comedian who publicly announces her pregnancy and subsequently her decision to terminate it: all of which is a narrative tool. As a person in public life, Astrid legitimises the voyeuristic gaze of the viewer who peers into the intimate relational life of this family.

Two experiences of pregnancy and familial relationships

The plot of both films is structured by the embodied temporalities of a pregnancy, the ambivalent intuitions of the individuals, and the complex consequences for familial and social relationships.

The story of *Week 23* starts with intimate images showing the love between Rahel and Ohad. It then leads us through expansive fields of hope and anticipation in the first months of pregnancy. The physicians have discovered that Rahel is pregnant with identical twins. There are actually two "little peanuts", as Rahel calls them, writing in her diary. "I didn't know where it would lead, and then we found out we had identical twins," says Ohad. "I come from a background of art as well as film, and the idea of identical twins sounded like a good concept for making art" (Ahituv 2016). However, soon afterwards, in week 23, a shock diagnosis changes everything: one of the twins has died in utero. Physicians tell the couple that the other twin carries a high risk of being severely disabled as a result of being together with the dead foetus. Doctors say that in the rare cases when the second foetus does not die immediately, it is almost certain to be born with severe brain damage and other disabilities. They are unanimous in recommending that the couple should terminate the pregnancy, because the risk of allowing the child to be born is too high. This places the couple in a critical dilemma. Rahel resists the physician's recommendation; her feelings are very clear. The journey that started with such hope turns into an emotional roller-coaster with no rescue in sight.

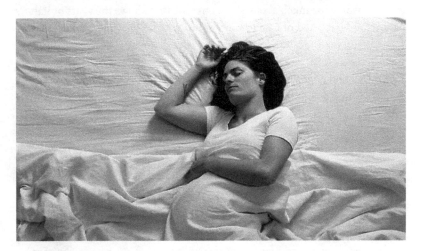

Still from Week 23 (2016) שבוע. © Ohad Milstein

Should they end the pregnancy by aborting the surviving foetus? Beyond her maternal instincts and her faith, she has – or so it seems to her, and within this social context – no rational argument for refusing an abortion. In the background of the two families there is however a conflict between different views on the morality of terminating the pregnancy. The families are rooted in two different cultural contexts in two different countries. Rahel's parents live in the German-speaking part of Switzerland, where she grew up in a protected environment, imbued with religion. Her father is a bishop. In their view, all life should be cherished: it comes from God and therefore has a right to be. We should not interfere in divine plans. Rahel's parents believe that even a child with disabilities is a child of God and should have a chance to live. They are very concerned about the pressure Rahel feels as a result of the medical counselling that she has received. Ohad's mother, on the other hand, lives in Israel, and cannot understand Rahel's reluctance to terminate in this situation. Her view is that if Rahel waits too long, it will be too late. It is self-evident that she should abort, since the child would be disabled for its whole life, and would suffer. This is not a question for her. In her earlier life, as she explains in the film, she has had abortions herself, has lived through the pain and probably also the moral quandaries accompanying them. Her own subjective strategy of normalisation is not to worry too much about abortions. The film shows the visits of Rahel's parents to Israel, and of Ohad's mother to Switzerland. The parents respectfully explain their ideas and thoughts to each other. Caught between different sides, Rahel is torn. She knows that Ohad wants a child with whom he can go swimming and diving, and that by keeping a child with disability she is likely to destroy this dream and burden the family. At the same time, she is acutely aware of her parents' position. In the end, it seems that she is not so much evaluating positions or the value of life, but rather has the strong intuition that her "little peanut" is actually fine. But does such intuition count?

The turning point comes when both Rahel and Ohad start to resist the power of measurements, tests and the physicians, and define the terms of the pregnancy for themselves. They resist medicalisation and take back control over their situation. The medical system is overwhelmingly powerful, and therefore resistance is very difficult, until Ohad discovers a significant mistake. Repeatedly scrutinising the medical papers they have received from the physicians, he checks the calculations. He discovers inconsistencies that can be explained only if numbers have been swapped. This discovery proves to Ohad and Rahel that the medical system is not perfect, or at least not as perfect as their self-confident physicians believed it to be. It promises to perfect procreation by identifying imperfection before birth, but the system itself is not perfect. Humans and human-made practices, including the work of physicians, are prone to fallibility and error.

In this situation, Ohad's mother too changed her mind. She concedes that it is now too late for an abortion. Rahel brings the child to term. The story ends in relief: a healthy baby is born.

24 *Wochen* is about Astrid's second pregnancy (see Absalon 2020; Institut für Kino und Filmkultur, no date). Astrid is a successful professional comedian, a person in public life. In sketches in front of large audiences, she laughs about her big belly. She is a bright, spirited person, and so is the atmosphere of the film. This does not change after a test reveals that the baby will be a boy – and he will have Down syndrome. She immediately obtains the information that there can be very mild forms of Down syndrome, and also that a late abortion is legally possible.

Sometime later in the pregnancy, and still in a state of uncertainty, Astrid and her partner Markus, together with their daughter Nele, go to a concert where the performers are young people with Down syndrome. The soft chant of the choir is contrasted with a hard, loud beat in a disco where Astrid goes the following night. Astrid and Markus decide to have their child, and also to announce it to everybody: "We want it!" ("*Wir wollen es!*") The response from family members and friends is mostly embarrassed silence. But Astrid's mother, Nele's grandmother, offers to help the young family in this difficult time, and moves into Markus and Astrid's house. But the situation is tense; the grandmother is too intrusive, and she later moves out again. Everybody around the couple seems to have an opinion. But then a second examination shows that the child will be born with a serious heart defect (two holes, no septum, one shared heart valve) that will require immediate surgery after birth and major open-heart surgery later on when the ventricles are large enough. This throws the world of the still-resilient parents out of equilibrium. During a visit to a neonatology ward, Astrid sees tiny premature babies in incubators and wonders whether it might be better for her child not to be. Two mothers recognise the famous comedian Astrid, whom they had heard on radio saying she wanted to keep her baby despite the disability, and praise her for this. But Astrid, who now knows about the heart defect and the future surgeries, is no longer sure. Her determination to keep the baby is dwindling and she decides to have a late abortion. In an emotional scene on the balcony, she confirms her decision by smoking a cigarette, something she had avoided during her pregnancy in order to protect the foetus. Then she screams out her emotion.

A midwife prepares her for the operation by graphically describing all the important details (injection of potassium chloride into the heart). It will be an ordeal for her. In the expectation of losing her child, she knows that it will be difficult to say goodbye to it. In a carefully worded dialogue Astrid asks the midwife what she would have decided in her situation. The midwife answers: "You can only make such a decision if you have to. No one can take it away from you, and no one is allowed to judge it."[1] Astrid says: "I would have liked to have made a different decision. – But I couldn't, I just can't. Maybe because I'm not strong enough, or too scared."[2] She hopes that her decision is the right one –

---

1   "So eine Entscheidung, die kann man nur treffen, wenn man sie treffen muss. Das kann einem keiner abnehmen und da darf auch keiner drüber urteilen."

2   "Ich hätte mich so gern anders entschieden. – Aber es ging, es geht einfach nicht. Vielleicht weil ich nicht stark genug bin, oder zu viel Angst hab."

for the child and for the family. The film ends with a second broadcast radio interview, and Astrid saying: "I don't know if it was right or wrong. I aborted my child in the seventh month."[3]

One of the most striking scenes in 24 *Wochen* is the moment when Markus realises that Astrid already has decided – against their previous agreement – to end the pregnancy. "Is it your decision or ours?" he asks. Astrid replies: "It's mine."[4] That is the only moment in the whole film where Markus loses his temper, smashing objects from a bookshelf. He feels excluded from what he had believed to be a family project. For Astrid, at the end of the day her pregnancy is hers alone. – This resonates with the end of the film, where the uniqueness of a woman's decision is emphasised. The midwife's words ("You can only make such a decision if you have to. No one can take it away from you, and no one is allowed to judge it.") echoes a societal attitude towards "medically" motivated abortions and to prenatal diagnosis in general: it is the woman's sole responsibility. She is in a highly personal conflict and resolves this conflict through the means of prenatal diagnosis and possible termination. The respect granted to the woman, the recognition of her right to autonomy, has a flipside: she is on her own, and others refuse to share responsibility. It is her decision and she has only herself to blame. Nobody else is allowed to judge it, not even her partner or other family members.

In contrast, the family in *Week 23* is highly judgemental. Through their Christian faith, Rahel's Swiss parents know the right thing to do. Terminating a pregnancy because the child is expected to have a disability is not, and never can be, a justified option for them. Ohad's mother, on the other hand, is very clear about her belief that under these circumstances, the pregnancy should be terminated. Her later agreement with the decision to keep the child – because she also thinks that it is now too late – is important for the couple. Harmony in the family is re-established. The ordeal that Rahel goes through is compassionately shared by Ohad, even though he follows his mother's opinion, at least at first. But soon he ardently contributes to the process of decision-making. He is the one who checks and rechecks the physicians' measurement protocols and discovers the mistake that stirs distrust in the medical prognosis.

---

3   "Ich weiss nicht, ob es richtig oder falsch war. Ich habe im siebten Monat mein Kind abgetrieben."

4   "Es ist deine oder unsere Entscheidung?" – "Es ist meine. "

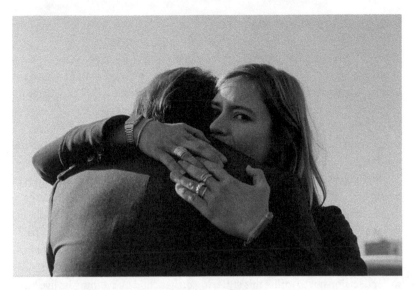

Still from 24 Wochen. © Friede Clausz / zero one film 2016.

While the morality of decision-making in 24 Wochen tends to rest on the woman's shoulders alone, but is shared within the family in Week 23, it is the German family that is presented as open and blatantly scrutinised in the public eye. Astrid is a public figure, tells her audiences about her pregnancy, gives radio interviews about her decision, and never claims to be right or justified. The story of Week 23 stays within the space of the family, and of the future parents' relationship. The family – both Swiss and Israeli – remains existentially important for the lives of Rachel and Ohad. Of course this family is also related to the two different socio-cultural contexts, but the feature film keeps it implicit, whereas in the documentary 24 Wochen this context is made excessively overt. The comedy show is a family enterprise, and so the family is an enterprise, and its moral intimacy is presented to the public. Yet this German family seems less integral to the overall process of how to decide.

Interrogating prenatal sociality

The two films could not provide a greater contrast in how they raise questions about anticipated familial relationships with the unborn. *24 Wochen* is an exemplary story of a model family, with a woman who takes a solitary decision that should not be judged by anybody; *Week 23* is an intimate story of a unique set of events, which does not in any way claim to be representative other than being real and authentic. But questions of fundamental human significance are present in both films.

Prenatal diagnosis is an advance attempt to get to know the child who is to be born. In this attempt to become capable of making a decision about continuing the pregnancy, the unforeseeable reappears. However medically informed (or as in Rahel and Ohad's case *mis*informed), the diagnosis is still only a guess at the chances of the surviving foetus. And it is not foreseeable how heart surgery will cause a child to suffer; the maternal compassion that leads to her decision not to inflict this suffering on her child by avoiding its live birth is not a reliable indicator of actual child suffering. The deal made between parents and fate under the promise of knowledge includes making hard decisions in conditions of uncertainty. Milstein's film *Week 23* does not simply investigate a difficult process of decision making but is, as the film-maker says in an interview, even more strongly about a disconnect between "parents' gut feelings and female intuition, on the one hand, and medical procedures that don't leave room for this. Moreover, Israeli society is wary of outliers. If you have an unborn child who may not be 100 per cent okay and you want to have it anyway, that's considered off the charts. Being weak and imperfect is shameful in Israel" (Ahituv 2016). Thus the film's themes are manifold: the disconnect between personal body experience and the medical apparatus, on the one hand, and on the other a society that tends to support selecting out a foetus with genetic aberrations or possible severe health problems. Within this context, a self-determined decision to keep a child with the prospect of disability goes virtually unsupported by family or society. This conflict is presented through the different attitudes of the family members. It is interesting and somewhat touching to see that Ohad's mother, who strongly supported an early abortion, relents in a practical but not unsupportive manner when she realises that the pregnancy will continue. "You should pursue the pregnancy, it's too late for an abortion."

The Israeli film, with its background of liberal policies towards prenatal diagnosis and termination if a condition has been detected in the foetus, focuses on the renunciation of a medically recommended termination; while the German film, with its background of restrictive policies towards prenatal diagnosis and termination if a condition has been detected in the foetus, highlights the pregnant woman's burdened – but in the end also confident – choice. The two films take no sides, nor can they be placed into categories of pro-choice or pro-life films about abortion (Köhne 2018).

Neither *Week 23* nor *24 Wochen* is a sober documentary about typical problems in pregnancy; both films demonstrate how extreme situations and difficult questions are embedded in familial and social relationships. The films show how a situation provoked by prenatal diagnosis may bring out special characteristics of people, shake up relationships, and insidiously influence our view of the world. The emotional shake-up is intensified by the familial and social context. In both films the pregnant woman is faced with a range of opinions about what to do. In *24 Wochen* the focus is strongly on how the couple makes their decision. Even though people in their close circle have opposing or supporting positions, the film rests on the couple's relationship, its conflicts and strengths. The observer in the film follows Astrid and Markus on their path of dealing with medical information, and having sudden insights into the opinions and attitudes of family members and friends towards disability. These are insights and expressed opinions we have not previously asked for, and which are mostly seen as taboo: for example, the outrage of the nanny of the existing daughter Nele, who suddenly quits her job because she finds the prospect of caring for a child with Down syndrome revolting. In the course of the film, the viewer learns quite a bit about the apparatus of medicine, the upsides and downsides of prenatal testing, and the possibilities of neonatological intensive care. Even though genetic disability can be tested for and may no longer be regarded as pure fate, it cannot be shut out of society or be isolated from family discussions. The film is therefore not just about late abortion, but even more about the conflicts between questions of prenatal genetic testing, what to hope for in future life, and how to count on family relationships. The issue of what to hope for in future life and in the family becomes apparent in both films. Yet how the individual opinions, intuitions and hopes are generated is rather different. In the film *Week 23*, it seems that the family is existentially involved in spite of all their differences, whereas in *24 Wochen* the family fundamentally provides the context. Both films depict the way that the pregnant women are caught between their personal intuition and the medical system. Whatever is decided in the end, the medical information that there is "something wrong" with the foetus is never innocuous and always concerns more than one being.

References

Absalon, Beate (2020): "Spätabbruch: Avenue." In: Wissenskultur 8, pp. 82–84. (https://avenue.jetzt/knappe_zeit/spaetabbruch/), accessed 16 June 2022.

Ahituv, Netta (2016): "The difficult pregnancy that spawned a beautiful documentary." In: Haaretz, June 29, 2016. (https://www.haaretz.com/israel-news/culture/2016-06-29/ty-article/.premium/a-difficult-pregnancy-that-spawned-a-beautiful-documentary/0000017f-e10b-d38f-a57f-e75b66ef0000), accessed 16 June 2022.

Berrached, Anne Zhora, interviewed by Patrick Wellinski (2016): "Abtreibungsdrama '24 Wochen': Verzweifelte Odyssee durch Ärztezimmer." In: Deutschlandfunk Kultur, September 17, 2016.

Köhne, Julia Barbara (2018): "Absentes vergegenwärtigen: Schwangerschaftsabbruch und Fötalimagologie in westlichen Filmkulturen seit den 1960er Jahren." In: Aylin Basaran/Julia B. Köhne/Klaudija Sabo/Christina Wieder (eds.), Sexualität und Widerstand. Internationale Filmkulturen, Vienna/Berlin: Mandelbaum, pp. 243–285.

Institut für Kino und Filmkultur (no date): 24 Wochen. (http://www.film-kultur.de/publikationen/24-wochen_kc.pdf), accessed 16 June 2022.

IV. Intertwining knowledge practice, epistemology and ethics

10. The Unconditionality of Parent-Child Relationships in the Context of Prenatal Genetic Diagnosis in Germany and Israel[1]

Hannes Foth

The relationships between parents and children are often characterized as being unconditional, unchosen or un-cancellable. All these descriptions are expressions of the fact that these relationships lack the leeway that would be normal in other relationships for choosing or rejecting them, or breaking them off – and they lack this leeway either completely or to a great extent. Adjectives of the absolute that refer to this certainly do have an empathic or poetic dimension, in that they often profess a *perceived* absoluteness, irrevocability or unconditionality. But this empathic dimension does not disqualify the expressions from being descriptive categories for parent-child relationships. Rather, as the following analysis is intended to show, they contain a kernel of truth which can be clarified by a differentiated analysis, and are also helpful in categorising and critically discussing numerous phenomena in the development of parent-child relationships and the founding of families.

The focus of this consideration will be on the category of unconditionality.[2] This, according to a first thesis, corresponds to a multidimensional, complementary and multilateral relational context, which may be present in varying configurations, and is largely moderated by models of good parenthood. Not least, the variability of the relational context of "unconditionality" can, according to a subsequent thesis, shed light on why unconditional relationships take different forms in different societies. While in the context of the German

---

1   This chapter was translated from German by Monica Buckland, including the quotations. Besides her, I would like to thank Christina Schües, who contributed most to its development, as well as my colleagues from the PreGGI project and the participants of the conferences where I had the opportunity to present some of its ideas.

2   On un-cancellable relationships, see Foth (2019).

debate about prenatal diagnosis, intact and loving parent-child relationships are often made dependent on the earliest possible and the prospective parents' most comprehensive love towards the child growing in its mother's womb, in the Israeli context the focus is more on safeguarding ideas of a fulfilling parent-child and family relationship by making arrangements before the child is born. These different approaches interact with reactions to the possibilities of prenatal diagnosis which are not completely distinct, but do display differences in emphasis and sometimes contradictory tendencies. For example, in the German controversy about the application of recent non-invasive prenatal testing (NIPT), concern about the overuse of prenatal diagnosis is ever-present, while the primarily professional discourse in Israel tends to pose the question of whether these tests contribute to a high standard of care.

New test methods offer important possibilities for reflecting on parent-child relations, as a recent quote by Braun points out:

> For a long time, but increasingly urgently, the question arises of how parent-child relationships are changing, as prospective parents are able to gain ever more knowledge about the probably genetic constitution of their future children (2016: 7).

Since 2011, the establishment of NIPT has been accompanied by both hopes and concerns (Hashiloni-Dolev/Nov-Klaiman/Raz 2019). As these tests only require a blood sample from the pregnant woman (through which cell-free foetal DNA can be obtained), they lack the risks associated with invasive methods such as amniocentesis. Moreover, they can be used early in pregnancy, from about the 8–9th week, and with the testing options constantly evolving beyond the initial focus on trisomies. Although their reliability still depends on the age of the pregnant woman and the objective of the test, many countries have considered their coverage by public health insurance, at least for trisomies 13, 18 and 21 (Löwy 2020). Increased use of prenatal testing thus becomes likely and justifies the concern about its impact on parent-child relations.

Methodologically speaking, the following reflections form an explorative philosophical essay, which is empirically inspired, but not yet adequately anchored in empirical terms. It emphasises a conceptual analysis, as well as reacting to tensions within comparative research into the social arrangements for childbearing, in order to draw initial conclusions.

Such a field of tension consists – in the first place – of a charged relationship between the vocabulary of unconditionality and the extension of prenatal diagnosis in combination with the possibility of abortion, i.e. with making the continuation of a pregnancy dependent on the expected state of the embryo, foetus or baby. A number of descriptive categories or conceptual framings have already been introduced into the debate for these reservations, such as the "tentative pregnancy" (Katz Rothman 1986), as well as the description considered to be often problematising, that of prenatal "selection", or the reverse, the euphemistic-sounding "selective reproduction" (Wilkinson 2010) and the less known "conditional parentage" (Efron/Lifshitz-Aviram 2020). This word-coining indicates both the descriptive and the more or less pronounced evaluative colouring of so-called thick terms, and thus already points towards the heated debates on prenatal diagnosis in bio(ethics), politics and society.

A further – second – field of tension arises out of the different (open ethical-political) discourses that refer to these developments, phenomena and categories. This applies, for one thing, to the discourse of concepts and ideals, particularly that of motherhood with feminist theory and care ethics; in these connections, unconditionality can easily be identified with categories of unconditional love or motherly love, although in feminist discourse these are treated with considerable ambivalence and are often associated with domestic self-sacrifice. On the other hand, particularly in Disability Studies and disability ethics, there are also demands for unconditional parenthood as the ideal of relationships for all concerned, or an important part of a culture of inclusion and welcome.

Finally – thirdly – there is the difficult question of what conclusions can be drawn from the coexistence of experienced or desired unconditionality and the contrasting reservations for the characterisation of different social arrangements for childbearing. For example, do (expecting) parents in some societies have a more unconditional relationship with their growing children – at least in the prenatal stage? Do others tend more strongly towards risking intact relationships? Or does the ostensible vocabulary of unconditionality conceal and burden the reality of parenthood, instead of illuminating and inspiring it?

This also shows how the comparison between Germany and Israel threatens to be both exciting and fraught with tension. Although public healthcare in both countries shows similarly high medical standards, there are significant differences in the way they handle the possibilities of reproductive medicine. But attempting to evaluate these quickly leads to the difficulties of judging, in which historical experiences play an important role for both countries, yet in very different ways. In reaction to the unparalleled crimes against humanity that were committed in so many areas of society, the successively evolved basic principles of German post-war policy and of many social movements include a desire to present a positive counter-model and, within the framework of what is possible at all, to make amends. More than to any other country we consider ourselves indebted here to Israel, the country that has become a homeland for many Jewish survivors of the Holocaust and their descendants.[3] Conversely, on the Israeli side, there is at least *one* important lesson of the Holocaust: developing one's own strengths (Hashiloni-Dolev/Raz 2010: 89, 97). The need to nip things in the bud, first and foremost in one's own country, driven by the extent of the crimes committed in Germany – this has no equivalent in the context of Israel, where the excesses and crimes were not committed by their own people, but suffered by them. Therefore, possible criticism from post-war German society is subject to particular difficulties[4]: for one thing, because the heirs of the perpetrators elevate themselves morally to become the critics of a society or political landscape that is, in a distinctive way, marked by the descendants of their victims; and for another, because they do it by virtue of a horizon of experience that these descendants do not share. Only a discussion that takes such differences into account, as well as the sensitive constellation of discourse, can be both critical and fruitful.

To be able to process these questions, irritations or even tensions, the first part of this essay undertakes a conceptual clarification of various levels and aspects of unconditionality, points out contrasting connections to it, and relates it to alternative concepts from prenatal care and prenatal diagnosis. The second part then addresses cultural-social variations in Germany and Israel, and finally discusses both descriptive and normative consequences of conceptual clarifications and comparative insights. Despite this superficially linear structure, the actual logic of thinking is cyclical, and returns repeatedly to particular issues and aspects of the topic rather than finalising them conclusively in each case.

1.1 Locating unconditionality and its counterparts

In a conceptual explication of unconditionality it is first important to specify what it does *not* mean. For example, it does not mean the unreasonable or naïve claim that something arises without pre-existing conditions, a *creatio ex nihilo*.

---

3   See Kloke (2005); and on scientific cooperation also Steinhauser, Gutfreund and Renn (2017).

4   Cf. the intoduction and chapter 12 of this volume.

Motherhood or parenthood, and the condition(s) of being born, of natality, are an age-old object of social and political concern and influence, framed by numerous parameters. Who becomes a parent, with whom, when, and how, are dependent on so many conditions and formed by so many perspectives that they demand their own treatises (Schües 2016; Schües/Foth 2019). But it is important to note that, despite all attempts to take control, pregnancy and the beginning of parenthood is a process with many unknowns that are not characteristic of or comparable to the development of other social relationships. In this comparative perspective on unconditionality, the term indicates the *characteristic absence* of particular reservations in the genesis, development and continuation of a relationship. Compared to the process of becoming friends, the genesis of the bodily parent-child relationship does not rest on gradually increasing affection for a concrete Other, a process driven by mutual sympathy. Such processes of becoming friends, or equally of romantic love, can swell to a *perception of unconditionality* in which the relationship to the other is no longer *subjectively* available for negotiation, or becomes the object of total devotion. In terms of society, however, both types of relationship remain subject to the *proviso* of continuing mutual affection and satisfaction, which enables disappointed friends and lovers to step back from their perceived unconditionality and continue the relationship under certain conditions only. The relationships between parents and children are different. Even if the developing child is the object of particular hopes, fantasies and expectations, the physical relationship which has already begun with the embryo/foetus in utero needs no agreements (so to speak) in order to develop further. At the same time, it is a relationship with an unknown human being about whom, despite any perceived closeness or attachment, little more is known than the story of its genesis, its anticipated human form, and initial processes that make themselves felt in the form of foetal movements.[5] Its more precise physical constitution is the object of sensations and only to a limited extent of knowledge. This (social-ontologi-

---

5   Mills puts this pointedly: "Except in rare cases of adoption of older children with already revealed and well-established personalities, the choice of a child is the choice of a pig in a poke. Gender, appearance, intelligence, talents, and temperament all appear to the parents as an unfolding surprise. Parents of two or more children are invariably astonished at the differences between individuals produced by the same parental genes and reared in the same family environment. We are still far away from the prospect of 'designer' children, tailormade to match parental expectations." (2003: 150–151)

cal) starting position is – or was – (objectively) largely one of unconditionality or the impossibility of controlling the course or the outcome of a pregnancy.

However, this starting point changes with the use of prenatal diagnosis which makes it possible for prospective parents to acquire more knowledge, or at least probabilities, about the constitution of their child, providing a basis on which to make decisions. It puts them in the position of knowing more about the developing child (the "glass belly", Hey 2012), such as its sex and its organic or genetic constitution, and the possible consequences of this for the child and its family. Prenatal diagnosis facilitates a focus on the technically measurable physical condition of the child as a basis for deciding whether to continue the pregnancy or not, provided there is the possibility of termination. In interaction with the law on abortion, or on tolerating it, prenatal diagnosis provides, alongside its therapeutic goals, the societal possibility to add a physical provision to the child's birth and in doing so to take a step back from unconditional parenthood. The subjective internalisation of this (objective) possibility is described by the term "tentative pregnancy".

In the triangular understanding of the parent-child relationship as the relationship of one parent to the child, the child to the parent, and possibly the parents to one another (in terms of the child), the physical reservation towards continuing a pregnancy lies on the level of the *responsivity of prospective parents*. This level should be differentiated from other sides of the multidimensional, complementary and multilateral relational contexts of unconditionality. It describes neither the level of an *irreversible* event (the causally irreversible biological-genetic-physical bringing about of one existence through another), nor the related social attribution of parenthood and childhood, with its often very limited exit opportunities. It is much more a form of pregnancy-related reaction and interaction of the prospective parents with the developing child, the complementary counterpart of which is the helplessness of the developing child (Schües 2016; Graumann 2010: 138). From the perspective of this being comes another dimension of unconditionality, which consists in the developing being having no choice but to be entrusted to this pregnant woman, or these prospective parents. The more opportunities are afforded to prospective parents, in order to make their reaction dependent on particular conditions, the more the social-ontological status of the possible child also shifts as a result of their decisions about whether to make use of these opportunities or not. Parental unconditionality is now no longer the reaction to the inevitability of how a pregnancy turns out, but a subjective decision, which might – and can – turn out differently. The social facilitation of prenatal diagnosis and the so-called "selective" termination of pregnancy implies in principle their permissibility, even if only within certain limits. Both factually and normatively, the unavailability of a particular outcome of a pregnancy is relativised, and thus the norm of the unconditional acceptance of any child is also made optional. But this means that even within the triangle of two possible parents and child, the internalisation of unconditionality between the prospective parents can turn out differently; if we take a step back from the narrow focus on the parent-child dyads, the reaction of possible further children in the family also becomes relevant, as does that of other members of the family and the social environment, which affirms particular norms or sends conflicting messages.[6] This is what I refer to when I describe unconditionality as "multilateral".

Now the physical reservation that prenatal diagnosis offers prospective parents, or even suggests to them, can be interpreted in different ways. For those who label it *prenatal selection*, which is usually critical and problematising in Germany, the reservation often implies a negative value judgement of a life with disability. From the assumed perspective of the possible child or its parents or family, the child's life, for itself or for others involved, is not considered sufficiently worth living to continue with the – originally wanted – pregnancy. The judgement that individuals make may be free or socially prejudiced, and either way results in the selecting out of foetuses with particular physical characteristics, i.e. it has eugenic dimensions as well.

Equating the physical reservation with (eugenic) selection is, however, also open to criticism (Foth 2021). Particularly in Germany, this term is strongly associated with mass murder driven by the state, and a particular, medically veiled contempt for humanity directed against people with disabilities, at times with especially drastic devaluations of their worth. There yawns a considerable gap between such judgements and the often complex motives of pregnant women and others involved in pregnancy, making use of prenatal diagnosis and contemplating a termination. Comparative studies of such motives demonstrate a wide spectrum of concerns and perspectives, which in many cases are about the compatibility of a child with special needs and one's own capabilities and wishes (self-care), as well as the perspectives of other

---

6   The documentary film *Week 23*, by the Israeli director Ohad Milstein, about the pregnancy of his Swiss wife Rahel, exemplifies how differences become apparent, both between the couple and in their families, and in the changing medical context (see chapter 9 in this volume).

family members (concern for third parties).[7] It may be that in such considerations, misleading views about disabilities and their conflation with suffering play a key role, and that, as some authors argue (Asch/Wassermann 2005), prospective parents often underestimate their own capacities. But this does not justify reducing a decision that is often difficult for one's conscience and one's life – the decision to end a pregnancy – to a negative value judgement. This, at least, is implied by the regulatory path that Germany has taken, which rejects disability as the ultimate justification for an abortion (embryopathic indication), and instead recognises only the possible impacts of a disability on the bodily or mental condition of the pregnant woman and her individual situation as a justification (social-medical indication). The individual perspective that leads to a particular abortion does not imply the generalised judgement that it would be better for other pregnancies as well to reach a similar decision.[8] Rather, it is precisely the cases of parents who – often after much agonising – use prenatal diagnosis in order not to have an additional child with special needs that show how complex such decision-making, and how open the results, can be.

From this perspective, deciding for or against a pregnancy does not automatically imply a particular value judgement, even though the risk remains of being drawn into making it, for example through an uncritical routinisation of prenatal diagnosis. It is also at the root of a scepticism towards the efforts of some liberal authors to use "selective reproduction" as an umbrella term for a whole series of procedures that influence how a pregnancy turns out, and discussing them as possibly welcome options in having children (Wilkinson 2010). In place of the sometimes overcritical and negatively loaded word "selection", the wording is now uncritical, reductive and downplaying (Rehmann-Sutter 2021), making it easy to lose critical distance from the logic of selection, which may not be (openly) eugenic in nature but becomes problematic in its consumer-orientation, or when it takes an economic or perfectionist stance. This is addressed in public discourse using phrases such as "the child as a product", "designer baby" or "perfect child". None of these wordings does justice to the phenomenal experiences of prospective parents, who do not understand

---

7   See chapter 8 of this volume.

8   As Asch and Wasserman make clear, opting for termination does not imply making a similar decision at a later point: "A woman may be willing to abort after eighteen weeks but not after twenty two; she may be willing to abort, but not to put an impaired newborn up for adoption." (2005: 194).

their willingness to terminate a pregnancy either as a negative, generalisable judgement or as a corrective on the path towards their plan of parenthood, but as a way out of an emergency in which they unexpectedly find themselves.

In the wake of the "selective reproduction" approach, the authors Yael Efron and Pnina Lifshitz-Aviram (2020) have suggested establishing the term "conditional parentage" for some of these phenomena. In addition to prenatal phenomena such as preimplantation diagnostics (PGD) and selective abortion, it also encompasses experiences of postnatal parenthood under reservation, particularly in the case of adoption. Using the examples of Israel, the United Kingdom and other European countries, the authors argue that in all of these fields, Western states enable and foster the right to make parenthood conditional on the constitution of the child. They describe this legal phenomenon, or the underlying wish of prospective parents, as "conditional parentage". It refers to the decision about "whether" to become parents and not "how" to parent, like so-called "conditional parenting" as a kind of guiding through conditional love and acknowledgement as part of bringing up a child. The authors themselves expend a lot of energy on presenting "conditional parentage" as an expression of contemporary and well-understood eugenics, which should be implemented cautiously so as not to repeat any mistakes of the past. The authors' other provocation consists in recognising and welcoming the conditionality of possible parents implied in granting and exercising rights to choose, as these serve valuable individual and societal goals. This signifies a strengthening of the conditionality of parenthood, which runs contrary to the idea and the ideal of unconditional acceptance of every child, and that makes it necessary to analyse the associated qualities more deeply. I will now undertake this analysis and return to consider the term "conditional parentage" as part of my conclusions.

1.2 Unfolding unconditionality

The descriptive-normative dual character of "unconditionality" is based on its assessment as an important prerequisite for parent-child relationships and for families, the loss of which should be mourned or – if possible – compensated for. This ambivalence is already clearly expressed in the term "tentative pregnancy". For Katz Rothman, the establishment of tentativity in pregnancy injects a fundamental conflict between the actual and often socially supported process of bonding with the developing foetus, and the willingness to break this bond if necessary, in reaction to a prenatal diagnosis.

> The problem, or one of the problems, with the technology of amnio-centesis and selective abortion is what it does to us, to mothers and to fathers and to families. It sets up a contradiction in definitions. It asks women to accept their pregnancies and their babies, to take care of the babies within them, and yet be willing to abort them. We ask them to think about the needs of the coming baby, to fantasise about the baby, to begin to become the mother of the baby, and to be willing to abort the genetically damaged fetus. At the same time. For twenty to twenty-four weeks. Women suffer in this contradiction of demands (1985: 190).

This conflict has direct potential for the suffering of ambivalent feelings and an ordeal for the persons concerned instead of a pregnancy that might otherwise have proceeded without any worries, alongside the possible indirect psychological repercussions of a decision to terminate or not. It could also mean a loss of or possible damage to the resulting parent-child relationships. This *reverberation* is feared by other authors too, either through a lasting weakening of the relationships and the attitudes and abilities of the parents that protect them – e.g. Sandel's true parenthood as a "school of humility" (2007: 85) – or as a latent cause of conflict in later relationships:

> A child who knew how anxious her parents were that she have the "right" genetic makeup might fear that her parents' love was contingent upon her expression of these characteristics (Anderson 1990: 428; cf. Kittay/Kittay 2000: 169, 182ff.).

These conflicts may not lie solely on the parent-child or child-parent levels, but may also be carried "socially invasively" into the parents' relationships, as one recent publication on NIPT in Germany suggests, and thus they raise both the direct and the indirect potential of suffering and breakdown (cf. Reinsch/König/Rehmann-Sutter 2021: 12).

The topos of a tentative pregnancy also serves to make clear some ambivalences in the feminist discourse that affect the way we deal with the vocabulary of unconditionality. Ultimately, tentative pregnancy accompanies one of the central achievements of feminist demands, the right to abortion. The watershed here is the already mentioned "selective" abortion, in which a basically wanted pregnancy is then terminated after all, under the physical reservation in response to a finding (cf. Waldschmidt 2006). While some authors defend this as extended freedom of decision, others, and particularly representatives of the disability rights movement and disability studies scholars, distance themselves from it. They demand that every possible child be viewed as a gift who deserves to be loved unconditionally and made welcome, also the family should not be an exclusive club, and its moral foundation consists precisely in its inclusivity, i.e. for the child to be accepted unconditionally and to be able to sense this for the whole of its life, knowing it and being able to draw strength from it (cf. Asch/Wasserman 2005: 202–203; cf. Kittay/Kittay 2000: 169, 182, 192).

Added to the feminist ambivalence towards selective termination is an ambivalence towards the category of unconditionality – above all if this is interpreted in the light of *unconditional motherly love*. The ambivalence towards this concept of love is built on its interconnection with particular ideas of motherhood (or womanhood) and the understanding of this as ideological (Mullin 2006; Schütze 2010; Diabaté 2015). Unconditional love approaches (prospective) mothers as a presumed *natural* requirement and justifies and explains their *sole or primary responsibility* for childcare and management of the household. It serves to exacerbate domestic self-sacrifice, dependency and exploitation. Instead, feminist voices demand an understanding of motherhood as part of a wider network of care, which assures mothers of the conditions in which they are able to continue along their personal and professional paths, or the conditions of their self-respect (Gedge 2011). Many authors fall back on other terms to describe parenthood (Mullin 2006). Parenthood then has the character of a commitment or a particular form in which the developing child is recognised (Schües 2016; Wiesemann 2015). Schües, for example, draws on the "gift" metaphor to illuminate the acceptance of a newborn irrespective of its conditions (for although, or perhaps precisely because, its vulnerability puts it at the mercy of its parents, it also makes a multitude of demands of them).

These considerations often take place in the horizon of ideas about parental care and responsibility. They specify how prospective parents' response or reaction might look if it is to represent an *affirmative* response to the child growing in its mother's womb and this child's needs.[9] They may serve to avoid the

---

9   This wording is inspired by Waldenfels' reflections on responsivity (1994: 75; 2012), insofar as prospective parents (have to) react to the course of the pregnancy, by taking or refusing to take decisions, they "respond" in a broad sense to the situation and the implied demands of the developing child; in a more narrow sense, however, respon-

abbreviations and distortions of the understanding of parental unconditionality laid down in the concept of unconditional love. For, in analysing what it is that in my view shows an unconditional parental response, four categories or groups in addition to love dominate: the most prominent expresses the unreserved decision in favour of this child (giving birth to it, and taking on parenthood), and terms such as acceptance, acknowledgement or welcoming stand for this, as also "that parents must appreciate [...] the uniqueness of their children" (Asch/Wasserman 2005: 209). The next emphasises above all the act of caring, attentive care, support, playing a protective role, and devotion up to the extreme case of self-sacrifice; a further category is best described as commitment, and expresses the responsibility and duty that prospective parents take on towards the children in their care, or the promise they make to them (Schües 2021; Wiesemann 2015); finally, temporal categories of duration point in two possible directions, i.e. to remain unconditional for as long as possible, or to commit as soon as possible, perhaps even at the point of wanting a pregnancy (cf. Asch/Wasserman 2005: 202). These five groups of categories and their different versions are at the heart of a conception of unconditional responsivity, while any further features that often form stumbling blocks for the feminist approach, such as its naturalness (which expresses the idea that an unconditional response is a biological mechanism, is self-rewarding and has some authoritative force) or exclusivity (which sees the mother or the parents in a unique or privileged position to provide these qualities), can be dissociated from it. Thus, it becomes clear how the possible aspects of unconditional responsivity can separate from one another, for example if a bond is felt in the sense of tender care, but commitment is withheld, or if there is a feeling of obligation but not of true joy about the pregnancy, or when earlier reservations are given up in the light of growing level of care (see above, Fn. 8).

By differentiating the possible dimensions of concepts of unconditional responsivity or parenthood in this way, it becomes clear how they can be challenging or all-encompassing to a greater or lesser degree, and how they can be intertwined in different ways with the ideals of parenthood.

---

sivity denotes accepting this situation and these demands, in contrast to the attempt to withdraw from them.

1.3 Gaps in the concept

The main problem of such concepts of unconditional responsivity, however, remains the lack of contextualisation, or their indeterminacy in the relational context of the individual, family and society. While it is clear that the form of responsivity is unconditional in the sense that it is not subject to the condition of the physical constitution of the foetus and is thus also independent of associated ideas of quality or performance, other aspects of decision-making by prospective parents remain unaddressed. These include the personal connection to professional or other biographical goals, or to the existing demands of the family or level of social support. Sometimes it is the parents who already have a disabled child and so can hardly be suspected of making value judgements about life, who are most torn between wanting to encounter unconditionally the child developing in a further pregnancy, and the worry that having another disabled child would be too much of a burden or would lead to competition for care (Nippert/Horst 1994: 39–44). Therefore, it is in fact the existing obligations that can cause a pregnancy to be called into question.

Nor does the notion of unconditionality offer a clear orientation for how to deal with anticipatory compassion, in which prospective parents paint a future bleak picture for a possibly disabled child, an existence full of suffering, and doubt whether it really is good for the child to be born. These considerations run the risk of underestimating their own capacities as well as the potentials of both society and of the child, and serve a kind of self-deception (Asch/ Wasserman 2005: 181). Additionally, in the context of Germany these considerations are burdened by the massive abuse of similar justifications during the Nazi-era "euthanasia" programme, and are therefore open to particular mistrust. Nevertheless, the fact is that this motive can play a significant role in prospective parents' thinking (Nippert/Horst 1994; pro familia Bundesverband 2018) and it appears questionable to assume that such cases generally involve a form of self-deception. In principle, what follows is the difficult situation of deciding to terminate a pregnancy on the grounds of a concern for the possible child as well (on this, see Hashiloni-Dolev/Shkedi 2007; DER 2013, Dissenting Position 2).

The gaps in the concept of unconditional responsivity, and the potentials for conflict, might perhaps be bridged by a concept of responsibility. As a normative category, responsibility is well suited to identifying complex or poorly defined areas that can only be grasped to a limited extent by explicit guidelines on how to act and how to be. In addition, there is a close conceptual relationship with the notion of responsivity. The concept of responsibility is however not established on unconditional responsivity, as becomes clear looking at the concept of prenatal "genetic responsibility", which often relates directly to reproduction (Lipkin/Rowley 1974; Leefmann/Schaper/Schicktanz 2017: 2). The concept demands that, in view of the possible presence of genetic deviations or defects, appropriate precautions must be taken either before a pregnancy commences or during its course. The idea of genetic responsibility has some roots in societies or communities where particular genetic diseases have or have had higher prevalence, and potential parents can have their carrier status tested in advance (on carrier screening, see Raz/Schicktanz 2016: 46ff.). The concept can however be generalised beyond this, and require prospective parents to check the genetic status of their offspring at various pre-birth stages and, if necessary, intervene to prevent the birth. Since the concept favours knowing over not-knowing, and the taking of extensive precautions rather than accepting a pregnancy and letting it happen, and since it can be associated with ideas of optimisation, the concept is particularly controversial in Germany – in contrast to Israel (cf. Remennick 2006: 48).

2.1 The example of Israel

Seen from Germany, Israeli society and the way it deals with pregnancy, birth and the family offers some unusual perspectives. For one thing, there is a strong "(pro)natalism", that is, a widespread fixation on having children and founding families (Gross/Ravitsky 2003: 251f.), which is reflected in the very high birth rates for a Western country (3.11 children per woman in 2016), even among secular Jewish women (Okun 2016), as well as in numerous other phenomena; these include the particular significance of shared sabbath meals in Jewish families (Münch 2017), and, to add some rather anecdotal impressions, the special child-friendliness of Israeli restaurants or the way people mention how many children and grandchildren they have when they introduce themselves. The traditional, historical, social and political reasons for this orientation have already been unpacked in numerous articles (Hashiloni-Dolev and others) and will not be repeated here. It is accompanied by a strong focus on the family, shown in comparatively frequent family contact and marked interdependence (Kagitcibasi/Ataca/Diri 2010, Hashiloni-Dolev 2018). The promise of happiness and the model of a good life associated with natalism and family orientation leads to a glorification of parenthood over the possibility of remaining consciously child-free, for women in particular (Donath 2015). It does not expect of prospective parents, particular mothers, to abstain from professional paths, but accepts the dual-earner household as normal, not least as a response to the high cost of living for many Israeli families.

> The basic assumption of Israeli women from all population categories, including the ultra-orthodox, is that family and outside work can be combined. Thus, the employment of mothers with young children is a rather common phenomenon in Israel (Lavee/Katz 2003: 204).

It is also taken as read that care tasks will be shared out among different members of the family (Lavee/Katz 2003). This family orientation is also very inclusive and open to the use of assisted reproductive technologies, single parenthood (with a sperm donor), same-sex parents[10] and, not least, late pregnancies at an advanced age. Even postmortem parenthood is made possible through the freezing of sperm and eggs.

For another thing, the State of Israel, with its genetic screening programmes and wide-ranging prenatal testing, strives to make the birth of children with genetic deviations or disorders preventable (Raz 2018). In contrast to Germany, the expansion of these programmes since the 1970s has been associated with the targeted prevention of heritable gene defects (Zlotogora et al. 2016) that occur frequently in particular Jewish or Israeli communities and that often have an indisputable potential to cause suffering. First and foremost is Tay Sachs syndrome, which as a result rarely occurs now, along with Betathalassemia. This has been implemented both through pre-conception carrier screening[11] and through prenatal screening programmes. In comparison with Germany, where prenatal screening programmes attract considerable mistrust, forms of state-supported gene tests are normal for Israelis, many of whom use them individually (e.g. before marrying). This willingness to undergo genetic tests continues with antenatal care, at least for the majority of the non-ultra-orthodox Jewish population for whom abortion is in principle an option.

---

10   This inclusivity refers to (assisted) pregnancy, but not to marriage (Knaul 2016), which in Germany is precisely the opposite.

11   Collected under the "national carrier screening programme for reproductive purposes", which is partially covered by health insurance funds (see Zlotogora et al. 2016).

Israeli women who question prenatal screening and advocate more natural and women-controlled models of childbearing are currently in a
minority, and their voice is seldom heard (Remennick 2006: 49).

Although the Israeli abortion law is strict *de jure*, in that the assent of a committee is necessary, *de facto* it shows a very high rate of acceptance and includes
embryopathic indications (Rimon-Zarfaty/Jotkowitz 2012). This kind of "selective" abortion based on a possible impairment of the child is not subject to
stigmatisation or public criticism (ibid.: 27). While the political and medical
provision of prenatal testing is based on the principle of informed self-determination, and the provision of medical information and recommendations is
supposed to be non-directive, the interplay of wide-ranging testing, a *de facto*
liberal abortion law, and social conditions in which providing care for a child
with a disability is difficult, combine to generate a clear preference for avoiding
having impaired children, even among the medical staff providing advice (cf.
Zlotogora 2014: 93; Efron/Lifshitz-Aviram 2020: 26). This applies to the secular,
liberal, middle class or upper middle class Jewish population at least; attitudes
are different, and terminations often not considered, among very religious or
ultra-Orthodox families and communities, as well as in Arab or other non-Jewish ethnic groups.[12]

Israeli disability rights groups have become more significant over the last
decade, and draw upon the UN Convention on the Rights of Persons with Disabilities, which Israel has also recently ratified.[13] However, these groups rarely
focus their criticism on the prenatal sector, and some even call for prenatal
testing to be expanded. There is no indication of a critical distance from official policy and medicine, even in the form of an inherited mistrust because of
a state extermination policy and its support from medicine, as in Germany.[14]
Criticism of rigid ideas of normality in medicine and society, or of equating
disability with suffering, are much rarer than in Germany, where they are part
of the official discourse surrounding prenatal diagnosis. It is hardly surprising

---

12   Ultra-Orthodox pregnant women often interpret termination to show a lack of faith in
      God and the task he has imposed, and is thus experienced as a spiritual crisis (Teman/
      Ivry/Bernhardt 2011: 78); prenatal unconditionality thus appears as the expression of
      unconditional trust in God, or a deeper level of relationship, i.e. with God, and thus
      enjoys appropriate recognition in the community.
13   On Disability, see chapter 6 in this volume.
14   Care for pregnant women is largely provided by hospitals; midwives are also trained
      nurses, and home births are rare (Raz 2008: 28; Brusa/Barilan 2018).

that the prevention of suffering (and not eugenic selection) is often named as a goal of the prenatal programme (and of the human geneticists involved) (cf. Hashiloni-Dolev/Raz 2010: 97).

The testing strategy also differs from that in Germany. In Israel, for example, a screening program for Down syndrome and other trisomies is well established (Zlotogora/Haklai/Leventhal 2007) and is covered by health insurance, through a mixture of non-invasive and invasive testing as part of the so-called "Health Basket". This basket also covers non-invasive first trimester screening (FTS) and invasive amniocentesis in combination with the chromosomal microarray (CMA) analytical procedure, which in contrast to conventional chromosome analysis is able to show even the tiniest changes (Müller-Egloff 2017: 458f.). As a result, Jewish children with Down syndrome are mostly born into the ultra-Orthodox community (Zlotogora 2014: 88). In Germany, although FTS is often used, and perhaps sometimes covered by the health funds – the data on this are not always clear – they are *not* an explicit part of health insurance cover, while CMA tends to be used very cautiously and is not recommended by the professional medical associations for routine use (Müller-Egloff 2017: 459). The routinisation of this testing in Israel indicates that the widest possible testing is encouraged, and the risk of miscarriage caused by higher rates of invasive testing is accepted in favour of gaining information (although it is argued that this risk through routinising the procedure is extremely small, which contradicts the figures circulating internationally). With this backdrop of established standards and priorities, the alternative of integrating NIPT, introduced in 2012, into the Health Basket (at current conditions in terms of costs, reliability and test spectrum), although certainly desired from many sides, does not appear attractive enough in terms of health policy. It could even be counterproductive, if to prevent the risk of miscarriage it were to result in recourse to a reduced and less reliable testing spectrum and thus "underprovision" of prenatal diagnosis.[15]

Three of the most important conflicts that the German regulation of the prenatal sector had to overcome are interpreted differently in the Israeli context, and are weaker. This applies first to the personification of the embryo or foetus, second to the danger of heteronomy (through family, state, society), and

---

15   This interpretation is based on the situation that NIPT has twice been proposed for the Health Basket and rejected, and on impressions from professional presentations at events in the PreGGI project (cf. chapter 3 of this volume).

third to the culture of welcome in society, which links the parents' decisions in individual cases with the social fate of people with disabilities.

Embryos or foetuses are not recognised in Israeli law as autonomous legal entities. At first they are considered to be part of the pregnant woman, and then gradually develop into a person, but formally it is only at birth that they acquire their own legal status (Rimon-Zarfaty/Raz/Hashiloni-Dolev 2011: 217). Although many Israelis perceive the foetus to be an autonomous organism as the pregnancy advances, and think of it more as its own person when its movements are felt by the pregnant woman, these attributions tend to occur later than in comparative studies from countries such as the USA or Australia (ibid: 222). Another comparison with European countries observes that "Israeli women were most likely to think that a developing baby acquires human dignity with birth and that a developing fetus is not yet a human being" (Fischmann 2011: 59). This might be reflected in the professional discourse, in stronger reservations about an unreflected way of speaking about an unborn life, baby or child. German abortion law's fundamental conflict between mother and unborn child therefore collapses, or is at least weakened. Both positions are rarely seen as being in need of protection against outside influence as well.

Unconditional parental affection towards the born child, in the form of unconditional love and being embedded within the family in a "system of mutual love and caring" (Hashiloni-Dolev 2018: 123), is certainly expected and highly regarded in Israel, and "conditional love" possibly understood as offensive (cf. Weiss 1994; Watzman 2005).[16] Nevertheless there appears to be a significant difference between the prenatal and postnatal phases, at least among secular Jewish Israelis.[17] The resistance to unconditional responsivity implied in the topos of a tentative pregnancy does not appear as a risk to the relationship between parents and children, but as a way to harmonise different desires, goals and interests. The final acceptance of the developing foetus as a future child and family member is held back; motives of anticipated compassion, as well as care and responsibility, also for other family members, may also play a role

---

16   According to Weiss (1994), the focus on healthy children without impairment is so widespread in Israel that it prevents many parents who unexpectedly have a disabled child from accepting them; the study, "Conditional love: parents' attitudes toward handicapped children" is however not uncontested (cf. Watzman 2005).

17   On divergent ideas of so-called "New Age" mothers, or religious but not ultra-Orthodox pregnant women, see Rimon-Zarfaty (2014).

here. In this perspective the physical reservation is not perceived as a threat to family cohesion, but rather as a possible way to generate it.

In combination with a reluctance to personify the foetus and accept it unconditionally, the widespread idea of "genetic responsibility" (Remennick 2006: 48) elevates preventing the birth of a child with a genetic impairment almost into a duty. The decision of the individual prospective parents is often linked to the idea that a disabled child will be a burden on the family and on society (Hashiloni-Dolev/Raz 2010: 97). So a social pressure becomes clear, which (prospective) parents may feel if they decide against using prenatal diagnosis and to accept any child unconditionally (see Rimon-Zarfaty 2014).

2.2 The example of Germany

The population of Germany is almost ten times as large as that of Israel and there are also ten times as many organisations that (want to) have a say in prenatal diagnosis. In comparison with Israel, prenatal diagnosis is disputed terrain in Germany. Not just because of German history and the above-mentioned tensions in regulating antenatal care and abortion, but also because of different paths of policy implementation. In Israel many competences are concentrated (vertically) in the Ministry of Health, while in Germany they are delegated (horizontally) to committees with a corporatist tradition, such as the German Federal Joint Committee (Gemeinsamer Bundesauschuss, G-BA).[18] As the process for the health funds covering NIPT demonstrated, these committees do not have access to reliable data on the status of prenatal diagnosis, so that the intended provision of the Maternity Guidelines cannot be compared to provision established in practice, nor can reliable scenarios be extrapolated from them (TAB 2019: 192). In addition to ethical and political polarisations, the discourse is thus conducted under dubious conditions (Scharf et al. 2019). Nevertheless, the G-BA has approved amending the Maternity Guidelines in favour of NIPT, setting the future course in several interesting directions. Foremost, there is increased individualisation of the indication for prenatal diagnosis. The classification of a "risk pregnancy", which justifies additional tests – long criticised for its tendency to spread and its unsettling effect – has been renamed "pregnancy with particular risks" and the indication for the newly

---

18   Neither implementation programme accords with the idea of a "republican discourse", which some call for (cf. Braun 2005: 44; see also chapter 5 in this volume).

added NIPT made dependent on the personal circumstances of the pregnant woman (cf. G-BA 2019; Rehmann-Sutter/Schües 2020). How practical limitations might make this focus on individual cases collapse back into routinisation remains to be seen.

In contrast to the Israeli discourse, concern about routinisation and overprovision of prenatal diagnosis is common (TAB 2019: 93–96). This is not just concern about externally determined overprovision, but also about the loss of a carefree, hopeful pregnancy (on medicalisation, cf. TAB 2019: 168f.) and the burden and conflicts of decision-making based on problematic and sometimes only probabilistic information (Petersen/Jahn 2008).[19] In addition, it appears that pregnant women who make use of prenatal diagnosis often do so without having already decided whether they would consider terminating in the event of a problem being found, or even that they have in fact ruled out termination and welcome non-invasive tests (with no risk of miscarriage) only to have certainty as early as possible and if necessary prepare themselves for the birth of a child with special needs (cf. Reinsch/König/Rehmann-Sutter 2021: 6). Similar motives can also be found among pregnant women in Israel, particularly those who are critical of prenatal testing, but this does not change the fact that the majority fully accept wide-ranging testing and some consider it just routine ("pregnancy is checkups", Nov-Klaiman/Raz/Hashiloni-Dolev 2019: 4, 9; Rimon-Zarfaty 2014).

It is uncertain whether similarly clearly marked groups can be seen in prenatal diagnosis in the German context. Many Israeli publications on genetic testing programmes or attitudes to them start out by differentiating population groups (e.g. differentiating the Jewish population into ultra-Orthodox, religious/conservative/traditional, secular mainstream vs. "New Age") between which marked differences have been observed for some time. Although in Germany religiosity is often mentioned as a possible factor in decision-making on prenatal testing possibilities or results (e.g. in TAB 2019: 73, 144), and religious institutions such as the churches exercise influence in the relevant debates and take up a clear position, differentiating pregnant women according to social, regional, cultural or ethnic origin plays no great role in reporting on the state of prenatal diagnosis, at least not in the recent reports of which I am aware such

---

19   Here, Petersen and Jahn (2008: 47) refer to the literature on the potential for physiological harm: "In fact, increased levels of maternal anxiety and stress can adversely affect the cognitive, behavioural, and emotional development of the child. One possible underlying mechanism can be found in the elevated maternal stress hormones."

as the TAB Report (2019: 129f.). It is therefore impossible for me to differentiate many general statements on the German discourse.

In comparison with Israel, Germany shows a markedly lower birth rate (although it has been rising since 2010), with 1.59 children per woman in 2016. Although childlessness polarises opinion in society it is widely accepted, and thus relativises parenthood and family as the main purpose in life and the model of a good life. In abstaining from having children, individualistic life-goals and the desire for autonomy sometimes play a role, but uncertainties and constraints are often mentioned too. This applies, for example, in terms of being unable to reconcile having children with a career, but also because of fears of not being able to live up to the demands of parenthood (Dorbritz/Diabaté 2015). With a view to reconciling work and family, traditional ideas of the division of labour and for mothers having the main responsibility for early childcare ("intensive mothering"), particularly in West Germany, compete with the acceptance of outsourcing childcare so that mothers can work full-time (more in East Germany) (Pfau-Effinger/Smidt 2011; Diabaté/Beringer 2018).

> East German women are more strongly child-oriented, but reject sole childcare through the mother more often than West German women. What these women have in common is considering bringing up children to be a challenging task, in which as parents it is possible to get a lot wrong. Here, those interviewed obviously share the same concerns (Schiefer/Naderi 2015: 168).

Mothers having jobs is mostly accepted in principle, as well as their own individual "self-care", yet there often remains an unresolved conflict with equally strong demands for their presence in the household. Even the international literature indicates this, with some fascination for the singular German expression (and stigma) of "Rabenmutter" (literally a "raven mother", defined by the Duden dictionary as an "unloving, coldhearted mother who neglects her children") (Heffernan/Stone 2021). For some time the model of "responsible parenthood" has meant that the high requirements for parenthood have grown (Ruckdeschel 2015). This model requires that people only become parents if they are able to offer the child a good future (the *whether* of parenthood) and to undertake everything necessary for that (the *how* of parenthood), with the possibly dual effect that although an intensive process of reflection about parenthood is undertaken, parenthood itself is increasingly perceived as a burden.

In the German discourse on prenatal diagnosis and NIPT, proper parenthood is a persistent motive and is also reflected in the relevant publications, such as the Report of the German Ethics Council (DER 2013: 143ff.) and the TAB report (2019: 167ff.).

Prenatal testing is associated not only with concerns about heteronomy – I cannot, unfortunately, go into detail here about preimplantation genetic diagnosis or in vitro fertilisation – but also with the fear of burdening pregnancy and parenthood, and deforming the bonds between parents and children. Although unable to make statements about their frequency, some interviews indeed demonstrate the worry of prospective parents about the effects of their decisions on their later child, other children in the family or other members of society (Reinsch/König/Rehmann-Sutter 2021: 11f.). This illustrates the conflicts that the possibilities of prenatal diagnosis, in combination with the ideas and norms of parenthood and family relationships, can really give rise to.

Whether the norms of unconditional parenthood really do still prevail in the German context and discourse, or whether they are necessarily equated with the (prenatal) acceptance of every possible child, appears unclear (to me). The relevant norms are often described in the literature, sometimes bound up with voices from discourses of recent decades, e.g. on preimplantation genetic diagnosis (Hashiloni-Dolev 2007; Hashiloni-Dolev/Shkedi 2007; DER 2013: 143–146), yet on the other hand, the now well-established procedures of prenatal diagnosis are already associated with a possible rethink. Sigrid Graumann's statement summarises this well:

> The unconditional acceptance, and thus recognition, of the child, without taking into account the characteristics and abilities that are expected of it, *has up to now been the prevailing societal norm.* It is important to note that a pregnancy is the most extreme form of the existential dependence of one person upon another. [...] Every unborn child is existentially dependent upon being accepted unconditionally by its mother. Prenatal diagnosis now opens up the possibility of making the acceptances of the child in advance dependent on its genetic constitution. *This changes the societal norm* (2010: 138, emphasis added).

The direction in which society's norms are changing (not just in the sense of common practice but also of common expectations), and how advanced this process is, appear nevertheless to be subject to contrasting interpretations. For example, representatives of the first dissenting opinion of the German Ethics Council make the following call:

Medical research and public health policy may not reinforce the *social pressure of expectation* that disabled children should no longer be born. On the contrary, they must counter it by giving a signal that every child, whether with or without physical or mental disability, is welcome. A social atmosphere of acceptance and encouragement may make it easier for parents to give love and care to a child which enriches their lives in another way from the children who lead their lives without physical or mental disablement (DER 2013: 168–169, emphasis added).

Meanwhile, the authors of the second dissenting position state:

Women who make use of prenatal diagnosis as a general rule wish to satisfy their general responsibility for the future welfare of the child. In certain circumstances this may mean from the viewpoint of the pregnant woman that in the last instance she decides against carrying the unborn child to full term. *Currently, such decisions are respected by a broad section of our society and also by the legal system* – in full knowledge of the associated serious moral dilemma, not least for the woman herself (DER 2013: 171, emphasis added).

In my opinion, such evaluations not only show that there are varying perceptions of the status quo, but also make clear an ongoing process of replication and reinterpretation of parental and family models, the interpretations of which have gained currency in parallel and in conflict with one another. This is also reflected in statements by organisations providing advisory services for pregnancy-related conflicts. For example, in answer to the question "Are parents in the crossfire of an ethical and medical debate?" pro familia NRW notes:

Much is said about the reaction of prospective parents after prenatal diagnosis has identified a problem, but they themselves rarely get a chance to speak in the debate. All too often it is assumed they will not want a child with a disability. Yet many consultations in recent years have failed to confirm this. Rather, upon receiving the diagnosis of an abnormality parents find themselves in one of the most difficult of life situations. Often this is a long-planned, wished-for pregnancy. The couples who come for advice after abnormal findings are struggling to make a decision that actually cannot be made. Deciding between not having their own much wanted child, or a life with a disabled child, presents an almost irreconcilable conflict. The decision to terminate the wished-for pregnancy is never taken lightly. Termination is associated with great pain and grief for those involved. And yet the fear of getting into financial difficulties, of being socially isolated, and not being able adequately to care for a child that will require a lot of support throughout its life, is too great. Many parents also worry that the child will suffer once it is born. *Most of those affected* articulate very clearly that they *believe society does not approve of either of these decisions.* This is often the reason why they entrust only a few people in their circle with their news (pro familia NRW 2018: 5; emphasis added).

There is now apparently a situation in which, depending on one's focus and the approach of those providing the information, social pressure, prevailing expectations and norms are perceived very differently (on this, see Schneider 2018: 244). These expectations and norms can, although they do not need to, reinforce the internal conflicts of prospective parents. But even if they do not feel such a conflict themselves, they are likely to experience tension in their environment, since social polarisation around the issue means they always have to reckon with rejection or criticism from one side or another. This applies not just to those who have a disabled child, but also those who decide against having one, although in different ways.

2.3 Concluding reflections on the comparison

Comparing the different ways societies deal with pregnancy and prenatal diagnosis can help in questioning one's own assumptions and distancing oneself from all too familiar pathways of thinking and feeling. It can make it possible to admit different interpretations of what is good, right or desirable, instead of assuming an apparently clear ideal. Unconditional parenthood stands for a central principle of human relationships, which when one looks more closely actually has space for possible interpretations, gaps and gradations.

While in the Israeli context there is an apparently more unconditional social "commitment" to becoming parents (of several children if possible), to the point of discriminating against or pitying (consciously) childless people in the light of a broadly shared view of what constitutes a good life, this commitment is linked, at the political and medical-administrative levels and throughout large parts of society, to making pregnancy manageable and to support for at least some prenatal reservations, i.e. about the kind of children. This commitment also implies rejecting the unconditional, earliest possible acceptance of any developing child. But I see no indication for support of parental reservations at birth or later, so that in principle this *caesura* also means that parental or family unconditionality is expected and encouraged (which might be described as a temporal gradation of unconditional responsiveness).

In the German context by contrast there are stronger reservations about becoming parents in the first place, or having several children. Medical-administrative procedures and social expectations tend to oscillate between positions that are critical of any interference in pregnancy and prenatal life, and that support the earliest possible acceptance of all developing children, at least in wanted pregnancies, and positions that accept and want to enable having reservations to different degrees. Across this spectrum the development of the parent-child relationship appears potentially conflict-laden and tensions are more expected to carry over into the resulting relationships.

Awareness of the concerns and ambivalences about prenatal diagnosis, widespread in Germany, focuses attention on the many vulnerabilities that its use can bring, despite its superficial alignment with the principle of non-directive counselling and the informed self-determination of pregnant women. Consciousness of these vulnerabilities produces a particular (and sometimes one-sided) caution about extending prenatal diagnosis. This caution is both justified and relativised by observing how prenatal diagnosis is handled in Israel. On the one hand, this observation strengthens concern about routinising prenatal diagnosis in a way, which let its intensive use in some population groups become so much a matter of course that is scarcely questioned, and accordingly places more pressure on pregnant women. On the other hand, the Israeli example also suggests that many fears about the disruptive effect of prenatal diagnosis are not compelling and that there are different paths to fulfilling family relationships.

The earliest possible unconditional responsivity of prospective parents appears to be neither a necessary prerequisite for nor a guarantee of the integrity of the parent-child relationship or intact family relationships, at least not in the context of Israel. Nevertheless, the parental affection and family acceptance *perceived* as unconditional by the born child are indispensable. Perceiving this unconditionality is however dependent on many factors, such as the safety and comfort actually experienced in a family and how family is appreciated and its cohesion[20] promoted by society; and how and in what climate decisions that affect one's own coming-into-the world and one's own identity are thematised in (later) relationships (on this, see e.g. Kittay/Kittay 2000).

In my opinion, it is in the interests of both societies to learn *something* from the example of the other. For the Israeli context this would mean recognising and valuing the possible alternatives (which are also covered by the principle of informed self-determination and non-directive counselling) of voluntary not-knowing, carefree pregnancy, and an unconditional decision in favour of a possibly disabled child, and therefore to create the practical conditions for this; in the German context, it would mean overcoming the situation of an apparently insoluble double stigmatisation and to enable free decision-making both *for* and *against* having a possibly disabled child, and to accept this decision as the expression of fully considered parenthood. The German Ethics Council recommendations state only:

> Society and the state should respect[21] the readiness of parents to give care, security and love to a child which will possibly suffer physical or mental impairments (DER 2013: 165).

How a decision for reservation or even termination should be treated is left open. According to Asch and Wasserman, this would still – though with every sympathy – be expecting people to feel some discomfort for their decision's implied indirect discrimination against people with the same impairment, and relativising the valuable model of unconditionality (2005: 209f.). This sounds more like tolerance than acceptance.

I think a central lesson to be drawn from this comparison in the German context is the need to counter the tendency towards an ever-greater escalation of pregnancy conflicts, such as when particular overloaded and overloading

---

20   Family cohesion also depends on "doing family" (Jurczyk/Lange/Thiessen 2014: 12), in particular the internal construction of community as a closely connected group with a shared identity, a working model of family, and a feeling of belonging together, as well as the external presentation and performance of the family, not least as part of a battle for recognition.

21   The official English version of this Opinion differs subtly from the German original, and loses important nuance. A closer translation might be: "The willingness of parents to give care, security and love to a child who might be *affected* by physical or mental impairments deserves the *admiration* [Wertschätzung] of society and the state" (2013, German version, p. 179). There is no mention of "suffering", and "Wertschätzung" implies something stronger than mere "respect".

ideas burden prospective parents with too much responsibility. For example, the implication that prospective parents' actions either have particular motives or carry messages, which could be stigmatising ("what you're doing is selection" etc.), should be avoided; and advocacy for unborn life should not lead to a personification of the foetus, counter to the wishes of the pregnant woman (cf. pro familia Bundesverband 2012); and finally, prospective parents should not be held responsible as guarantors of social inclusion in place of the State. A willingness to terminate a pregnancy after a prenatal test result does not imply a rejection of unconditional affection for other children in the family, with or without disability, and neither does it necessarily bring with it any baggage for these relationships.

Rather, I suggest that the parents' prenatal decisions can *retrospectively* be the source of both identification and rejection, and which it is depends on numerous contextual factors, in the light of which parenthood can (later) be viewed. Adult children, particularly those who are themselves becoming parents, could identify with their parents' decisions and handle things in the same way, or at least find them reasonable. There appears to be potential for conflict primarily when the parent-child relationship is already experienced as difficult, strained or burdened, and information about the prenatal chapter of the relationship fits into a pattern of perceived lack of love or acknowledgment. Although finding out that one (i.e. the child that one would have become) would have been accepted by one's parents in any case, may give one a special feeling of reassurance (which one would like to pass on to one's own children), it is by no means certain that similarly strong feelings of security might not be engendered just as well in other ways, such as through parental love that is always *experienced* as being unconditional, or strong family cohesion. The potential for retrospective damage is greatest when it interacts with elements of the parents' characters that would always be problematic, such as the inability to cope with diversions or disappointments.

The key question of course is whether such parental characteristics are reinforced by the increased provision of prenatal diagnostic methods. Do they weaken the fundamental standards and ideals of parenthood? I think that they have potential to do so as ever more characteristics can, through the use of prenatal testing, be made the object of reservations. Whether this actually happens depends on many factors. Theoretically prenatal diagnostic methods are a gateway to the expression of prospective parents' more self-centred motives that are not to the benefit of the children or the resulting parent-child relationships (e.g. consumer mentality, desire for control, intolerance, or overambition). There will certainly be such cases, although I cannot say anything about their frequency or any significant increase. My impression up to now is that, in both Germany and Israel, most prospective parents try to act responsibly towards their children and to bring this responsibility into harmony with their (equally legitimate) personal aspirations and desires. Responsibility is however interpreted in different ways. In the German context, the norm of "responsible parenthood" always contains the option of *not* becoming parents, if the demands appear too great. However, there are competing interpretations of these demands, between the poles of the most encompassing responsivity towards the developing child, and more or less recognised reservations reflecting individual situations and family constellations. In the Israeli context on the other hand, abstaining from parenthood receives little approval, but at the same time, there is a widespread willingness or even expectation to adapt pregnancy to the individual or family situation. What would need to be shown is that these forms of responsibility have been misdirected or corrupted (for example, through egocentric or heteronomous motives or a sense of responsibility for achieving the best possible result that steers prospective parents towards thoughts of optimisation even before birth). The theoretical approaches that I know of, sometimes using case studies, criticise the (prenatal) loading of parenthood with unnecessary worries, conflicts and attributions of responsibility, or concerns about harm to an inclusive society and its members, but provide less illumination of their consequences for lived parenthood and family after the birth.[22] At least Asch and Wasserman, who connect (almost) all reservations on the part of prospective parents with "an impoverished conception of parenthood and families" – but have some sympathy for those reservations in a societal context that presents extreme difficulty to parents of children with disabilities (Asch and Wasserman 2005: 202) – appear to believe that these kinds of relationships approach a liberal understanding of family as an interest group of individuals, who cannot achieve the depth and quality of unconditional relationships. This is surely based upon the idea that prenatal reservations are translated into lasting reservations within the relationships, or that exercising choice in building the relationships may translate into a willingness

---

22   On this, see also Remennick's criticism of increased "genetic anxiety" in connection with the provision of prenatal diagnosis in Israel (2006: 37), or for Germany, Samerski's diagnosis of a "decision trap" in human genetics counselling (2010), as well as the review by Beckermann, which is critical of both "fear as big business" (2010: 4–5), and Samerski's generalising comments.

of parents and children to distance themselves from one another in future. In the Israeli context of a strong family orientation, however, such a development appears unlikely. I therefore find it hard to see clear indications of (impending) negative changes in relationships between parents and children.

Does it then follow to say that, at least before the child is born, the parents' dependency on conditions and prenatal reservations can be an alternative model? This is the position taken by Efron and Lifshitz-Aviram. As a reminder, these authors have three main theses: first, that in Israel and other Western countries we can observe a legal or underlying political and sociomedical phenomenon that enjoys widespread recognition and which they call "conditional parentage"; second, that this is a form of modern eugenics; and third, that conditional parentage (as a new, welcome form of eugenics) should be carefully regulated to serve the interests of parents, families, and society.

This overt demand to re-establish the term "eugenics" (positively), although it can only be a divisive "red cape" (Hashiloni-Dolev/Raz 2010: 90), appears to me to be neither promising nor right. Because in the light of historical experience the term is quite rightly a "red flag" – an indicator of danger. But even without the reference to eugenics, affirming "conditional parentage" remains difficult. The core of this, which I consider questionable, lies in the strength of state and society support for parental choices, whether negative (ruling out particular conditions) or positive (targeted selection or causation of particular conditions) as the expression of parental autonomy in harmony with the values of family and society. Although the authors themselves note the danger of collapsing these measures into particular negative trends, their own description already seems susceptible to misinterpretation and an idea of responsibility for optimal results. I would highlight one sentence: "All prospective parents wish for a healthy offspring with maximum potential to succeed in life" (Efron/ Lifshitz-Aviram 2020: 49). I doubt very much whether all prospective parents would phrase their wishes for their offspring in this way. The problem is not the desire for good health expressed here – although "health" can of course be understood in different ways – but the superlative vocabulary at the end of the sentence. I believe that many prospective parents would rather speak of their children being happy or able to lead a normal life, rather than adopt the language of the optimum. Already because of this tendency (to slip from fundamental concerns about health to the maximisation of life chances), I consider the assertive support of parental reservations to be wrong.

Prospective parents' reservations are plausible where they are the expression of justified concern (about themselves, the possible child, and the situation of the family). I therefore consider it wrong to equate the responsibility and concern of prospective parents straightforwardly with (the earliest possible) prenatal unconditionality. Parental unconditionality, whether before or after the birth of a child, is a powerful and important model (or part of the model) of good parenthood, but models interpreted (too) one-sidedly always risk appearing overpowering, or skewing one's view of the diversity of cases. Ideals or models often prove themselves in bringing together several issues that are significant in themselves, and so ordering a field of human practice in a convincing way. Prenatal unconditionality can be placed at the service of three distinct issues: carefree and hopeful pregnancy, the birth and affirmation of any child, and fulfilling family relationships. Of these three concerns the birth and affirmation of any possible child (and the indirect result of a more inclusive society) is the centrepiece, for which unconditionality appears indispensable. But this is different from both carefree pregnancy and fulfilling family relationships: these concerns can be realised in various ways, depending on the circumstances of the prospective parents. Pregnant women who would basically consider, with both their head and their heart,[23] terminating the pregnancy if test results are positive, can also draw reassurance from the (earliest possible) exclusion diagnostics and then, at least in this limited sense, enjoy their pregnancy. If this takes place in unity with the other parent-to-be and without ambivalent feelings, for instance, due to a previous, unconditional pregnancy, prenatal testing need not become socially invasive. Furthermore, the semantics of a *restrained* bonding with the foetus need not imply its complete absence, but often its persistent growth, so that despite initial reservations a felt unconditionality can sooner or later develop on its own, especially in a pregnancy that is much wanted by the family circle (in a society that is crazy for children). Here, there is also obviously the possibility of compensation for withheld feelings of bonding. Thus, intact and fulfilling family relationships are not dependent on prenatal unconditionality. At the same time, the appeal to the earliest possible unconditionality has the advantage of already naming that on which it finally depends, namely that love, care and unconditionality are authentically experienced in the family.

---

23   The fear that prenatal diagnosis primarily addresses a rational calculation and distracts from what feels like certainties but is arguably more difficult to articulate, runs through their critical commentary; see Katz Rothman (1985: 190), Reinsch/König/Rehmann-Sutter (2021: 2), and Stadelmann (2018: 75).

References

Anderson, Elizabeth S. (1990): "Is Women's Labor a Commodity?" In: Philosophy & Public Affairs 19/1, pp. 71–92.

Asch, Adrienne/Wasserman, David (2005): "Where is the Sin in Synecdoche? Prenatal Testing and the Parent-Child Relationship." In: David Wasserman/Robert Wachbroit/Jerome Bickenbach (eds.), Quality of life and human difference: Genetic testing, health care, and disability, Cambridge: Cambridge University Press, pp. 172–216.

Beckermann, Maria J. (2010): Review of Silja Samerski, "Die Entscheidungsfalle: Wie genetische Aufklärung die Gesellschaft entmündigt", 17 October, (https://arbeitskreis-frauengesundheit.de/2010/10/17/die-entscheidungsfalle-von-silja-samerski/), accessed 20 July 2022.

Braun, Kathrin (2005): "Not just for experts: The public debate about reprogenetics in Germany." In: Hastings Center Report 35/3, pp. 42–49.

Braun, Kathrin (2016): "Aussenansicht: Aussieben von Leben." In: Süddeutsche Zeitung, 6 September, (https://www.sueddeutsche.de/politik/aussenansicht-aussieben-von-leben-1.3150256), accessed 20 July 2022.

Brusa, Margherita/Barilan, Yechiel Michael (2018): "Childbirth in Israel: home birth and newborn screening." In: Hagai Boas/Yael Hashiloni-Dolev/Nadav Davidovitch/Dani Filc/Shai J. Lavi (eds.), Bioethics and Biopolitics in Israel: Socio-Legal, Political, and Empirical Analysis, Cambridge: Cambridge University Press, pp. 180–201.

DER (Deutscher Ethikrat) (2013): "The future of genetic diagnosis – from research to clinical practice.", (https://www.ethikrat.org/en/publications/kategorie/opinions), accessed 20 July 2022.

Diabaté, Sabine (2015): "Mutterleitbilder: Spagat zwischen Autonomie und Aufopferung." In: Norbert F. Schneider/Sabine Diabaté/Kerstin Ruckdeschel (eds.), Familienleitbilder in Deutschland: Kulturelle Vorstellungen zu Partnerschaft, Elternschaft und Familienleben, Opladen/Berlin/Toronto: Barbara Budrich, pp. 207–226.

Diabaté, Sabine/Beringer, Samira (2018): "Simply the Best!? – Kulturelle Einflussfaktoren zum 'intensive mothering' bei Müttern von Kleinkindern in Deutschland." In: Zeitschrift für Familienforschung 30/3, pp. 293–315.

Dorbritz, Jürgen/Diabaté, Sabine (2015): "Leitbild und Kinderlosigkeit: Kulturelle Vorstellungen zum Leben ohne Kinder." In: Norbert F. Schneider/Sabine Diabaté/Kerstin Ruckdeschel (eds.), Familienleitbilder in Deutschland: Kulturelle Vorstellungen zu Partnerschaft, Elternschaft und Familienleben, Opladen/Berlin/Toronto: Barbara Budrich, pp. 113–132.

Donath, Orna (2015): "Regretting Motherhood: A Sociopolitical Analysis." In: SIGNS: Journal of Women in Culture and Society 40/2, pp. 343–367.

Efron, Yael/Pnina Lifshitz-Aviram (2020): "Conditional Parentage is the New Eugenics." In: Child and Family Law Journal 8/1, pp. 19–50.

Fischmann, Tamara (2011): "Distress and Ethical Dilemmas Due to Prenatal and Genetic Diagnostics: Some Empirical Results." In: Tamara Fischmann/ Elisabeth Hildt (eds.), Ethical Dilemmas in Prenatal Diagnosis, Dordrecht: Springer, pp. 51–64.

Foth, Hannes (2019): "Kontaktabbrüche und Unkündbarkeit bei Eltern-Kind-Beziehungen im Erwachsenenalter." In: Simone Dietz/Hannes Foth/Svenja Wiertz (eds.), Die Freiheit zu gehen: Ausstiegsoptionen in politischen, sozialen und existenziellen Kontexten, Wiesbaden: VS, pp. 153–193.

Foth, Hannes (2021): "Avoiding 'selection'? – References to history in current German policy debates about non-invasive prenatal testing." In: Bioethics 35/6, pp. 518–527.

G-BA (Gemeinsamer Bundesausschuss) (2019): "Mutterschafts-Richtlinien: Nicht-invasive Pränataldiagnostik zur Bestimmung des Risikos autosomaler Trisomien 13, 18 und 21 mittels eines molekulargenetischen Tests (NIPT) für die Anwendung bei Schwangerschaften mit besonderen Risiken." In: Bundesanzeiger, AT 20.12.2019 B6, (https://www.g-ba.de/bes chluesse/3955/), accessed 20 July 2022.

Gedge, Elisabeth (2011): "Reproductive choice and the ideals of parenting." In: International Journal of Feminist Approaches to Bioethics 4/2, pp. 32–47.

Graumann, Sigrid (2010): "Pränataldiagnostik und Fragen der Anerkennung". In: Hartmut Remmers/Helen Kohlen (eds.), Bioethics, Care and Gender: Herausforderungen für Medizin, Pflege und Politik, Osnabrück: V&R Unipress, pp. 133–145.

Gross, Michael L./Ravitsky, Vardit (2003): "Israel: Bioethics in a Jewish-Democratic State." In: Cambridge Quarterly of Healthcare Ethics 12/3, pp. 247–255.

Hashiloni-Dolev, Yael (2007): A Life (Un)Worthy of Living: Reproductive Genetics in Israel and Germany, Dordrecht: Springer.

Hashiloni-Dolev, Yael (2018): "The effect of Jewish-Israeli family ideology on policy regarding reproductive technologies." In: Hagai Boas/Yael Hashiloni-Dolev/Nadav Davidovitch/Dani Filc/Shai J. Lavi (eds.), Bioethics and Biopolitics in Israel: Socio-Legal, Political, and Empirical Analysis, Cambridge: Cambridge University Press, pp. 119–138.

Hashiloni-Dolev, Yael/Nov-Klaiman, Tamar/Raz, Aviad (2019): "Pandora's pregnancy: NIPT, CMA, and genome sequencing – A new era for prenatal genetic testing." In: Prenatal Diagnosis 39, pp. 859–865, (https://pubmed.ncbi.nlm.nih.gov/31161621/), accessed 20 July 2022.

Hashiloni-Dolev, Yael/Raz, Aviad E. (2010): "Between social hypocrisy and social responsibility: professional views of eugenics, disability and reprogenetics in Germany and Israel." In: New Genetics and Society 29/1, pp. 87–102.

Hashiloni-Dolev, Yael/Shkedi, Shiri (2007): "On new reproductive technologies and family ethics: Pre-implantation genetic diagnosis for sibling donor in Israel and Germany." In: Social Science & Medicine 65/10, pp. 2081–2092.

Heffernan, Valerie/Stone, Katherine (2021): "# regrettingmotherhood in germany: Feminism, motherhood, and culture." In: SIGNS: Journal of Women in Culture and Society 46/2, pp. 337–360.

Hey, Monika (2012): Mein gläserner Bauch: Wie die Pränataldiagnostik unser Verhältnis zum Leben verändert, Munich: DVA.

Jurczyk, Karin/Lange, Andreas/Thiessen, Barbara (2014): "Doing Family als neue Perspektive auf Familie: Einleitung." In: Katrin Jurczyk/Andreas Lange/Barbara Thiessen (eds.), Doing Family: Warum Familienleben heute nicht mehr selbstverständlich ist, Weinheim, Basel: Beltz, pp. 7–49.

Kagitcibasi, Cigdem/Ataca, Bilge/Diri, Aysesim (2010): "Intergenerational relationships in the family: Ethnic, socioeconomic, and country variations in Germany, Israel, Palestine, and Turkey." In: Journal of Cross-Cultural Psychology 41/5–6, pp. 652–670.

Katz Rothman, Barbara (1985): "The products of conception: The social context of reproductive choices." In: Journal of Medical Ethics 11, pp. 188–193.

Katz Rothman, Barbara (1986): The Tentative Pregnancy: How Amniocentesis Changes the Experience of Motherhood, New York: Norton.

Kittay, Eva/Kittay, Leo (2000): "On the Expressivity and Ethics of Selective Abortion for Disability: Conversations with My Son." In: Erik Parens/Adrienne Asch (eds.), Prenatal Testing and Disability Rights, Washington, DC: Georgetown University Press, pp. 165–195.

Kloke, Martin (2005): "40 Jahre deutsch-israelische Beziehungen." Bundeszentrale für politische Bildung, 7 July.

Knaul, Susanne (2016): "Queer-Familien in Israel: Das Recht auf Kinder." In: TAZ August 27.

Lavee, Yoav/Katz, Ruth (2003): "The family in Israel: Between tradition and modernity." In: Marriage & Family Review 35/1–2, pp. 193–217.

Leefmann, Jon/Schaper, Manuel/Schicktanz, Silke (2017): "The concept of 'genetic responsibility' and its meanings: A systematic review of qualitative medical sociology literature." In: Frontiers in Sociology 1/18, (https://www.frontiersin.org/articles/10.3389/fsoc.2016.00018/full), accessed 20 July 2022.

Lipkin, Mack/Rowley, Peter T. (eds.) (1974): Genetic responsibility: On choosing our children's genes, New York: Plenum.

Löwy, Ilana (2020): "Non-Invasive Prenatal Testing: A Diagnostic Innovation Shaped by Commercial Interests and the Regulation Conundrum." In: Social Science & Medicine: 113064.

Mills, Claudia (2003): "Duties to Aging Parents." In: James M. Humber/Robert F. Almeder (eds.), Care of the Aged. Biomedical Ethics Reviews, Totowa, NJ: Humana Press, pp. 145–166.

Mullin, Amy (2006): "Parents and Children: An Alternative to Selfless and Unconditional Love." In: Hypatia 21/1, pp. 181–200.

Müller-Egloff, Susanne (2017): "Methoden der invasiven Pränataldiagnostik." In: Alexander Strauss (ed.), Ultraschallpraxis in Geburtshilfe und Gynäkologie, Berlin/Heidelberg: Springer, pp. 441–459.

Münch, Peter (2017): "Geburtenrate: Warum in Israel so viele Kinder geboren werden." In: Süddeutsche Zeitung, 6 January, (https://www.sueddeutsche.de/leben/geburtenrate-warum-in-israel-so-viele-kinder-geboren-werden-1.3320566), accessed 20 July 2022.

Nippert, Irmgard/Horst, Jürgen (1994): "Die Anwendungsproblematik der pränatalen Diagnose aus der Sicht von Beratenen und Beratern – unter besonderer Berücksichtigung der derzeitigen und zukünftigen möglichen Nutzung genetischer Tests. Gutachten im Auftrag des Büros für Technikfolgen-Abschätzung beim Deutschen Bundestag." TAB-Hintergrundpapier 2, Bonn.

Nov-Klaiman, Tamar/Raz, Aviad E./Hashiloni-Dolev, Yael (2019): "Attitudes of Israeli parents of children with Down syndrome toward non-invasive prenatal screening and the scope of prenatal testing." In: Journal of Genetic Counseling 28/6, pp. 1119–1129.

Okun, Barbara S. (2016): "An investigation of the unexpectedly high fertility of secular, native-born Jews in Israel." In: A Journal of Demography 70/2, pp. 239–257.

Petersen, Juliana/Jahn, Albrecht (2008): "Suspicious findings in antenatal care and their implications from the mothers' perspective: a prospective study in Germany." In: Birth 35/1, pp. 41–49.

Pfau-Effinger, Birgit/Smidt, Maike (2011): "Differences in women's employment patterns and family policies: Eastern and western Germany." In: Community, Work & Family 14/2, pp. 217–232.

pro familia Bundesverband (2012): "Das Recht der Frau auf selbstbestimmte Entscheidung: pro familia Position zum Schwangerschaftsabbruch", Statement, May 2012, (https://www.profamilia.de/ueber-pro-familia/stel lungnahmen), accessed 20 July 2022.

pro familia NRW (2018): "Zulassung des Nicht invasiven Pränataltests (NIPT) als GKV Leistung für Risikoschwangere", Statement, 19 December, (https: //www.profamilia.de/fileadmin/landesverband/lv_nordrhein-westfalen/ profa_NRW_Stellungnahme_Zulassung_des_Nicht_invasiven_Praenatalt ests_2017.pdf), accessed 20 July 2022.

Raz, Aviad (2008): "Disability, Genetics and Tradition – Socio-Cultural Aspects of Genetic Practice in Israel." In: Simone Ehm/Silke Schicktanz (eds.), Der Einfluss von Religion und Kultur auf die Biomedizin: ein Deutsch-Israelischer Dialog, Frankfurt: Dokumentation des evangelischen Pressedienstes 24, 3 January, pp. 26–31.

Raz, Aviad E. (2018): "Reckless or Pioneering? Public Health Genetics Services in Israel." In: Hagai Boas/Yael Hashiloni-Dolev/Nadav Davidovitch/Dani Filc/Shai J. Lavi (eds.), Bioethics and Biopolitics in Israel: Socio-Legal, Political, and Empirical Analysis, Cambridge: Cambridge University Press, pp. 223–239.

Raz, Aviad/Schicktanz, Silke (2016): Comparative empirical bioethics: Dilemmas of genetic testing and euthanasia in Israel and Germany, Berlin: Springer.

Rehmann-Sutter, Christoph (2021): "Should prenatal screening be seen as 'selective reproduction'? Four reasons to reframe the ethical debate." In: Journal of Perinatal Medicine 49/8, pp. 953–958, (https://doi.org/10.1515/jpm-2 021-0239), accessed 20 July 2022.

Rehmann-Sutter, Christoph/Schües, Christina (2020): "Die NIPT-Entscheidung des G-BA. Eine ethische Analyse." In: Ethik in der Medizin 32, pp. 385–403, (https://doi.org/10.1007/s00481-020-00592-0), accessed 20 July 2022.

Reinsch, Stefan/König, Anika/Rehmann-Sutter, Christoph (2021): "Decision-making about non-invasive prenatal testing: women's moral reasoning in the absence of a risk of miscarriage in Germany." In: New Genetics and Society 40/2, pp. 199–215.

Remennick, Larissa (2006): "The quest for the perfect baby: Why do Israeli women seek prenatal genetic testing?" In: Sociology of Health & Illness 28/1, pp. 21–53.

Rimon-Zarfaty, Nitzan (2014): The influence of new medical technologies on perceptions of the "fetus" and "parenthood" among Israeli parents. PhD Dissertation (In Hebrew). Ben-Gurion University of the Negev.

Rimon-Zarfaty, Nitzan/Jotkowitz, Alan (2012): "The Israeli abortion committees' process of decision making: an ethical analysis." In: Journal of medical ethics 38/1, pp. 26–30.

Rimon-Zarfaty, Nitzan/Raz, Aviad E./Hashiloni-Dolev, Yael (2011): "When does a fetus become a person? An Israeli viewpoint." In: Journal of Family Planning and Reproductive Health Care 37/4, pp. 216–224.

Ruckdeschel, Kerstin (2015): "Verantwortete Elternschaft: 'Für die Kinder nur das Beste'." In: Norbert F. Schneider/Sabine Diabaté/Kerstin Ruckdeschel (eds.), Familienleitbilder in Deutschland: Kulturelle Vorstellungen zu Partnerschaft, Elternschaft und Familienleben, Opladen/Berlin/Toronto: Barbara Budrich, pp. 191–206.

Samerski, Silja (2010): Die Entscheidungsfalle: Wie genetische Aufklärung die Gesellschaft entmündigt, Darmstadt: WBG.

Sandel, Michael (2007): The case against perfection, Cambridge, MA: Harvard University Press.

Scharf, Alexander/Maul, Holger/Frenzel, Jochen/Doubek, Klaus/Kohlschmidt, Nicolai (2019): "Postfaktische Zeiten: Einführung von NIPT als Kassenleistung. Eine vorläufige Bilanz." In: Frauenarzt 12/19, pp. 778–782.

Schiefer, Katrin/Naderi, Robert (2015): "Mütter in Ost- und West-Deutschland: Wie wichtig sind regionalspezifische Leitbilder für Elternschaft?" In: Norbert F. Schneider/Sabine Diabaté/Kerstin Ruckdeschel (eds.), Familienleitbilder in Deutschland: Kulturelle Vorstellungen zu Partnerschaft, Elternschaft und Familienleben, Opladen/Berlin/Toronto: Barbara Budrich, pp. 155–170.

Schneider, Diana (2018): "Nicht-invasiver Pränataltest und elterliche Entscheidungsfindung. Herausforderungen und Lösungsansatz." In: Florian Steger/Marcin Orzechowski/Maximilian Schochow (eds.), Pränatalmedizin: ethische, juristische und gesellschaftliche Aspekte, Freiburg/Munich: Karl Alber, pp. 230–251.

Schües, Christina (2016): Philosophie des Geborenseins, 2nd edition, Freiburg: Karl Alber.

Schües, Christina (2021): "Das Versprechen der Geburt." In: Olivia Mitscherlich/Rainer Anselm (eds.), Gelingende Geburt in der Diskussion, Berlin: DeGruyter, pp. 149–172.

Schües, Christina/Foth, Hannes (2019): "Elternschaft." In: Gottfried Schweiger/Johannes Drerup (eds.), Handbuch Philosophie der Kindheit, Stuttgart: Metzler, pp. 90–98.

Schütze, Yvonne (2010): "Mutterbilder in Deutschland." In: Psychoanalyse: Texte zur Sozialforschung 14/2–3, pp. 179–195.

Stadelmann, Ingeborg (2018): Die Hebammen-Sprechstunde, 3rd edition, Wiggensbach: Stadelmann.

Steinhauser, Thomas/Gutfreund, Hanoch/Renn, Jürgen (2017): "A Special Relationship: Turning Points in the History of German-Israeli Scientific Cooperation," 2nd edition, Berlin: Forschungsprogramm Geschichte der Max-Planck-Gesellschaft.

TAB (Büro für Technikfolgen-Abschätzung beim Deutschen Bundestag) (2019): "Aktueller Stand und Entwicklungen der Pränataldiagnostik." Arbeitsbericht 184, (https://www.tab-beim-bundestag.de/de/untersuchungen/u2 0810/ab184_Z.html), accessed 20 July 2022.

Teman, Elly/Ivry, Tsipy/Bernhardt, Barbara A. (2011): "Pregnancy as a proclamation of faith: Ultra-Orthodox Jewish women navigating the uncertainty of pregnancy and prenatal diagnosis." In: American Journal of Medical Genetics Part A 155/1, pp. 69–80.

Waldenfels, Bernhard (1994): "Response und Responsivität in der Psychologie." In: Journal für Psychologie 2/2, pp. 71–80.

Waldenfels, Bernhard (2012): "Responsive ethics." In: Dan Zahavi (ed.), The Oxford handbook of contemporary phenomenology, Oxford: Oxford University Press, pp. 423–441.

Waldschmidt, Anne (2006): "Normalcy, bio-politics and disability: Some remarks on the German disability discourse." In: Disability Studies Quarterly 26/2, (https://dsq-sds.org/article/view/694/871), accessed 20 July 2022.

Watzman, Haim (2005): "Furor at Hebrew U. leaves noted anthropologist in limbo." In: The Chronicle of Higher Education, 28 January, (https://www.c hronicle.com/article/furor-at-hebrew-u-leaves-noted-anthropologist-in-limbo-120851/), accessed 20 July 2022.

Weiss, Meira (1994): Conditional love: Parents' attitudes toward handicapped children, Westport, CT: Greenwood.

Wiesemann, Claudia (2015): "Natalität und die Ethik von Elternschaft und Familie." In: Zeitschrift für Praktische Philosophie 2/2, pp. 213–236.

Wilkinson, Stephen (2010): Choosing tomorrow's children: The ethics of selective reproduction, Oxford: Oxford University Press.

Zlotogora, Joël (2014): "Genetics and genomic medicine in Israel." In: Molecular genetics & genomic medicine 2/2, pp. 85–94.

Zlotogora, Joël/Grotto, Itamar/Kaliner, Ehud/Gamzu, Ronni (2016): "The Israeli national population program of genetic carrier screening for reproductive purposes." In: Genetics in Medicine 18, pp. 203–206, (https://doi.org/10.1038/gim.2015.55), accessed 20 July 2022.

Zlotogora, Joël/Haklai, Ziona/Leventhal, Alex (2007): "Utilization of prenatal diagnosis and termination of pregnancies for the prevention of Down syndrome in Israel." In: The Israel Medical Association Journal 9/8, pp. 600–602.

11. Can Not Wanting to Know Be Responsible?[1]
Conceptual Analysis and Meanings of Not-Knowing in Israeli and German Prenatal Genetic Practices

Christina Schües, Stefan Reinsch, Aviad Raz and Christoph Rehmann-Sutter

> Granted, we will truth: why not un-
> truth instead? And uncertainty? Even
> ignorance?
> Friedrich Nietzsche, *Beyond Good and
> Evil*, I/1.

What we know about who is about to be born, what we do not know, and what we should know, has become an essential part of the parental relationship and parental care. Currently, prenatal screening and prenatal tests imply that parental care is organised according to a binary code of knowing / not knowing, and is accompanied by information, counselling, public debates, moral and ethical discourse, professional guidelines and laws. These different facets and levels constitute the practice of prenatal testing. It involves personal decision-making in families, for which the pregnant woman is assumed to take the ultimate responsibility, in the name of what is often termed "reproductive autonomy" (Johnston/Zacharias 2017). Not wanting to know what one could possibly know about the future baby can have morally charged meanings, and can even be considered as wrong or irresponsible.

In this context, not-knowing appears in the horizon of knowing that one *could* know something, while not yet knowing it, having no access to the testing tools, or having decided not to use them. The decisions about the options

---

1   We like to extend our gratitude to Tamar Nov Klaiman who conducted the interviews in Israel, selected for us an appropriate sample of interviews, and supported this text with her interpretations and helpful comments.

of genetic testing are complex: they imply the possibility of a termination and therefore involve difficult existential, social and ethical questions about what we want for ourselves and for our family, or about what we owe to our future children. Laura Völkle and Nico Wettmann have identified seemingly paradoxical temporal references in this practice of knowledge: "Prenatal diagnostics seem to be mainly prognosis of the postnatal, whereas (non-)parental projections of biographies and life plans primarily determine what the current prenatal entity is" (2021: 2).

Prenatal genetic testing provides a distinct set of information that not everybody wants to have. It is a form of information some people find desirable, but others do not. This form of information is defined and limited by the arrangement of available biomedical tools: information about selected health-related traits of the future child. Information provided by a prenatal genetic test therefore suggests knowledge about the future, which can be reassuring for some people but not for others.[2] Such kinds of information often bring new uncertainties. Much of the information is about probabilities, rather than definitive knowledge about life with the future child. Sometimes it is even difficult for future parents to know *what* they want to know. Both the availability of testing and the (presumed) future knowledge that the test is assumed to bring have implications for the present. Some people feel good when they find out something about their unborn child that is reassuring, while instead others feel more insecure in the light of such possible knowledge. The possibility of knowledge itself might be a burden. The theme of not-knowing is especially interesting in the case of non-invasive prenatal tests (NIPT), because unlike with amniocentesis, arguments against testing are not based on concerns about iatrogenic pregnancy loss.

Prenatal diagnosis is always predictive. As such it is written into an "expectation arc" (Völkle/Wettmann 2021: 2) that constitutes the situation of a (wanted) pregnancy. Prenatal diagnosis can serve interests that may be contradictory: life and health interests of the foetus, the future child, the pregnant woman, her family, or society. The practice of testing, with its peculiar timing, rhythm and necessary waiting intervals, as well as the knowledge offered

---

2   The terms "information" and "knowledge" are not the same; there are subtle differences between them. For our context, "information" refers to the analysed medical data, while "knowledge" is taken to be the result of relevant information gained through learning, experiences or reflective processes of understanding. Knowledge is grounded on information, but information does not necessarily lead to knowledge.

by the results, provides new possibilities of responsible choice, but can also unsettle, frighten and even burden the woman or the couple. Prenatal testing followed by "abnormal" findings can imply the discontinuation of foetal development, since such pregnancies are often terminated. However, the ethics of abortion after a diagnosis, or the complicated questions of the moral status of foetal life in different discourses[3] in Israeli and German society, are not the subjects of this chapter.

In bioethical discourse and in lay people's discussions, particularly in Israel, it is often held that the (future) mother or parents have the responsibility to acquire genetic information relating to the future child. It may be considered irresponsible *not* to test and *not* to gain such knowledge. But the correspondence between the possibility of genetic testing, the care for the child and the responsibility to obtain genetic knowledge is not always taken for granted. In the chapter 2 of this book on genetic responsibility, Christina Schües explored different questions that emerge around the concept of "genetic responsibility". One of them is straightforward: Does *not testing* mean being irresponsible?

This chapter discusses how to understand *not knowing* and *not wanting to know* the genetic dispositions of the foetus. After introducing the "right not to know", we first discuss this issue by looking at the philosophical meanings of not-knowing, non-knowledge, and ignorance. How can we draw conceptual lines between them? How can we evaluate *not*-knowing with regard to certainty, relevance or responsibility? In addition to conceptual considerations, we discuss empirical material that we have collected in our comparative qualitative study. We asked women in Israel and Germany who had been pregnant about their reasoning for not wanting to know, or for regretting the decision to test for a trisomy. In the interviews, women retrospectively reconsidered the decisions they made during their pregnancy. Most of the interviews included in this analysis were with women who either decided against NIPT and did not regret it, or who had opted for more comprehensive testing, such as amniocentesis, possibly with chromosomal microarray analysis (CMA). Among our interviewees were two Israeli women whose NIPT gave them false negative results, so the regret they experienced was for not having had amniocentesis. We did not encounter any women who had NIPT with true negative results who regretted having them.

---

3   See chapter 7 of this book.

We start the conceptual discussions with some reflections about the right not to know, as is often addressed in bioethical discussions about genetic tests.[4]

1.   The right not to know

Claiming a *right not to know* implies an obligation to respect the freedom of not wanting to know something. With regard to genetic information, we can argue that (i) genetic information is personal, and (ii) there can be no obligation to test or to know results of a test if the person at risk prefers not to know. In some situations, knowledge might be unhelpful, even burdensome. In such situations, therefore, everybody should be entitled to reject this knowledge. This reflects common sense, as in poet Thomas Grey's famous line: "where ignorance is bliss, 'tis folly to be wise" (Grey 1742).

The right not to know one's own genetic status has been internationally recognised in emerging biomedical law (Andorno 2004). It is a special right in the context of medical practice, which is based on the view that, in a relationship of genetic counselling, voluntariness is one of the overarching ethical principles (Soniewicka 2016). Thus, the disclosure of health risk information to the person affected needs justification (as well as non-disclosure), and this again requires the recognition of the free will of the counselee (Chadwick 2009). There are exceptions, as in the case of a foetus or a child who cannot (yet) make a decision, which will be discussed below. There are, however, diverging views about how far into the field of genetic diagnostics this right should reach (Duttge/Lenk 2019). For instance, there is currently an international controversy about whether and how to return incidental and secondary findings of genetic tests to patients and research participants (Flatau et al. 2018).

In Germany, the right not to know one's genetic status is provided explicitly (Genetic Diagnostics Act of 2010: §9,5). In Israel it is not explicitly stated, but is implicit in the requirement to obtain informed consent, based on a pre-test explanation (Genetic Information Law of 2000; cf. chapter 3). This right not to know is directed at a field of not-knowing that is reasonably well defined. The German Ethics Council (Deutscher Ethikrat 2013) has extensively dealt with genetic diagnostics. The Council endorsed the view that detailed consultation is mandatory and the "right not to know" should be granted as an individual

---

4   Legal aspects are considered in the section II of this book.

right. The Council stressed that not every form of knowledge promotes agency and self-determination. Genetic predictive or prenatal tests are not a duty, and neither is it obligatory to find out the results of any tests one has had.

Generally, the governance of predictive genetic testing to foresee a person's future illness or physical or mental limitations is based on the following four principles: (i) voluntary consent to testing is required; (ii) the person concerned has a right not to know, (iii) there is a right to self-determination over whether to collect genetic or other data, and which data to collect if so; (iv) the particular psychological or social situation of a person at risk of illness, either for herself or another person, needs to be carefully considered in a genetic counselling session. Genetic testing of a foetus follows basically the same four principles. However, the foetus is placed into the charge of the pregnant woman, since its consent cannot be sought. There is no discussion in either country as to whether the former foetuses should be asked later, as adults, whether they want to know genetic information that had been obtained from a prenatal test.

For many people in both Germany and Israel, prenatal genetic tests are conducted with the intention of deciding about terminating the pregnancy should the result be positive. Women who have the test are usually shocked and sad if they receive results indicative of a trisomy. Unless they had already previously decided to keep the child regardless of the result, they are then confronted with difficult choices about ending the pregnancy. The imagined link, and often practised connection, between NIPT and abortion leads some women to decide against having the test in the first place. These women do not want to know because they do not want to be faced with such a decision, or because they do not want to abort regardless of the result. They seem few in number, but sure about their feelings and reasoning; for them, a test result would not be desirable because it gives them *useless knowledge*. We found examples of this reasoning among our interviewees in both countries.

Nora, a 36-year-old German mother of a healthy child, who works as a political disability advocate, was in her second pregnancy at the time of the interview. She criticised the wording of the information leaflets about NIPT as being one-sided and overwhelmingly pro-testing. In her view, the materials given to the women did not provide impartial information and therefore tended to restrict their freedom to decide. She was highly critical of this, referring to the "right not to know" as a protective shield and the disadvantages of knowing certain things:

> But I think it's just as legitimate to write more about the right not to know and what the disadvantages are of getting a result, so to speak, and what the advantages of not testing are. And how do people with Down syndrome live, so to speak, because the thing that really jumped out at you was: "you should avoid it." (GE 2018, Nora)

There could also be other reasons why not-knowing about the foetus' genetic characteristics can seem preferable to some women. For instance, a parent may prefer not to know information about susceptibility for late-onset diseases, something the foetal DNA can be searched for in principle (although it is illegal in Germany); even if it is not considered relevant for termination, parents may prefer not to burden the child's youth with the prospect of a disease later in life.

In prenatal situations however, knowing or not-knowing and their connections to the future life of the child and the family, to feelings of certainty and responsibility, are often less obvious.[5] We shall now discuss different ways in which not-knowing something can *manifest*, referring to selected literature from philosophy and bioethics, and using the empirical interview material that we collected in Germany and Israel as examples.

---

5   A right not to know may be insensitive to considerations of responsibility connected to that knowledge. If there is a right not to know, the person may exercise this right even in a situation where it would be important for that person or others to seek and accept this knowledge. If another person has an interest in knowing about the genes of the first person, perhaps because medical treatment depends on it, her or his right to know would need to be considered to take precedence over the first person's right not to know. Anneke Lucassen has described a complicated ethical dilemma within a family, where Jane's preventive mastectomy could only be avoided by having information about the precise mutation that caused her aunt Phyllis' cancer. However, Aunt Phyllis, whose feelings toward her family are hurt for other reasons, does not want anybody in the family to know about her cancer and cannot therefore be asked to take a genetic test (Lucassen 2005). A right not to know presumes a possible wish of the person to avoid certain knowledge and provides that this person is entitled to be protected from that knowledge. A right not to know does not, however, presume that the right is always exercised for ethically sound reasons. Thus, in certain special situations it can be ethically irresponsible to exercise a right not to know despite being legally entitled to do so. But in most cases we see it as an act of responsibility to respect a person's right not to know. This is relatively easy to see, if we assume that knowledge is simply either present or absent.

2.   Concepts of not-knowing

Contrary to the assumption that not-knowing is only a notion of deficiency, i.e. a negative phenomenon, we now want to explore its complex and meaningful presence. Not-knowing therefore has its own epistemic qualities within the realm of experience. In trying to explain this epistemic constellation we need to look closely at the lived experience of not-knowing, and how not-knowing *manifests* itself in people's experiences and in social contexts.

2.1 Traditional thinking: Not-knowing as deficiency

In the context of the modern belief in the continuous progress of knowledge, which is leading humanity to ever-better living conditions, not-knowing is primarily negative and has always had a precarious status. Knowing always seems to be better than ignorance or not-knowing. As Michael Smithson (1989:1) puts it: "Western intellectual culture has been preoccupied with the pursuit of absolutely certain knowledge, or, barring that, the nearest possible approximation to it." The knowledgeable person is the better one, not the person who refuses to know, or who is unable to understand. In this explanatory context, not-knowing something is at best provisional: we do not know it *yet*.

Not-knowing in this sense denotes a specific field of lacking knowledge: a kind of not-knowing where a person does not yet know something but has the urge to know or the feeling that she *should* know, or thinks she may benefit from the knowledge. In this case not-knowing comes as a deficit that demands compensation, i.e. striving for knowledge. In other instances, absence of knowledge may mean a field of knowledge that a person now believes they know, but at some later point in time, will retrospectively acknowledge not to have known in full. Or, to imagine a third constellation, absence of knowledge may mean knowledge that one believes one has, but this later on proves to be wrong. In such cases the lack of knowledge is a not-known or non-knowledge.

Throughout Western history, people have flirted a little with not-knowing and ignorance. Standing on the market square of Athens, Plato's Socrates confidently and eagerly showed his dialogue partners that they actually did not know what they thought they knew. During the trial in which he had to defend himself for blasphemy and corrupting youth, he reflected that he actually knew that he was – adjectivally speaking – not-knowing. As translator Grube renders it: "I am wiser than this man; it is likely that neither of us knows anything worthwhile, but he thinks he knows something when he does not, whereas when I do not know, neither do I think I know; so I am likely to be wiser than he to this small extent, that I do not think I know what I do not know." (Plato, Apology: 21d) This reference indicates an ambiguity between being a not-knower and the verb (not-)knowing, which lies at the root of the history of not-knowing. This ambiguity paves the way for the modern ontological and epistemological differentiation of *knowing what* and *knowing how*: What we think we know, we always know in the horizon of not-knowing. This is how we know what we think we know. In Socratic dialogues, this thesis about not-knowing is regarded as a key motive for philosophising. Insight into and consciousness of one's own not-knowing is the first step on the path to knowledge. And the last steps on this path invite us to submit the (supposedly) gained knowledge to the *logos* that provides a strict argumentative test, which can fail and may expose the "knowledge" to be a "mere wind-egg" (Plato, Theaetetus: 151e). Central to the Platonic approach to knowledge is the idea that the knowledgeable person – and even more so, the wisest person – is the most ethical one.

Partially following the pattern of using not-knowing as an epistemic motive and as a new justification for the legitimisation of knowledge, Descartes presented a methodological form of scepticism as a path for establishing the foundations of knowledge. Everything I see around me and feel within me can be illusionary – I can know nothing for sure – except that I am thinking, even when I am doubting the truth of my perceptions. As the only form of reliable knowledge, he proposed the evident insight of the *cogito*. What is not proven, we do not know, but only believe. However, Descartes also saw not-knowing as a deficiency and as undesirable. It could therefore function as a motive to strive for knowledge. It seems that the search for epistemic certainty and security, as (rhetorically) proclaimed by most providers of prenatal genetic testing, is deeply rooted in the history of Western thought. Knowledge and the sciences that provide it are rated more highly and considered to be more valuable than the lack of knowledge, ignorance, and mindsets that reject knowledge. Against the background of this way of thinking, which is typical and constitutive of modernity, the justification of wanting to remain ignorant must always be stronger than justifying the pursuit of knowledge. The burden of proof is on the ignorant, not on the person who seeks to know.

For scientists, not-knowing has a positive function in the research process: it is a research opportunity, a defined lacuna, inviting us to fill it. In scientific publications, a state of knowledge is very often described and the research question is shaped (and justified) by the aim to provide insight that we do not yet have. Conversely, in technology assessment, not-knowing seems problematic if technology entails risks, such as risks to human health or the environment. It seems we should know about them. Decision-making under such conditions of uncertainty is considered a challenge (Böschen et al. 2006). However, in other life contexts, not-knowing can also be valued positively: it may protect privacy and confidentiality; or provide security for society, e.g. in the case of bomb-making instructions, genome sequences of deadly synthetic viruses, security gaps in computer software, or methods of suicide. But ignorance can also be at the root of epistemic injustice, for example, when a witness is not believed because of her gender or skin colour, or when simply the vocabulary for describing a fact is not understood because of prejudice (cf. Fricker 2007; Schües 2018).

Thus, ignorance is not only a political problem, as in the case of disinformation campaigns, but may be also an issue in medical discourse with regard to the lifeworld of women, families, or people with disabilities. We think it is important to keep this in mind in transcultural studies, because white ignorance or Eurocentric ignorance, or related forms that are influenced by prejudice, may become a hidden driver of interpretation. In the general practice of daily life, ignorance can be used as an excuse for not being able to decide, or for not having acted as one should have, but it may also protect against excessive moral demands and so against being paralysed when having to decide or to act. In this essay we mostly use the notion of not-knowing, and the term "ignorance" only in specific contexts.

Following the Thomistic distinction between *scientia* and *opinio*, it is not enough merely to have an opinion about something. To count as knowledge, a claim must be based on some version of the "scientific method", i.e. on reliable evidence and sound argument. An opinion that happens accidentally to be true can therefore not be counted as knowledge in this sense. Not-knowing – traditionally defined as a lack of knowledge – may either mean general ignorance about unspecific and undefined areas in the world or ignorance about a more defined field of (possible) knowledge. However, there are good reasons to believe that not-knowing has, at least for some people or in some situations, a value of its own as well, and therefore its own meaning and sense-constituting power. Not wanting to know cannot be reduced to mere deficiency; it reflects a subjective process of deliberation, weighing up the pros and cons.

In the case of prenatal genetic testing, for instance, the right not to know refers to a field of information that is not necessarily well defined, but limited, namely information about the genetic make-up of the foetus. To decide not to know in the context of prenatal testing, whether by invasive methods (e.g. amniocentesis) or non-invasive methods (NIPT, ultrasound), refers to a defined field of not-knowing when an expert (human geneticist, genetic counsellor) or a physician, i.e. obstetrician or gynaecologist (ob/gyn) offers to find something out that the pregnant woman might not want to know while she is pregnant.

2.2 Manifestations of not-knowing

Phenomenologically we can distinguish between different manifestations of not-knowing by bringing out the differences between knowledge and not-knowing on the one hand, and between known and unknown on the other. There is *known* knowledge and *known* not-knowing, while there is also *unknown* knowledge and *unknown* not-knowing. The table in four quadrants reveals both an asymmetry and an intertwining between knowledge and not-knowing. Focusing on the manifestations of not-knowing with regard to knowing or not-knowing that one is ignorant, we need to consider the epistemic, social and ethical contexts, that both not-knowing and knowing always have.

category / character	knowing	not-knowing
known	known knowledge	known not-knowing
	(1) knowledge that is known, but not apparent	(2) knowledge that we know we do not know
unknown	unknown knowledge	unknown not-knowing
	(3) knowledge that we do not know that we have	(4) knowledge that we not (yet) know that we do not know

Table 1 Manifestations of not-knowing.
Adapted from Wilkesmann 2019: 213–216.

Table 1 illustrates the four different ways that not-knowing can manifest itself, either in somebody's mind or in a discursive situation (cf. Wilkesmann 2019: 213–216; Bammer et al. 2008). It is a map of four different kinds of knowing and not-knowing, construed in a phenomenological perspective. Not-knowing never appears alone but always in relation to some knowing. Knowing and not-knowing are asymmetric, but also "symbiotic" (Kerwin 1993:

172). Table 1 is not based on a scientist's presumption that not-knowing is mainly relevant for gaining knowledge. It does not represent the (possible) transformation of not-knowing into knowing. Our explanation focuses on how not-knowing may manifest itself in terms of both knowledge and the lack of knowledge.

Since the manifestation of not-knowing can be specific in different scientific, medical or social fields, we will first give some general ideas to clarify what is meant in this category, and then provide examples from the practice of prenatal diagnosis.

1. Known knowledge. It might at first sound counter-intuitive to look under this heading for a manifestation of *not*-knowing. If, for example, Jack knows that Jill is pregnant, in Jack's mind not-knowing about Jill's pregnancy is not intermingled with this knowledge. He just knows it and is conscious of his knowledge. Whether *Jill* knows or believes that Jack knows that she is pregnant is another story.[6] Here is why we think that even from Jack's point of view not-knowing can still be involved in "known knowledge": Known knowledge is not just knowledge that one knows one has. We can know something but not really "have" it in the sense of being aware of it. This manifestation of not-knowing applies to knowledge that has the characteristic of being known, but is not apparent as such. We know that we know something but we cannot grasp it. Jack, for instance, in a situation where Jill's pregnancy is not evident, may know that Jill is pregnant, and can even be sure about it in the depths of his heart, but still answer honestly, in all good conscience: "I don't know, I am not sure." We see two kinds of situations where this might happen, one about knowing how, the other about knowing what:

a.   NIPT are tests that most patients know are available. NIPT is today an established method in the practice of prenatal care, a tool that can be used to identify chromosomal variations in the child to be born. But sometimes the test is not used, whether for ethical, social or simply practical reasons. Thus, even though the know-how is present, i.e. the person knows how to

---

6   A similar example from ordinary language can be found in Smithson (1989: 2), who refers to Peter Unger's book *Ignorance: A Case of Scepticism* (1975: 93) in which he claims that "no one ever knows anything to be so". This thesis and its further debates are far from our concerns about prenatal genetic practice, yet the example might illuminate the concept of known knowledge.

acquire information about a genetic disposition, for some reason this is not made apparent. Hence, a couple might ignore their knowledge about NIPT, or refuse its application. Refusing a test falls under the right not to know. Formally, an individual can only rely on the right not to know with regard to a knowledge that is generally known or can be retrieved in principle.

b. The second category might include the problem of really knowing what a piece of bioinformation will actually mean. There is a difference between data and knowledge; knowledge can also have degrees of concreteness. Obtaining knowledge of the test results (data) might still not mean knowing what one wants to know about the future child (concrete knowledge). Women see genetic test results as information, although this does not tell them how life will be for a child with Down syndrome, for example. One German woman, herself a physician, who has a younger sister with Down syndrome and who did not want to have the test during her own pregnancy, commented on the lack of information given to women being confronted with decisions about testing or not testing:

> I think it's ABSURD that this explanation is given without even explaining to the people which symptoms it actually refers to, and what it actually means, okay? That Down Syndrome is NOT AT ALL just Down syndrome, right, that there are HUNDREDS of different degrees of how severely people are affected. (GE 2018, physician)

This woman distinguishes between information about the chromosomes and the knowledge that relates to a person's life. Thus, as explained above, we have here a further example showing that knowledge and information are not the same.

2. Known not-knowing, or known unknowns is a common epistemic category in science studies: knowledge that we know that we do not know. This is an obvious and explicitly circumscribed instance of not knowing something. Researchers specialise in different specific fields of study and leave to one side others about which they know little. Or scientists know that there is a specific lacuna of knowledge that they decide to address.

In prenatal genetic diagnosis this might refer to the possible expansion to further fields that could be included in NIPT. In consequence, women will not be confronted with the possibility of knowing every genetic detail about their foetus via NIPT. The information leaflets should be clear about the fact that this test delivers particular information, and not everything (perhaps) possible. For a pregnant woman who considers but refuses testing, the known not-knowing also represents the constellation of knowing that there is a test that could possibly show a specific genetic disposition. While she knows about the how, i.e. about testing, she might decide that she does not want to receive that particular piece of knowledge about the foetus. Not wanting to test (or, after testing, not wanting to learn the test results) means not wishing to know a specific kind of knowledge that could in principle be known. It is therefore a known unknown.

3. Unknown knowledge   is a type of not-knowing when somebody, despite knowing something, actually does not know that she knows it. This would be the case when someone cannot reflect upon or formulate what she knows. This form of knowledge has been called tacit knowledge (Polanyi 1958). Such a constellation of not knowing that one knows something is realised, for instance in intuitions ("I *knew* it but did not know why I knew it"), or in care-giving situations, when a caregiver *simply knows* what to do without being able to explain it.

In the realm of pregnancy and motherhood this type of not-knowing represented by unknown knowledge occurs rather often, for instance when mothers intuitively act appropriately with regard to their child. Or while giving birth, when a woman feels that her body "knows" what to do and what comes next. Intuitive knowledge about what will be good for the family (and for herself) is also important in decision-making about prenatal genetic testing, when the previously established "risk" is only one factor that motivates her to decide about testing. For example, in Ohad Milstein's documentary film *Week 23*, the protagonist Rahel, who is diagnosed with a high-risk pregnancy, *knows* at some point that everything is "ok" with the baby and she stops worrying.[7] This believed "knowledge" that everything is ok with the baby does not, however, always prove true.

4. Unknown not-knowing   is applied to a kind of knowledge that we do not know that we do not have. Unknown not-knowing can only be discovered retrospectively, i.e. after we realise that, at a previous point, we did not yet realise that we did not know what we happen to know today.

With regard to pregnancy and birth, this category can refer to the detection of a trisomy that was there without being recognised, and the possibility of its presence (and the corresponding non-knowledge) was not something parents

---

7   See chapter 9.

thought or worried about. Or this kind of unknown not-knowing might also occur in the situation of false-negative or false-positive results, when parents see that their child actually does (or does not) have a disposition they believed to be otherwise.

We interviewed Anna-Lena when her son with Down syndrome was 10 months old. She told us that she had a carefree pregnancy after receiving a falsely negative result from NIPT. After the birth they could not believe what they started to realise:

> [...] the boy had, *mhm*, he opened his eyes and I was puzzled, because you could see it in his eyes a bit. We weren't sure, because we thought, well, I saw it, my husband saw it too, um, we thought "OK, now we're seeing something that isn't there!" (GE 2017, Anna-Lena)

In light of these distinctions between different manifestations or kinds of not-knowing, it does not seem at all convincing to consider not-knowing things about the genetic constitution of the foetus as a simple opposite of knowing. Not-knowing does not mean simply the deficit or the lack of knowledge; rather, knowing and not-knowing are two non-exchangeable poles that lie on different levels, and are therefore in *asymmetric* opposition towards one another. The implication of this finding is: not-knowing has a particular and constitutive role on its own. The observation that both knowing and not-knowing have their own constitutive status is shown in the observation of uncertainty about the test results and the corresponding ideas about their certainty and security.

In the next section we will examine questions of certainty and security in the light of interview data that we gathered from women who had made a decision about using or not using NIPT. This will show that the decision not to learn about the genetic make-up of their offspring can be supported by a range of different reasons and feelings.

3.   Uncertainty and insecurity

The interpretation of these interviews and the following conceptual thoughts were guided by the overall question about the relation between not-knowing and responsibility. The above chapter about "genetic responsibility" has tried to explain the meaning of responsibility and irresponsibility in prenatal genetics and for care for a future child in a societal context. However, the interviews show that responsibility is not the only issue involved. Furthermore, the relevance of the genetic test, the way the procedure and consultations take place, and issues of empowerment, uncertainty or insecurity very much influence the experience of pregnancy. Therefore, before we explicitly refer to aspects of responsibility and irresponsibility, we need to focus on different meanings of not-knowing for the people concerned. These different meanings are accompanied by impressions of the standard procedure of NIPT and its informational context, and feelings of empowerment, uncertainty or insecurity that may accompany knowing or not-knowing.

3.1 Standard procedures and future retrospective view

When testing becomes standard or is routinely offered to particular groups of pregnant women, it may be harder for them to decline and justify their wish to avoid the associated knowledge. This concern has been voiced by a great many critical observers of prenatal genetic practices (Suter 2002; Nuffield 2017; Rubeis et al. 2020). As we argue elsewhere (Rehmann-Sutter, Timmermans, Raz, submitted ms.) routines can differ considerably in how much emphasis they place on fair and comprehensive information and free decision-making. Although well-intentioned, some contexts or constellations where the testing itself becomes routine practice without thinking, may fail to provide space for women to deliberate, or even to feel the desire to do so.

The following examples from women's reports show how the "standard procedures" of explanations, information about women's right not to know, and free and informed decision-making about testing may be neither useful nor appropriate for all people concerned. This aspect is important for those who retrospectively consider that they did not really want the test.

Maja, a 28-year-old mother and primary school teacher from southern Germany, had two pregnancies: she had the test in the first but not in the second. She said that in her first pregnancy she had not given much thought to NIPT but agreed to have it because it was suggested by the ob/gyn. Although, as she firmly states, "money wasn't the main reason for us to take the test", she suspects her ob/gyn proposed she have the (then) new NIPT, namely the HarmonyTest, because of her insurance status: since she was on private health insurance, her insurance company would be likely to cover the costs, she was told. She and her long-term partner "didn't think long about having the test", but just followed the physician's suggestion.

I: Was there a counselling process? I mean somehow when you got the leaflet.

M: Well, not from her, actually, no. I mean, as I said, she did explain briefly, in about five minutes, and really no more than was on the leaflet. Basically, that there was no danger for me, or my child either, because it's just a matter of taking blood. [...]
And otherwise, it's actually quite a while ago, but what I've got in my head is that there wasn't much information given.

I: And the information you were given, would you describe that as neutral?

M: In retrospect, I'm finding it quite difficult, I mean, at that time I definitely thought it was neutral, and I think it's good, or I think so at any rate. I mean, knowing that it's there and not somehow [...] coming across it myself, let's say, doing something like this.
But despite that, I mean especially with hindsight, I also view this critically.
[...] Because – and now we're getting to the point – where do you distinguish it?
I mean, what do I get out of the result, or what do I do with it afterwards, and I think [...]
So, retrospectively, I gave much more thought to it than beforehand, to be perfectly honest. (GE 2018, Maja)

Maja also now believed that she and her husband were a bit naïve to think everything would be "ok" anyhow. In their discussion following the test while awaiting the results, the couple decided they would not consider an abortion if a trisomy were detected. So, during the second pregnancy, at the time of the interview, the couple decided not to have NIPT.

What would be the consequence of it for us? [...] after all we said: well, if we do have it, it wouldn't actually change anything. [...] I don't feel: oh, I could know that [...] What's the *use*, well, the *added value* is simply not there, and it's not that I'm afraid of it, either." (GE, 2018, Maja)

After deciding not to have NIPT, she felt much more relaxed and able to "enjoy" an "unburdened" second pregnancy. It was not only her own actions that Maja questioned and evaluated. She was also critical about the way she was put into a situation where she was tested without having thought twice about the consequences of obtaining the information.

This perception is rather different from what women in Israel said. One Israeli woman, Nira, who had NIPT in two pregnancies, said that she was given a checklist of tests at the beginning of each. This was a schedule she perceived she needed to follow:

> That pregnancy – I really did it by the book. Like – how should I describe it – like when a baby is born you receive a detailed vaccination plan that needs to be given each week: in the hospital – this one and that one; a week or a month after – another one; and then three and six months later and so on – this is exactly how I was during pregnancy. I was completely on top of it. It was by the book. My doctor told me: "These are the tests" – I had a plan. I did everything without exception. [...]

> I: Did you ever stop and ask yourself or him why you even need all these tests?

> No, I just went for it. I didn't ask why at all. It is clear to me that he's the authority here. Just as I don't ask about the vaccines. Some people ask why to vaccinate or why have this combination of vaccines together and some split them. I don't. This is what I was instructed – so this is what I do. That's what I did. (IL 2017, Nira)

Nira told us proudly that she did everything "by the book", and that that was fine with her, while other women had second thoughts, and did not want parts of a testing plan – as Maja explained. Maja's evaluation in her second pregnancy, being more alert to what follows, was that she simply did not want to know: "What's the use?" Nira's reasoning, however, was that she wanted to have done everything correctly so that in retrospect she would not blame herself for things she had left undone. Like a vaccination plan, the physician's plan was – in her judgment – the most trustworthy guidance on that course of action.

3.2 Empowerment and insecurity

Genetic tests generally yield a special kind of bio-information, the collection and status of which are controversial because of the far-reaching prognostic implications of genetic data for the life of a person (Rehmann-Sutter/Müller

2009). Knowledge about the genome can, under certain circumstances, contribute to a feeling of security, but it can also create new insecurities. Knowledge can empower people, and can also make them powerless. What they may wish for in a prenatal test may be security, but genetic knowledge is just a means of obtaining this security. The lack of information would then be judged not so much from a cognitive point of view (as ignorance, not-knowing something) but from the point of view of security, which having had a test may bring.

Some future parents find the information that comes from prenatal test reassuring and beneficial. The reason can be that the information is empowering. Tehila, for instance, an Israeli mother of four children, 31 years old, a modern religious woman who works at a bank, has had different tests in each of her pregnancies. At one point in the interview she talked about her decision to have amniocentesis plus chromosomal microarray analysis instead of NIPT:

> I: Please tell me about this move that led you to have a test, which is an invasive test and entails a risk, when you were actually not given a recommendation to do so. What were your considerations pro and con the test? What determined the decision?
>
> T: Peace of mind. Knowing that everything is ok in that respect. [...] There is great uncertainty around the entire pregnancy. No matter how many tests you had, you are still afraid. If it isn't about the foetus, it could be during the delivery. A thousand issues. So at least if there is one thing I can get a stamp on [i.e. a guarantee] – then I take it. (IL 2018, Tehila)

Tehila is concerned about a thousand things, and wants to lower the number of open questions. The field of not-knowing is too large and too uncertain for her. "Peace of mind", what she is striving for, is achieved in reducing the field of the unknown, and she finds even a small fraction beneficial. For Tehila, the medical information is like putting a reassuring "stamp" on an unclear and confusing situation. Since this stamp is something she gets from experts, she does not need to decide for herself that "everything in this respect is ok". It is somebody else's judgment, that of an expert.

For another set of women, in addition to being reassuring the genetic information was also empowering. Sarah, a 41-year-old Israeli woman who did not have NIPT, explained:

> As far as I understand, the genetic chip [i.e. the CMA] is far broader than all other tests. So I thought that if I am having a test – and I was going

to have amniocentesis because it is funded – then I might as well have the reliable, most precise and broadest test. (IL 2018, Sarah)

She saw the information yielded by genetic tests as empowering:

I: So, what are your feelings when you receive medical information?

S: First, it lowers my anxiety. Second, it empowers me. It gives me the power to choose. Power in general. In my view, knowledge is power. (IL 2018, Sarah)

Sarah is a modern religious Israeli woman in her third pregnancy after two miscarriages, who had all the routine tests as well as amniocentesis and CMA. She agreed with her husband that they would terminate a pregnancy diagnosed with genetic disorders. The reason for this is her daily acquaintance with the suffering caused by disability due to her job as a physiotherapist, where she treats disabled people. Power for her means being able to choose – so she is a good illustration of the citizen who takes autonomous decisions.

But there is also the other side. The meaning and the value of testing is not always clear for everyone. How much can a person's choices rely on such tests? Genetic information seems to provide prognostic information, i.e. insight into the future, but is such prognostic information already "really" knowledge? Here, the differences between information and knowledge might loom large. And in the context of genetic knowledge as well, there is the challenge of information overload. It might be that lack of clarity about the meaning of information provides a reason for preferring not to know. We found an example of this type of reasoning in the interview with Maja in Germany, quoted above.

Some people also fear the misuse of bioinformation. Although the disclosure of genetic data to third parties in is prohibited most countries, there is still concern that insurance companies or employers could have an interest in genetic data. Thus, the voluntary transfer of data would not eliminate the possibility of "genetic discrimination" (Lemke 2013; Rehmann-Sutter 2003) against risk carriers by employers or insurers.[8]

Furthermore, there is the difficulty that originates in the ambivalence of bioinformation itself. On the one hand, more security and self-determined life planning could be enabled if a disease/disability risk can be clearly determined,

---

8   There is a concern that certain persons with a positive test result would be charged a higher insurance premium. (Mieth 2001: 105–108; Breyer / Bürger 2005).

especially if possible therapy exists for the health problems that sometimes accompany disability. On the other hand, there is the threat of *more uncertainty*, or "enlightened powerlessness" (Lemke 2004: 72: "*aufgeklärte Ohnmacht*"), because the conditions associated with many genetic findings cannot be altered. A positive result can only be interpreted in the context of personal imagining about the future as a mother/parent and the family, as well as one's own means of caring for a child, not knowing how much support it will need. Those who decide in favour of a test then have perhaps more information, but at the same time more uncertainty and not-knowledge. But this can also be said about those who do not have the test despite being aware that the pregnancy might be abnormal.

Knowing and not-knowing are temporally contextualised, and they are not value-free. Imagining is prospectively informed about the future child, and considering such knowledge retrospectively can show the participants that (a) any information is transformed when it is seen within the personal and social context; hence (b) good information gives security and bad information gives insecurity, even though there might be the wish that it would have been better not to know; (c) knowing something or not-knowing something is re-evaluated when reflecting retrospectively how life has turned out.

3.3 What non-knowledge and not-knowing mean

A sociological perspective observes different ways in which non-knowledge is recognised, defined and dealt with in various "cultures of non-knowledge" (Böschen et al. 2006; cf. Wehling 2001; 2006). The recognition of non-knowledge is often tacit, its definitions are often indirect, and how people deal with it is often implicit (Böschen et al. 2006: 296). When we speak of *not-knowing* we always think of people who do not know certain things, whereas when we speak of *non-knowledge* we have in mind the absence of knowledge in certain circumstances. Smithson, followed by Böschen et al., defines ignorance in a more specific way referring to knowledge that could theoretically be present but is actually absent. In Smithson's words: "A working definition of ignorance, then, is: "A is *ignorant* from B's viewpoint if A fails to agree with or show awareness of ideas which B defines as actually or potentially valid" (Smithson 1989: 6). Ignorance thus implies the possibility of knowing. It is a form of not-knowing that is theoretically regarded as unnecessary, and therefore potentially reversible. We can however also fail to know, and even know that we do not have this kind of knowledge, without implying that it would be possible to know it.

As we have stressed earlier, the concept of not-knowing is rather dispersed and heterogeneous. Depending on whether knowledge or not-knowing is considered with regard to the natural sciences, medicine or social science, it is construed and also understood differently. As laboratory sociologist Karin Knorr-Cetina has pointed out, the epistemic cultures of non-knowledge differ between scientific disciplines. She studied high-energy physics and molecular biology. While high-energy physicists actively deal with the edges and limits of knowledge and are attentive to disturbances, distortions, errors or unexpected events, and treat them as interesting phenomena in their own right, she found molecular biologists to be less interested in the limits of their knowledge. Instead, they tend to vary the conditions of an experiment, for instance in genetic engineering, in order to produce the kind of outcome they are interested in (Knorr-Cetina 1999; cf. Böschen et al. 2006: 296). In more practical contexts as well, for instance in medicine, the dimensions and types of not-knowing have different meanings and impacts.

In order to understand what people say when they speak about not-knowing, we therefore need a more precisely specified conceptual basis. Böschen et al. (2006: 296) have convincingly suggested distinguishing between three dimensions that characterise specific cultures of non-knowledge: awareness, intentionality, and temporal stability of non-knowledge. The authors understand these terms thus: (1) Awareness means knowledge about non-knowledge. It "spreads between full awareness of nonknowledge (we know what we don't know) and complete unawareness ('unknown unknowns')"; (2) the intentionality of not-knowing "contrasts unintended non-knowledge with the conscious refusal of certain cognitions"; (3) temporal stability of non-knowledge means the extent of its reducibility. It "extends from what is not yet known, but (presumably) does not present any substantial difficulties to cognition, to the entirely 'unknowable' and therefore uncontrollable." We can also use this to specify the general field and meaning of not-knowing in prenatal genetic testing, and in particular NIPT. Each of the dimensions suggested by Böschen et al. has degrees of intensity. Awareness can be fully recognised or be not recognised at all; not-knowing can be unintended or knowledge can be consciously refused; temporal stability can refer to reducible ignorance, when something is not yet known, or it can refer to something that is entirely unknowable. We therefore propose to place each of the dimensions in a table into three degrees of intensity: strong, partial and low.

dimensions / degrees	(1) awareness or knowledge of not-knowing *field*	(2) intentionality of not-knowing *Agent*	(3) temporal stability of not-knowing *time*
strong	specified ignorance, clear non-knowledge	actor decides not to know, rational ignorance	something is impossible to know, ignorance is irreducible
partial	intuition, anticipation	actor is ambivalent, insecure	ignorance is disputable, unclear, uncertain
low	unknown unknowns, total ignorance	actor is unaware of the possibility of knowing	something is not yet known, ignorance is reducible

Table 2 Dimensions and degrees of not-knowing or non-knowledge.
Cf. Wehling 2006; Böschen et al. 2006; Heidbrink 2013.

The distinction between different dimensions and grades of not-knowing provides an ordering that can, on the one hand, be useful for comparing the not-knowing of a test such as NIPT for trisomy, with a genetic test that can do a lot more. On the other hand, specifying the particular dimensionality and degrees of not-knowing helps to identify different meanings of not-knowing for non-users of NIPT, as well as for users of NIPT who wished retrospectively that they had not used it, for example where the test has failed to detect "an issue" and created false reassurance. It will thus become apparent that knowing and not-knowing are not value-free. They are linked to particular feelings and attitudes, which may change according to the temporal perspective, i.e. between a prospective and a retrospective view.

The difference between knowing-what and knowing-how is important in practical contexts for a differentiated understanding of the use and not-use of a test in its function as access to knowledge. *What* is known refers to a field, a subject, or a theme of knowledge: that something is, or is not, the case. Knowing *how* refers to using a test as epistemological access to gaining knowledge or information about something.

In the following, we ask how these dimensions apply (i) to the field in which not-knowing occurs, (ii) to the agential perspectives involved, and (iii) to temporality in the lives of parents and families.

i.   The relevant *field* of knowledge and non-knowledge is primarily medicine but, no less importantly, social understandings of this technology. Medically speaking, NIPT is known as a technique; thus, the knowing-how is quite clear, and medical professionals know well what type of knowledge can be given by particular forms of NIPT (today, chromosomal aneuploidies plus a few other common conditions). NIPT has been more or less well introduced into a number of societies, and many people have at least a rough idea about what it means, and what the issues are. Particularly in Germany there have been numerous discussions in wider society, e.g. the question of whether testing should be financed by health insurance was hotly debated in newspapers, on radio, TV and on the internet. In Israel, however, there was rather little debate on these themes. Public opinion, place and time influence a decision to test or not to test. The field of knowledge is certainly intertwined with the agent who is knowing or not-knowing.

ii. The degrees of intentionality of not-knowing refer to one or more *agents* or agential perspectives who engage more or less intensively in forms of knowing or not-knowing. Intentionality encompasses several volitional possibilities, including the will not to know (protected by the right not to know), the suppression or the suspension of deciding to know or not to know, or even a general ignorance. The special focus of this chapter is about intended ignorance, deliberate not-knowing, which is often related to the question of accountability and responsibility because it is commonly believed that deciding and acting responsibly requires and therefore presupposes appropriate knowledge. But interviews show that this is not so clear.

iii. Not-knowing has a *temporal* dimension in the lives of those involved, insofar as some not-knowing is actually not-yet-knowledge that will be transformed into a known within a particular timeframe at a later stage of pregnancy. It might be relevant to mention here that NIPT has an inherent ambivalence or partiality of knowing since it is not diagnostic, and a positive test result needs to be confirmed by amniocentesis. The other pole of not-knowing as not-yet-known would be the never-known, which is a form of non-knowledge that agents do not know about, and hence cannot care about. Epistemology and philosophy of science are primarily concerned with not-knowing as not-yet-known. The transitions from one stage to another cannot be explained by objective scientific criteria. On the one hand, they "remain disputable and dependent on epistemic possibilities and resources" (Wehling 2006: 146). Yet on the other, the agents' wish or will to know (or not to know) are influenced by scientific developments and driving forces from their families or wider society.

The question of what sorts of not-knowing relate to NIPT can, we hope, be better understood by using table 1 of different manifestations, together with the dimensional table 2. We can differentiate the interviews with women who said "No" to NIPT into roughly four groups. Two groups were following routines. The first followed religious routines, i.e. they said "No" to NIPT because their religion prohibits abortion; a second group followed medical routines, i.e. they said "No" to NIPT because the medical routine does not require it. Both had what table 2 calls a "specified ignorance". Ignorance was decisive and more or less irreversible. Two other groups also said "No" to NIPT, but not because they followed routines. They reasoned out of their personal position: the first were non-users of NIPT in Germany, and Ultraorthodox women in Israel, who declined NIPT to avoid "knowing something that would burden their pregnancy." This can be seen as an instance of "rational ignorance". In contrast, a significant group of Israeli non-users of NIPT were secular women who sought more knowledge about their pregnancy, and therefore preferred the more comprehensive and reliable invasive diagnostic tests (amniocentesis + CMA). This amounts to "reducible ignorance".

Some people feel that more knowledge may not just be reassuring, but also lead to uncertainty. There is, we believe, a qualitative difference between not-knowing und uncertainty. This difference cannot be reduced to a graduation between uncertain and unknown knowledge. Uncertainty can be the consequence of knowing; knowledge can itself create uncertainty. It is a characteristic of uncertainty that it is often attached to knowledge that concerns the future by way of statistical probabilities and/or information about a risk that cannot easily be translated into daily life. Uncertainty includes a "probabilistic evaluation" (Heidbrink 2013: 122) of a risk process or, in our case, the manifestation or the realisation of a genetic disposition. Thus, uncertainty might emerge not just because of the absence or lack of knowledge, but can also be brought about by knowledge itself. Knowing about a genetic disposition means being uncertain about its concrete implications for the life of the person affected. Without knowing the genetic disposition, the questions about uncertainty of the future manifestation of a disease might never come up. This connection lies within the horizon of expectations or attention because it is bound to the limited frame of observation and information, and also because it has no further socio-cultural system of reference. What a diagnosis for trisomy 21 really means for the life of the person and the family is not predetermined and certain. If a pregnant woman and her partner do not know that DS can also mean a fulfilled life for the individual and her family, the decision to have an abortion is unsurprising. Yet some women or couples also choose NIPT in order to prepare for a life with a disabled child. Evidently, once such information is known, an agent cannot successfully pretend not to know. Thus, in distinction to not-knowing, the choice to know cannot be reversed.

However, a lack of knowledge may also lead to feelings of insecurity, as Ateret told us in her interview. She is a mother of two, 31 years old, religious, works in an organisation that teaches Jewish tradition in primary schools, and lives in an Israeli city. Ateret had all the routine tests. In her second pregnancy, she was recommended to have amniocentesis following the result of her second-trimester screening test. After a great deal of contemplation she decided not to have amniocentesis or NIPT, and to put her trust in God.

> The birth was overcast by some fear. We wanted to be done with it already and know that everything is ok. I went to the delivery room with mixed emotions. [...] If I had the test [NIPT] and it came back normal, perhaps I would have come to give birth feeling more peaceful and calmer and not as fearful. (IL 2018, Ateret)

Insecurity can be caused by a lack of knowledge, like a blind spot or an abyss, and it may or may not result in a search for knowledge. The compensation for insecurity would be measures of protection against the dangers or the particular risks identified, but also interpersonal phenomena such as trust and promise (or hope).

4. The reasoning behind deciding not to know: The issue of responsibility

With regard to German and Israeli prenatal genetic practices and discourses, the options of knowing and not-knowing become an issue of varying intensity and complexity. Certainly, the questions about how we test and what we should know about the foetus expand the medical realm and are intertwined with the *social realm*. The ob/gyn and the pregnant woman (and her partner, her family, a rabbi, church leader, friends or other persons) may consult about medical tests. They may have opinions about life in general and the concrete life with a child affected by trisomy. The deliberation circles around questions of what can be known, what should be known, and what must be known. It also includes questions of responsibility. Generally, most interviews show the conviction that testing is reasonable and, hence, a responsible thing to do. This is illustrated by Israeli woman Inbar, age 43, who did have the test and believes that not testing was not an option:

> In my case, it would have been irresponsible. Even if I weren't a single mum [...] I don't know how you could [raise a disabled child]. It is irresponsible to give birth and then reject the child. But if you are capable of raising the child and you have the means and the energy – then very good. (IL 2018, Inbar)

In Inbar's first pregnancy, DS was diagnosed and she terminated. In her second pregnancy, she had NIPT alone and, as she puts it, gave birth to a "healthy" child. In her third pregnancy, she had amniocentesis and CMA, and another healthy child was born. For her it was very clear: "all these tests exist in order to prevent." She reasons as follows for the need to know:

> I see no reason to bring a child into this world when you know beforehand that there is something wrong. It isn't a missing finger or something like that, which you can live with. It isn't a congenital problem that can be fixed. It is something that will never change. It would mean condemning her to a life that is not [...]. It isn't an option in my view. (IL 2018, Inbar)

Although the word "responsibility" is not explicitly said, Inbar does opt for genetic knowledge and acts in what she considers to be the only responsible way.

However, it seems too simple to *necessarily* bind responsibility to knowledge and irresponsibility to not-knowing when discussing genetic testing. In our interviews we found very different feelings, concerns, and attitudes of responsibility relating to the scope of genetic knowledge towards the foetus, the family, society, culture's values, the time to come, and where one lives. The refusal to test may still involve a form of non-responsibility that is not equivalent to irresponsibility. While irresponsibility denies responsibility for no reason or for bad reasons, non-responsibility would be, as Schües argues in chapter 2 on genetic responsibility, a decision that involves declaring oneself not responsible for the realm of *genetic* decision-making, but nevertheless assuming responsibility for devoted care and nurturing of a child with whatever genetic disposition. This form of reasoning for a non-responsibility in such cases denies the transformation of a general moral responsibility to care into a genetic responsibility for a biological genetic disposition. However, even though the decision not to test may not be seen as irresponsible, that does not mean that it should be interpreted as a right or good decision.

In order to be attentive to different dimensions of responsibility that are inherent in women's (and couples') attitudes to prenatal screening, we first look at an *existential or personal dimension*, and then at her (or their) understanding of the *inter-generational relations*, i.e. of the relationship to her future child; and we also look at the relationships within the family as part of *society*. Since our interviews were conducted after testing (or declining to test) they are set in a retrospective context. This allows us to address temporal aspects such as feelings in the past, during the pregnancy, and also later on. First, we briefly introduce the three interpretative dimensions:

1. The *existential dimension* encompasses the personal life, feelings and attitudes of the person (and her partner) confronted with the test. In the interviewees' answers they may refer to themselves, to the family, to society in general, or to particular others. The existential dimension concerns the woman herself with regard to her past and present, and her possible future feelings and thoughts. How does she see her feelings and reasons about genetic testing with regard to her own life?

2. The *intergenerational dimension* refers to the vertical structure within the family and society with regard to the relationships between generations. The next generation is brought into the world having been tested (or not). How do pregnant women relate to their foetus or their future child? What sort of "generative" bond is created? How is the responsibility between the generations considered?

3. The *social dimension* denotes the horizontal structure within the family and society. People who are with us in the world, those with whom we live and those we have to deal with, those with whom we share particular norms and at least parts of a value system, and those who are family members, friends, acquaintances, simply our fellow humans. What is the social situation from the point of view of the interviewee? How do they feel about being responsible or being irresponsible towards their family members or further contemporaries?

When we looked at the reasons women gave to explain their decision not to have NIPT, we essentially found four types of most common reasons:

a. Not wanting to know
b. Not wanting the immediate consequences of tests
c. Feeling ambivalent
d. Considering the test to be useless.

Only the first type however addresses the theme of not wanting to know directly. We will first list the four types of reasons for not testing in a rather idealised manner, and then elaborate on them according to the existential, intergenerational and social dimensions. In order to give a richer account of not-knowing we have also included women who had a test but later wished they had not.

a. *No testing because of not wanting to know.* Some women reasoned that knowing the genetic information has unwanted consequences, i.e. becoming responsible for aborting a child with a disability. For the German woman Maja, Down syndrome is no problem. Sabine would not want an abortion. And Lisa said that, if the child had a trisomy, s/he would "be there anyway". These women did not want to bear this responsibility for a decision. Not having the test because they did not want to know also includes religious non-users who were unable to reconcile testing (and abortion) with their conscience and religious beliefs.
b. *No testing because of unwanted immediate consequences of tests.* Some women did not want to have the test because they felt that the "pregnancy would be less burdened" (GE 2018, Maja) if they did not have to wait for results. Other women, like Sabine, did not want to test because they were afraid of making a wrong decision should the test result be a false positive, and aborting a healthy child.
c. *No testing because of feelings of ambivalence.* Other women, like Sabine, felt ambivalent about testing. They would have taken the test (perhaps) if it were covered by insurance, i.e. if it were a standard medical procedure. An illustration can be found in the interview with an Israeli woman, Libi (IL 2018): "If it [NIPT] were free – yes. I would have done it. I think the financial aspect is the main thing that prevented me."
d. *No testing because the test is considered useless.* Some women said "No" to the test because they did not see a reason for it. Hence, they saw no use in it.

Sabine was relieved after nuchal translucency measurement in ultrasound and considered NIPT useless since she would not have amniocentesis anyway, and would not abort the child she had seen in the ultrasound ("five fingers, a little leg, a nose"; GE 2018, Sabine). Another non-user of NIPT, the anaesthetist Anina, felt great confidence in her partner, which left no room for doubts, and hence saw "no point" in it and considered NIPT unnecessary (GE 2018, Anina).

We now relate these types of reasons for saying "No" to NIPT to the three dimensions of responsibility that we have described before. We intend to detect meanings of not-knowing that contribute to how women and couples can make sense of their situation. If we can find such contributions, we have reason to claim that there is a particular sense-constituting role of not-knowing and of some of the reasons and feelings behind it.

4.1 Existential dimension

When a person refers to reasons of type (b) – not wanting to test because of unwanted immediate consequences of testing – a defined area of potential knowledge is excluded from the knowledge a person wants to acquire, because they fear existential burden or harm. Heidi, a 37-year-old mother of a healthy child who worked as an assistant in a property management company in a small town in eastern Germany, told us that for her, not-knowing was a form of protection from knowledge that would be harmful for her. After losing two pregnancies, she decided to have the best possible examination in her third pregnancy, which eventually led to the birth of her child in 2017. She took several prenatal tests, such as ultrasound, but not NIPT (or other genetic tests). Although her partner wanted to have the security of NIPT, she did not so they decided against it. Her reasoning was that she did not want to be confronted with the need to make a decision about continuing the pregnancy should the result of the NIPT be positive. The regular special check-ups made her feel safe, and she was glad that the nuchal translucency was "relatively fine", meaning they reduced the likelihood of Down syndrome. So she felt no other tests were necessary. This is also because she would not have known how to react. Heidi has explained it as follows:

> This is, you can't just make a blanket recommendation or not. I think every woman should know that this [NIPT] is really an examination,

whether the child is healthy or not, that it isn't just a film show ("Baby-Kino"). Full stop. And it's just, that it's an examination whether the child is healthy or not, and that maybe you'll face this question at some point, even in the middle of your pregnancy: are you going to keep the baby, or do you get rid of it? (GE 2018, Heidi)

For her, knowing a positive test result could lead to uncertainties, worries and anxieties because of the knowledge; we have already discussed some of the aspects involved in the section above. Part of these are the concerns whether or how much the baby's health is/will actually be affected. Out of this uncertainty within the knowledge, the wish may later emerge. And at this point knowledge can no longer be undone; it is transformed into an existential weight.

This observation of being existentially affected is in line with a common attitude that emerged from many interviews with Ultraorthodox women in Israel. For some of them, receiving abnormal results would mean burdening the pregnancy (reason type b), while they can do nothing about it, since termination is mostly not morally acceptable even though some rabbis give permission for it (Ivry/Telman 2019; chapter 7). Some women claimed such knowledge would result in harming their attachment to the baby, and they did not want to burden the pregnancy with testing. Thus, not wanting to test might not necessarily mean not wanting to know. Testing means that the pregnant woman or couple has to wait for the result, and the result may consist in another likelihood that may cause new uncertainties and anxieties. For some people this waiting for information is felt as a burden and as holding off on a relationship with the foetus.

For Tanja, a 42-year-old German lawyer, the decision-making process for the Harmony Test and the ensuing amniocentesis was accompanied by an intensive search for information. The wait for the results of the first Harmony Test took one week, and they then came as "invalid" ("gar nicht auswertbar"; GE 2018, Tanja). The second attempt turned out to be a 98 per cent probability for Down syndrome. The result was communicated by telephone: "The earth opened up beneath me." The ensuing amniocentesis confirmed the result. All in all, the diagnostic process was a time filled with a lot of waiting, a lot of worrying, but in the end, time had "absolutely played on the child's side":

There is an incredible lack of time, you know. Well, it all comes down to that, even if we now say that the prenatal testing or Harmony Test or whatever is brought forward to the 12th week of pregnancy, and for everyone, hmm [...] then no-one will take their time to give the women good advice on how to deal with a diagnosis like that. Because they simply won't have the time any more. Then in a case of doubt it's a race against the clock, checking that they don't miss this 12th week, until when, er, the indication solution is possible, you see. (GE 2018, Tanja)

Her "connection to the child was cut from the moment of the ultrasound", i.e. independently of the NIPT, and she describes her pregnancy then as one of the "hidden pregnancies" (English in the original). Later on, after she had cancelled the abortion, her belly bulged out, and she felt the child's movements and heard its heartbeat. Thus, we see here that the temporality of the testing practices, the decisions and worries, existentially influence the bodily being of the pregnant woman.

An interview with Adva (age 34), an Ultraorthodox mother of four children, the third with Down syndrome, gives a reasoning that refers to the untoward effects of testing:

I am happy I didn't know during pregnancy. Very happy. Because I think it would have made it a difficult pregnancy. You don't know what's going to happen, what's going to come out. [...] It seems to me like a very unpleasant experience. Both for you and the foetus, and the foetus feels it. It feels if it is wanted or not. I think the fact that my child felt all through the pregnancy that it was wanted, it's meaningful for the rest of his life. (IL 2019, Adva)[9]

Testing would have made her pregnancy "difficult", an "unpleasant experience".

An example of reason type (d), mixed with (b), i.e. not wanting to know since knowledge is considered useless, is the interview with Hodaya, a 24-year-old Ultraorthodox mother of two children, the older one with Down syndrome:

I think it [testing] is unnecessary for our community, since we don't have abortions anyhow, and it just provokes stress and worries during the entire pregnancy [when abnormality is detected]. You carry fear and depression much more. (IL 2018, Hodaya)

A similar reason was given by Anna, a 30-year-old German archaeologist who considered herself an atheist, with two children, both born during her studies at the university, the second child with Down syndrome. She also explained her

---

9   This quote has been also discussed in Nov-Klaiman et al. (2019).

decision not to have the test in terms of the irrelevance of such information at this stage in the pregnancy:

> And we didn't have the tests because, firstly, you can see that after it's born, you would still see it, and secondly, they wouldn't have had any consequences for me anyway, I wouldn't have aborted the child, regardless of whether it had a trisomy or not. (GE 2018, Anna)

Genetic information was not needed for this group of women because it would not be used to prompt the decision to have an abortion. For some of them, like Anna, it would also be useless as preparation. The impression that they were receiving useless information is not connected to religious conviction. The reasons may be manifold, but this group of women claimed that they would not abort, regardless of the test result. Furthermore, it seems that in an existential dimension, as understood in light of these interviews, the issue of responsibility seems less prominent.

4.2   Intergenerational dimension and the relationship with the child

Not knowing in relation to the intergenerational dimension touches several difficult aspects, such as insecurity, which thus endangers the relationship to the child. In the following example, Sophie-Louise was called upon by her ob/gyn to accept her responsibility and seek information, which she refused. For her, the abstract genetic information is different from lived knowledge that would include the prospect of what it is like to live with a disabled child. She felt that genetic knowledge would endanger her relationship with the child. Instead of medical reassurance, she was looking for a more beneficial kind of security in being accompanied and supported. Sophie-Louise is a 29-year-old mother of two, one with Turner syndrome (6 y), the younger child normal (3 y). She worked as an educator (*Erzieherin*) and lived in a major city in eastern Germany. She was also an activist who blogged about Turner syndrome, and had written a book on the subject. For her, what she called "the diagnostic voyage" began with an enlarged nuchal skin fold that was detected in the first routine ultrasound in week 10 of her pregnancy. Because of the suspected Down syndrome, the ob/gyn arranged a clinic appointment for her with a prenatal diagnostician, ending the consultation, as she recalled, with the words "You do know what Down syndrome means" (GE 2018, Sophie-Louise)

We may say that the ob/gyn assumed that Sophie-Louise wanted to know. Under this assumption she was acting on behalf of her patient, in her best interests. However, the physician also called upon her to take responsibility for knowing about the possible diagnosis. Here, the physician was in line with Sophie-Louise's husband, who had multiple sclerosis with associated visual impairments. His own disability led him not to want a child with a disability, and he was afraid that he would become a wheelchair user and unable to care for a disabled child. The husband here did not see himself as able to take the responsibility for a child, because he feared losing control of his own life. Sophie-Louise told us in the interview how she remembered her decision. She rephrased how she told it to her husband: "No, we're doing that now! It's *here* and I was *so* happy, and it *will be ok!*" (GE 2018, Sophie-Louise).

Even though she did not once use the term "responsibility" during the interview, we think that is what she actually described: against her physician's and her partner's calls to be responsible in the sense of having the test, she took responsibility in another sense – responsibility for the child that comes, no matter how it comes.

The decision that was expected or even imposed upon her by her partner has "left traces that never went away," although ultimately he "supported the decision" (GE 2018, Sophie-Louise). The couple eventually split up. Despite her initial resolution to go along with what comes, after the prenatal diagnostician told them it might be something other than Down syndrome, something rarer, and advised her to have amniocentesis, Sophie-Louise wanted to know everything at this point, as she explained:

> I have to admit, on the one hand I wanted to know everything, but on the other I was very, very naïve and somehow, I was very sad and [...] somehow, I didn't feel like that, that I could have just gone home and let things go on as they were. Because then, because there was such a – well – a bad feeling there. (GE 2018, Sophie-Louise)

With regard to our list of possible reasons not to know, we see in Sophie-Louise's statement reason type (c) – ambivalence – even though in the end she decided to know. The confirmatory amniocentesis then indicated Turner syndrome. It was in week 20 and she personally was happy that she heard the confirmation after the end of the first trimester, because she did not want to face a conflictual decision about an abortion (GE 2018, Sophie-Louise: "because I didn't want to enter into this conflict at all") – reasoning that may be understandable morally, but is not juridically valid since in Germany, abortion for medical reasons after amniocentesis is permitted with no time limit.

The information that she received about Turner syndrome was "not very humane", as she put it, since it was essentially saying that "life expectancy is reduced by five per cent" (GE 2018, Sophie-Louise). In our typology of reasons for not-knowing, in her retrospective evaluation this would come under (d) – useless knowledge. Being opposed to "prenatal selection" she said that in her view: "I don't think [these statistics] create knowledge in a form you would want. They open the door to so many uncertainties" (GE 2018, Sophie-Louise). Sophie-Louise considers prenatal diagnosis in general "superfluous" and "endangering the relationship with the child" (GE 2018, Sophie-Louise). The information from prenatal diagnosis was superfluous for preparing to live with her child, because the child was not as the literature had predicted, and diagnosis after birth would have sufficed (GE 2018, Sophie-Louise).

However, she learned this only with time. Here we see a second facet of the temporal dimension: knowledge that emerged later in life and that led to a different way of taking responsibility in a subsequent pregnancy. This is what she did. During her second pregnancy, Sophie-Louise chose to have only minimal diagnostics, underlining her "right not to know", and wishing for a different kind of security, through the midwife's emotional support. Sophie-Louise thought NIPT has a negative side-effect because it creates an expectation of false security that everything will be fine. Furthermore, she criticises how the test is used and how people make sense of results, in that they contain an ableist attitude:

> [...] and the test said there's nothing there, *thank God*. Because I see this hostility towards the disabled in that, because it doesn't have to be "thank God". (GE 2018, Sophie-Louise)

Another reason that has been raised against testing was the message such an act (testing) would send to a sibling with the condition tested for. As Ilanit, an Israeli mother of a child with Down syndrome, put it:

> Having this test (NIPT) put me in a situation of an inner conflict. Having this test – what does it mean? What does it say about my child who is alive? [...] What am I saying as a mother who has a child with Down syndrome and who is thankful for that? What am I saying? That actually I am not thankful [to have this child]? My arguments were complex. On the one hand, it is very important to know and to prepare and to know

what it really means. On the other hand, it puts me in a place of "what am I really saying about my child who is already alive?" (IL 2018, Ilanit)

Ilanit was a mother of three, the first child with Down syndrome. She was 35 years old, religious, a PhD student. In her third pregnancy she had NIPT and said that in the current situation, when they already had one child with DS, termination was not out of the question if abnormality were detected.

In retrospective interviews, as we conducted them, the timing of both the interview and the test results are important to bear in mind when we consider the evaluation women reported. Women who had a negative NIPT later mainly reported being reassured. However, although most women with a positive result reported being burdened by the result for the remainder of their pregnancy, we did encounter the opposite scenario. For example, one Israeli woman, who – following "abnormal" findings in the nuchal fold test – decided to have NIPT, in the hope of getting an early answer about the foetus' condition, without needing to wait for amniocentesis. The test detected trisomy 18. She recalled: "It helped me make the 'cut' and say: ok. An abnormal pregnancy. I must make an emotional cut and be done with it and only later [after the abortion] mourn it." She was strongly in favour of the test, even in this case which revealed an abnormality. (IL 2017, Ilanit)

This being said, for some women it is just important to know in order to be able to face the future, by reducing uncertainty about what is about to be born (Löwy 2017: 1). As has been shown in the literature, reducing not-knowing and creating "reassurance" is the most prevalent reason for women to use NIPT (Lewis, Hill & Chitty 2016). While for some women this would include the option of an abortion, others just want to know without necessarily wanting to abort in case of a positive result. Some couples would "welcome any child" (we found several examples); thus for them not-knowing may be preferred because knowing would not lead to an action and would be useless anyway (reason type d).

4.3 Social Dimension: Setting the discourse

The social dimension intersects with the intergenerational dimension. We observe a rich picture regarding genetic testing and responsibility. In Israel we observed that some women transfer their responsibility to the physician or to the rabbi, preferring to trust their judgement. Other women "took the lead" and had tests even though these were not recommended by their physician.

Yet other women did not have the test despite their physician's recommendation. Both scenarios can accord, in a way, with taking responsibility for the future child and the family. It seems that in Germany, responsibility tends to be placed on the pregnant woman who wants to decide, and is (socially) assumed to do so. She is supposed to take responsibility about what should be tested. In either context, following a physician's recommendation is not necessarily a manifestation of refusing responsibility in an unreflective way. Likewise, since there are very different ways of realising responsibility as well as irresponsibility, not following the recommendations can easily be regarded as either being responsible or as being not responsible or even as being irresponsible. This observation accords with the assessment that there is no consensus on whether genetic testing or not testing, knowing or not-knowing itself is considered to be either responsible or irresponsible. This ethical discussion therefore needs to take account of this.

In Israel, it is commonly perceived that responsible parents have a duty to prevent suffering for a future child and the entire family. Since disability is often considered a source of suffering, this responsibility begins in pregnancy, with prenatal testing. Testing during pregnancy seems a necessary tool for detecting disability and for allowing the termination of an affected pregnancy based on abnormal results (cf. see chapter 6 in this book).

To illustrate this, we quote from the interview with Efrat (age 38), a mother of two children, the younger with Down syndrome. She had a false negative result from NIPT:

> A friend of mine was pregnant around the same time I gave birth to my child and she decided not to do the tests, and I remember that in my view it was "How can you be a friend of mine, see what happened to us and decide not to perform the tests?" It was extremely irresponsible in my view. [...] The message I receive both verbally and non-verbally is "how could you be so irresponsible and not do amniocentesis and how did it happen that you have a child with DS?" As if he has no right to exist in this world. (IL 2018, Efrat)[10]

The question of whether the mother expresses a view that is held generally in Israeli secular society is not the only issue here. We also want to indicate the reproach of irresponsibility is not trivial; it is strong and affects close, familial and social relationships.

---

10   This quote had also been discussed in Nov-Klaiman et al. (2019).

In Germany, disability was not found to be connected with suffering in the same way as in Israel. The triangle of "disability, responsibility and testing", as we have explained above in the chapter 6 on "disability", has different meanings in Israel and Germany. A common German rationale articulated by women who already had a child with Down syndrome was that testing enables disability to be detected, which is necessary for (prospective) responsible parents of a child with special needs to prepare – both emotionally and practically. However, this is not representative of German society in general: most women who receive a diagnosis of Down syndrome in amniocentesis decide to terminate the pregnancy.

A majority of both German and Israeli interviewees stressed that performing prenatal diagnosis was a decision for the individual or the couple. They explicitly refused to make any recommendations or judgments. In line with this was Laura, a German woman, who used prenatal diagnosis in two pregnancies, which led to abortions in both cases, and who told us that her own family and her partner's were supportive of any decision she and her husband took regarding prenatal tests and a potential abortion, or about raising a child. However, she told us that in the second pregnancy, her ob/gyn made her feel that if she "did not have the tests, [she] would be a bad mother" (GE 2018, Laura). She reported the ob/gyn's reasoning was "to be extra sure". For those women who experience such strong social expectations, the issue of becoming a responsible mother in the eyes of the professionals may be an important factor in their own decision-making.

5. Conclusion

In this chapter, we explore the question of the reasoning of women who did not want to know the genetic disposition of their foetus or who actually tested because they had a strong feeling about the issue of not-knowing. In order to form a better understanding of the phenomenon of not wanting to know, we analyse the philosophical underpinnings of not-knowing and narratives of people who have experienced a decision-making situation about genetic information. The philosophical tradition and lay understandings privilege knowledge and tend to link knowing with responsibility, and not-wanting to know primarily with irresponsibility. Not-knowing is therefore treated as inferior, and there needs to be a "good and convincing" reason not to know. Yet, briefly stated, we found in the empirical study of the women who did not want to test or who wished that they had not been informed about their foetus' genetics, that some perceived genetic test information as overwhelming and leading to anxiety and burdening of the pregnancy. Thus, not wanting to know does not necessarily lead to ignorance, in the same way that wanting to know does not always lead to certainty. The relationship between genetic information and responsibility is strongly influenced by different feelings, such as uncertainty and insecurity.

Since all interviews were conducted retrospectively, the theme of not wanting to know also needs to be interpreted temporally. Time makes a difference, and the relevance of information given may change over time and with new situations. A *phenomenology of pregnancy* (Bornemark/Smith 2016; Völkle/Wettmann 2021) shows the different phases and times of waiting. What may seem right before testing during pregnancy can appear different later on when a test result is known, a baby born, or just when time has passed. As explained above (Section 3.1), prospective and retrospective perspectives are very different and produce different questions. The retrospective question "what would I rather not have known?" cannot be posed earlier but may lead to some of the insights we found in the interviews and have presented in this chapter.

A conceptual analysis of not-knowing with regard to empowerment, uncertainty and responsibility, which we present in the theoretical sections of this chapter, is challenged by experiences and reflections of people who actually grappled with these questions. What can we learn from this? Here we summarise the insights that seem to us most important:

i.   The philosophical conceptualisation of not-knowing has proved more complex than the empirical material. We have generated theoretical categories of different forms and intensities of manifestation of not-knowing and dimensions of how not-knowing is relevant. With regard to attitudes of responsibility and irresponsibility, as well as feelings of certainty and uncertainty, security and insecurity, the empirical material has nevertheless enriched the philosophical considerations. We suggest that particular rationales for not-knowing are more prevalent in one country than another and, hence, reflect different philosophical premises. In Germany, the rationale was by and large a construction of responsibility involving autonomy as individual self-determination. Prenatal diagnosis and NIPT are seen as a decision for the individual or the couple who explicitly refuse to give or be given any recommendations or judgments.

In Israel, the decision involved relational decision-making as informed by religion, following the recommendations of rabbis and family members. Here we found that the women either test and abort after a positive test result, or they simply do not have the test at all and leave it to fate. Contrastingly, our interviewees also included secular women (including some who rejected NIPT and amniocentesis), who explained that they are "settling" for the routine (and funded) tests. In other words, without abnormal findings from the routine tests and without a clear recommendation from their doctor, they saw no reason to risk the pregnancy with an invasive test or to spend a lot of money on a private test like NIPT.

Despite a common secular tendency to favour having as much information as possible, and thus testing, settling for the routine tests is not uncommon among secular Israelis. Rina, for instance, did not have NIPT or amniocentesis.

To be honest, I'm not so sure if it was so clever or not [not to test]. I was simply optimistic. In our family we don't have many [...]. There is one relative who has a genetic condition, but he isn't a close relative. It seemed to me like "nice to have", but not something that I really needed. [...] We already had healthy kids at home, so we saw no reason why this time there would be a reason to test. (IL 2018, Rina)

ii. Not-knowing has a constitutive meaning of its own and has been explored on an existential, intergenerational and social dimension. It is not simply a negative derivative of knowing as a lack of knowledge; not-knowing can itself have a sense-constituting role. Not-knowing in terms of NIPT primarily concerns a *known unknown*, i.e. a particular field that someone does not want to know. Different feelings or reasons may accompany the refusal of genetic testing and its information, such as the fear of having to decide should the test result be positive. Still, some women wished retrospectively that they had not been informed because they felt overburdened, uncertain or insecure with the result. In certain circumstances – as was particularly found in the German interviews – not knowing can even mean something positive for the woman, for instance allowing a pregnancy to be experienced as unburdened and full of confidence.

iii. Some interviewees mentioned the judgment that not to test would be irresponsible. Yet the overall relation between genetic information and responsibility is far more complex than assumed in an interview or in public discourses. Our interviews show that genetic information is not always accompanied by responsibility, security and certainty of judgment. The issue of the relationship between knowledge and responsibility, or of not-knowing and irresponsibility, is still philosophically and ethically debated. Thus, the question of when and why is it responsible to be ignorant about (genetic) information is still open.

Comparing Israel and Germany highlights the versatility of cultural and social ways of feeling, thinking and acting, and also emphasises not-knowing as a form of *responsible* decision-making that avoids information (rather than knowledge) for various reasons. While in Israel it is perfectly normal to do prenatal genetic testing, such self-certainty cannot be observed in Germany. The two countries seem not to differ greatly in terms of the decision to abort after a positive test result. When women decide against testing and do not want to know the genetic disposition of the foetus, there are some differences in the reasoning between Israel and Germany – yet in both countries, a woman who refuses to have the tests may be called a "bad mother". The focus on saying "no" to genetic information brings out different ways of reasoning according to their existential, cultural and social settings.

References

Andorno, Roberto (2004): "The right not to know: an autonomy based approach." In: J Med Ethics 30, pp. 435–440.

Bammer, Gabriela/Smithson, Michael/the Goolabri Group (2008): "The Nature of Uncertainty." In: Uncertainty and Risk. Multidisciplinary Perspectives, Abingdon/New York: Earthscan, pp. 289–304.

Böschen, Stefan/Kastenhofer, Karen/Marschall, Luitgard/Rust, Ina/Soentgen, Jens/Wehling, Peter (2006): "Scientific Cultures of Non-Knowledge in the Controversy over Genetically Modified Organisms (GMOs). The Cases of Molecular Biology and Ecology." In: GAIA 15/4, pp. 294–301.

Bornemark, Johanna/Smith, Nicolas (2016): Phenomenology of Pregnancy, Stockholm: Södertörn Philosophical Studies.

Breyer, Friedrich/Bürger, Joachim (2005): "Biopolitik," In: Leviathan Sonderheft 23, Wiesbaden: VS Verlag für Sozialwissenschaften, pp. 71–96.

Chadwick, Ruth (2009): "The right to know and the right not to know – ten years on." In: Christoph Rehmann-Sutter, Hansjakob Müller (eds.): Disclosure Dilemmas. Ethics of Genetic Prognosis after the "Right to Know/Not to Know" Debate, Farnham: Ashgate, pp. 9–24.

Deutscher Ethikrat (2013): Die Zukunft der genetischen Diagnostik: von der Forschung der klinischen Anwendung. (http:///www.ethikrat.org/dateien/pdf/stellungnahme-zukunft-der-genetischen-diagnostik.pdf), accessed 26 July 2022.

Duttge, Gunnar/Lenk, Christian (2019): Das sogenannte Recht auf Nichtwissen. Normatives Fundament und anwendungspraktische Geltungskraft, Paderborn: Mentis.

Flatau, Laura/Reitt, M./Duttge, Gunnar/Lenk, C./Zoll, B./Poser, W. (2018): "Genomic information and a person's right not to know: A closer look at variations in hypothetical informational preferences in a German sample." In: PLoS ONE 13(6), e0198249, (https://doi.org/10.1371/journal.pone.0198249), accessed 26 July 2022.

Fricker, Miranda (2007): Epistemic Injustice. Power and the Ethics of Knowing, Oxford and New York: Oxford University Press.

Grey, Thomas (1742): Ode on a Distant Prospect of Eton College (http://www.thomasgray.org/cgi-bin/display.cgi?text=odec), accessed 26 July 2022.

Heidbrink, Ludger (2013): "Nichtwissen und Verantwortung. Zum Umgang mit nichtintendierten Handlungsfolgen." In: Claudia Peter/Dorett Funke (eds.): Wissen an der Grenze. Zum Umgang mit Ungewissheit und Unsicherheit in der modernen Medizin. Frankfurt a.M.: Campus, pp. 111–140.

Ivry, Tsipy/Telman, Elly (2019): "Shouldering moral responsibility. The division of moral labor among pregnant women, rabbis, and doctors." In: American Anthropologist 121/4, pp. 857–869.

Johnston, Josephine/Zacharias, Rachel L. (2017): "The Future of Reproductive Autonomy." In: Just Reproduction: Reimagining Autonomy in Reproductive Medicine, special report, Hastings Center Report 47, pp. 6–11.

Kerwin, Anne (1993): "None Too Solid. Medical Ignorance." In: Knowledge: Creation, Diffusion, Utilization 15/2, pp. 166–185.

Knorr Cetina, Karin (1999): Epistemic cultures. How the sciences make knowledge, Cambridge: Harvard University Press.

Lemke, Thomas (2004): Veranlagung und Verantwortung. Genetische Diagnostik zwischen Selbstbestimmung und Schicksal, Bielefeld: transcript Verlag.

Lemke, Thomas (2013): Perspectives on Genetic Discrimination, London: Routledge.

Lewis, C./Hill, M./Chitty, LS. (2016): "A qualitative study looking at informed choice in the context of non-invasive prenatal testing for aneuploidy." In: Prenatal Diagnosis 36 (9), pp. 875–881.

Löwy, Ilana (2017): Imperfect Pregnancies. A History of Birth Defects & Prenatal Diagnosis, Baltimore: Johns Hopkins University Press.

Lucassen, Anneke (2005): "Families and genetic testing: the case of Jane and Phyllis." In: Case Analysis in Clinical Ethics, Cambridge: Cambridge University Press, pp. 7–18.

Mieth, Dietmar (2001): Die Diktatur der Gene. Bioethik zwischen Machbarkeit und Menschenwürde, Freiburg: Herder Spektrum.

Nov-Klaiman, Tamar/Raz, Aviad E./Hashiloni-Dolev, Yael (2019): "Attitudes of Israeli parents of children with Down syndrome toward non-invasive prenatal screening and the scope of prenatal testing." In: Journal of genetic counseling 28(6), pp. 1119–1129.

Nuffield Council on Bioethics (2017): Non-invasive prenatal testing: ethical issues, London. (https://www.nuffieldbioethics.org/wp-content/uploads/NIPT-ethical-issues-full-report.pdf), accessed 12 April 2022.

Plato (2000): Apology, trans. G.M.A. Grube in Readings in Ancient Greek Philosophy: from Thales to Aristotle, 2nd ed. Indianapolis: Hackett Publishing Company, pp. 112–130.

Plato (2018): Theaetetus, transl. by Benjamin Jowett, Adansonia Publishing.

Polanyi, Michael (1958): Personal Knowledge, Chicago: University of Chicago Press.

Rehmann-Sutter, Christoph (2003): "Die Ungerechtigkeit genetischer Diskriminierung." In: Realismus und Utopie. Zur Politischen Philosophie von Arnold Künzli. Zürich: Rotbuch 2003, pp. 247–265.

Rehmann-Sutter, Christoph/Müller, Hansjakob (eds.) (2009): Disclosure Dilemmas. Ethics of Genetic Prognosis after the "Right to Know / Not to Know" Debate, Farnham: Ashgate.

Rehmann-Sutter, Christoph/Timmermans, Danielle/Raz, Aviad (under review): Routinized prenatal screening with NIPT: Free and informed decision-making as a key criterion for the ethical evaluation of testing routines.

Rubeis, G./Orzechowski, M./Steger, F. (2020): "Non-invasive prenatal testing as a routine procedure of prenatal care. Perspectives and challenges regarding reproductive autonomy." In: Ethik Med 32, pp. 49–63.

Schües, Christina (2018): "Phenomenology and the political – injustice and pre-judges." In: Rethinking Feminist Phenomenology: Theoretical and applied Perspectives, London/New York: Rowman & Littlefield, pp. 103–120.

Smithson, Michael (1989): Ignorance and Uncertainty. Emerging Paradigms, New York: Springer.

Soniewicka, Marta (ed.) (2016): "The Moral Philosophy of Genetic Counselling: Principles, Virtues and Utility Reconsidered." In: The Ethics of Repro-ductive Genetics – Between Utility, Principles, and Virtues, New York: Springer, pp. 1–37.

Suter, S. (2002): "The routinization of prenatal testing." In: American Journal of Law & Medicine, 28, pp. 233–270.

Unger, Peter (1975): Ignorance: A Case for Scepticism, Oxford: Oxford Univer-sity Press.

Völkle, Laura/Wettmann, Nico (2021): "The Process of Pregnancy: Paradoxical Temporalities of Prenatal Entities." In: Human Studies (https://doi.org/10 .1007/s10746-021-09588-1), accessed 12 April 2022.

Wehling, Peter (2001): "Jenseits des Wissens? Wissenschaftliches Nichtwissen aus soziologischer Perspektive Beyond Knowledge? Scientific Ignorance from a Sociological Point of View." In: Zeitschrift für Soziologie 30/6, pp. 465–484.

Wehling, Peter (2006): Im Schatten des Nichtwissens. Perspektiven einer Sozi-ologie des Nichtwissens, Konstanz: Universitätsverlag Konstanz.

Wilkesmann, Maximiliane (2019): "Zum professionellen Umgang mit Nichtwissen im Krankenhaus." In: Das sogenannte Recht auf Nichtwissen, Münster: Mentis, pp. 211–231.

12. Comparison through Conversation
Thinking with Different Differences

Yael Hashiloni-Dolev, Aviad Raz, Christoph Rehmann-Sutter, Christina Schües

We have used NIPT as a lens to investigate the social practices of prenatal diagnosis in two distinct but culturally and historically related places. We compared the two countries we chose, Germany and Israel, to develop a better understanding of the plurality of perspectives and social realisations of genetic responsibility in reproduction. Some of the patterns we found were similar, while others were strikingly different. This final chapter discusses some of the meta-issues that we encountered and that we find important for clarifying the comparative methodology, on the basis of how we used and problematised it. We will therefore not "do" more cross-cultural and transnational comparisons in this chapter, but will use some examples from comparisons mentioned previously, in order to *reflect on* their methodological, epistemological and ethical implications. Some of the thoughts are aimed at transnational comparative work in general, but others have emerged specifically from this special pair of countries on which we focused – Israel and Germany – and on the understanding and the features of their very special relationship that made our work so fascinating.

One of the things we have learned and want to emphasise particularly here is that "comparison" alone has, for a series of reasons, proved insufficient. We shall explain why. The chapter argues for an idea of "conversation" as a wider approach that *includes* comparisons of different sorts and on different levels but goes beyond merely comparative work. It should not just observe what is common and what is different, but bring the two countries (and some of their representative groups and voices) into a mutual and ongoing process of learning and dialogue. Learning from each other includes commenting and questioning, and being in conversation with one another. (This, as the introduction says, is also the main purpose of the book as a whole.)

In the first part, we elaborate on the concept of "conversation" that we have in mind and explicitly relate it to comparison as a research strategy, distinguishing it from cross-cultural comparative methodology. A series of different methodological approaches to comparison in social anthropology are relevant here, and they need to be briefly reviewed in this context. In the second part, we start from some personal experiences that caused productive friction and made us think more distinctly about what we are doing while conducting the project. In the last part we reflect on the meaning of "differences" and of "different differences" that arise when the questions asked are not the same on both sides, but contextually adapted to make sense in one national context or the other.

1.   On philosophical conversation

1.1   From multinational comparison to transnational conversation

Multinational comparative research on prenatal testing and screening is a well-established and growing field. Several recent studies report how NIPT has been introduced in different healthcare systems; how it is offered in maternal care; what counselling needs it has generated and what resources are available; how it is regulated, financed, and discussed publicly. They include Perrot/Horn (2021) on England, France and Germany and Ravitsky et al. (2021) on Australia, Canada, China and Hong Kong, India, Israel, Lebanon, the Netherlands, the United Kingdom, and the United States. We ourselves have previously published a comparison between Israel and Germany (Raz et al. 2021), and an explicit comparison of NIPT policies in these countries is part of this book (chapter 2). It is certainly important to know how a new technology such as NIPT is spreading around the world, and what challenges it raises in different sociocultural, legal and economic contexts. Such investigations are an important step in advancing the ethical and policy debates about NIPT in different countries. However, the approach taken in multinational comparisons is also limited, and its limitations are linked to methodological challenges. In cross-cultural comparisons certain general themes or axes for comparison must be defined in advance and applied to all the countries compared, if a comparative picture is to be produced (top to bottom). Some nuances will be lost, in particular those which are more important in a single context, because they cannot produce general comparative themes. And deeper investigations into the background of the themes being compared are often impossible.

However, comparative researchers do not usually have all their comparative questions at the outset. Particularly if a smaller number of countries (two or three) is involved, some comparative themes can also be identified later on in the analytical process. These can then represent views from all the countries involved, instead of comparing the situation in one or more countries "abroad" with the situation "at home". Estrid Sørensen (2010) has described this procedure as a "multi-sited comparison". In her view, comparability is not given, "due to intrinsically comparable characteristics, but because comparability is established through interaction with the research object" (43). "Inside descriptions" of the special topic of comparative research need first to be produced. However, as Sørensen insists, they are "not a result of the researcher's perspective or interpretation, but of mutual involvements or *intra*-actions" (44, our emphasis). The researcher defines a common quality of the objects of comparison, a *tertium comparationis*, according to which they are then compared. Transcending the special constellation of ethnography, as a relationship between "away" and "home", and instead of having only one movement from home to away, in a multi-sited comparison researchers have "spatiotemporal overlapping and varying involvements in field sites" (54) between multiple sites at multiple places that are each simultaneously both "away" and "home". The questions for comparison originate at diverse sites, bringing the contexts into a set of perspectives from all sides. A classic statement by George Marcus (1995: 55) sees the inside description, the *tertium comparationis*, and thirdly the ex-post approach as essential for a multi-sited comparison: "[T]he ex-post approach means that we cannot prior to the study define the *tertium comparationis* of a multi-sited ethnography." This approach has to be found across and bottom-up during the study and needs to be based on multiple inside descriptions. Ethnographic methodology is inductive and often richer than a comparison according to a set of predefined themes of interest, such as attitudes to disability or equity of access to NIPT. And, as Sørensen has clearly pointed out, ethnographic descriptions are not just observations "of something" but are true productions that are generated in intra-active procedures together with actors in the field(s). Indeed, in the steps that lead to "inside descriptions", i.e. descriptions from the internal perspective of one side that form the basis of comparisons, communicative interaction and social construction are already involved, and researchers need to be aware of this. In an ethnographic study, bioethics, as it is done in a location, is part of the field; in our interdisciplinary study we have been observers and interpreters, as well as participants in the discourses that we were studying. This generated a rather complex epistemic situation that we needed to reflect on critically.[1]

Based on our experience of the NIPT study of Israel and Germany, we want to make the conversational elements of comparative research even stronger. Our interest was not solely ethnographic, even though ethnographic and qualitative work was part of what we did. We were also interested in the philosophical perspectives that can provide an understanding of the underlying ethical conflicts in the practices we studied. We were therefore not solely interested in descriptions and comparisons between descriptions, but were always engaged in the field as well, in our roles as philosophers and ethicists contributing to the discourse.

In order to clarify the most important implications of this, we start with the simple picture of a comparison. Comparison is, as Condillac has written, basically a double attention.[2] The comparative mind is attentive to one thing while looking at the other; and then it is attentive to the other thing while looking at the first. One's attention moves back and forth. Differences may appear between two coins for instance, or two paintings by the same painter, without knowing the *tertium comparationis* in advance. Similarities also appear in the same way. A comparison – if this simple explanation is valid – is then essentially a judgment about similarities and differences between two or more things that are considered comparable. The *tertium comparationis* is a *result* of the double attention that *observes* some differences and sees similarities. In Sørensen's considerably more nuanced approach to comparison in ethnography, this observation is focused on an interactive process between observer and the observed – "intra-action", as she calls it. But the aim of a comparison is still a judgment about similarities and differences in certain regards between two or more sites of interest.

Countries, societies, even groups of people or traditions are however not like coins or paintings that can be set next to each other. The resulting com-

---

1　The discourse about methodological reflexivity in comparative social anthropology has produced a rich literature in the last two decades. The term "comparative methods in anthropology" is used in radically new ways that, as Richard Fox and Andre Gingrich have stressed in the introduction to their collection (Gingrich/Fox 2002), today reclaim a variety of qualitative methodologies. See also Candea (2018), Scheffer/Niewöhner (2010).

2　Monnin (2004 : 231) cites Condillac (1795) : "La comparaison n'est donc rien d'autre qu'une double attention."

plexity and the infinity of possible comparative points of view and the impossibility of straightforward comparisons is an insight that is frequently stressed in the anthropological literature about comparison. One popular quotation is this phrase by Evans-Pritchard from 1963: "There's only one method in social anthropology, the comparative method – and that's impossible."[3] Comparing countries, even with regard to a technology such as NIPT, is basically impossible, since the meanings attached to a technology in a given socio-cultural context can be so different from the meanings attached to the same technology in another socio-cultural context that it is difficult to see how the "same" technology is contextualised differently in different countries. The meaning and practice of technology (such as NIPT) *is* not the same in both sites. We are then comparing the incomparable, as if the sameness of the technology and of its description in biomedical language produces a similarity and comparability of its socio-cultural meanings. These meanings are of special interest to cross-cultural comparison.

While comparative judgments are supposed to bring out existing similarities and differences, a conversation involves commenting on one another, questioning each other and challenging each other's views, with the aim of perceiving the familiar in one's "own" place less unquestioningly. The familiar becomes unfamiliar, the unquestionable becomes questionable. The process of turning the familiar into the unfamiliar is an achievement that takes conversation partners beyond their own horizons of beliefs and certainties. A conversation is therefore necessarily an ongoing process, not something that can be done once and for all. A conversation has to be continued, since new points of view can always emerge.

We can conceive of "conversation" in an even wider sense. It is a form of a dialogue that makes it possible to thematise those aspects which are not reducible to the views of one of the conversational partners. In a true conversation, new aspects can emerge that neither of the partners knew before. A conversation is essentially a creative process, not just a descriptive or an analytical endeavour. Therefore, the conversational approach is more congenial to the aims of philosophical understanding and ethical reflection than the ethnographic. It can however *include and involve* ethnographic material and ethnographic insights, and also anthropologists as reflective persons who *do* reflexive anthropology.

---

3   Quoted in Needham (1972: 364), in Scheffer/Niewöhner (2010: 8) and in Candea (2018: 29).

1.2 Conversation explained

We now want to give a more concrete explanation of "conversation". What did we as researchers actually do and experience when we entered the empirically complex, yet philosophically inspiring and challenging interdisciplinary and transnational collaboration of discussing NIPT in a transnational philosophical and cross-cultural study between Israel and Germany? How can we understand our own approach, the experiences that accompanied it, and how are these experiences tied to the interpretations we offer? Looking back at about five years of collaboration here, the first thing that comes to mind is that in order to make the project work we ourselves needed much conversation, sometimes about very practical things such as the bus system in Jerusalem, how to get around on Shabbat, or what shoes to wear in Germany's wintertime, but also on other, deeper levels of culture or politics. Who is the poet or politician after whom this street is named? What do her poems tell us about the Israeli (or German) views on the world? We noticed that the notion "conversation" captures many aspects of our project that go beyond research practicalities. Here are three aspects of conversations that reach deeper:

(1) Conversation became a *doing* in the sense that there was a lot of exchange about the research questions, the study design and the methods among the researchers who worked on the project or participated in our workshops and conferences.

It should come as no surprise that being in an interdisciplinary and international team meant that first impressions, methodological habits, feelings about communication and what each individual may consider "normal" could not be taken for granted. Thus, conversation helped us to work together and to follow up on our task of understanding and comparing our findings and thoughts about our own practices and ways of thinking. During this process, we came to realise that our ways of "seeing the world" have something to do with where we are situated and where we live.

(2) Conversation became a *form* of self-reflection that provoked us into questioning the standpoint of our own research approach and our own social and cultural horizon that might be blinding us to the overall picture, i.e. the details hidden in presuppositions or prejudices regarding oneself or the Other.

(3) Conversation became a *method of interaction* with the Other; however, "own" and "Other" cannot be always clearly distinguished. Israel and Germany are

entangled in an overlapping history; texts by Israeli and German, Jewish or non-Jewish philosophers, ethicists and sociologists are encountered in transnational discussions, which are in turn influenced by Anglo-American discourses. Traditionally, the tie between Israel and European nations/cultures is strong, as Levinas argues in *A l'heure des nations* (1988), a collection of essays about Talmudic texts, about thinkers of the Enlightenment, and conversations about Judaism. From him we learn that it is special to the Jewish ethic-religious heritage that when people stand up to it they live the riddle of otherness. The riddle of otherness means acknowledging the other in her otherness before using reason to formulate a judgement; it means also accepting, perhaps still wondering, about the fact that the other in this cultural context is not the "radical Other", but one who is always also in oneself, yet remains both a stranger and someone familiar. In a project about the beginning of life, prenatal diagnosis, and concerns about offspring and the family, the question about the other human is always an issue. Let the other be the future child, the family members, or the colleagues in their disciplinary, perhaps cultural otherness. Being a researcher, being human means even more to owe a justification to the other and to take on responsibility for her.

In our project the bi-national tie, the tie between others, is built by way of reference to Jewish thought, by readings of Western literature, and by practices as a matter of course – and this holds for people from both Germany and Israel. Thus, conversation can never mean just conversing between nations. Whatever people do, whether they are Israeli or German, researchers or future parents concerned with prenatal diagnosis, their practices are never just German or just Israeli. Every person is situated, every belief is situated. This situation remains ambivalent, as we felt throughout the period of research.

The conversations were transnational insofar as they took place between people who live in their respective cultural and social contexts. In conversation, the narratives of the people concerned, i.e. those who had been interviewed, were part of the transnational setting. Conversation requires someone to be given a voice in order to describe a decision or explain a feeling. These descriptions and explanations by the interviewees or by other people spoken to in the project thus gained a life of their own and created a conversational space. They brought in comparisons and made them possible, but they also brought elements that might not be easily comparable as well.

These three basic dimensions of conversation have been meaningful both for our interdisciplinary work and towards developing a transnational perspective.

1.3   A word about the tasks of philosophy

A word is necessary about the role of philosophy in an interdisciplinary team. Our interdisciplinary team consisted of empirical social scientists, bioethicists and philosophers (with multiple roles). While the people doing the empirical work focused primarily on conducting and interpreting qualitative interviews with users and non-users, experts and biopolitical activists, the philosophers in the team did conceptual work in a historical and systematic perspective. Philosophers question the main concepts involved and issues that are taken for granted, e.g. parenthood, responsibility, or the status of life. They explore these concepts with regard to the history of ideas, questions about their meaning conditions and their relationships with each other. Thus, the philosophers tried to understand how the practices of prenatal testing in Israel and Germany were constituted and became meaningful in terms of, for instance, our understanding of the self and others, or the body and society; and they re-read the intellectual heritage of Jewish and German philosophy as well as current bioethical publications on the project's topic. Since the project involved researchers from different disciplines as well as from different countries and their respective historical and socio-cultural horizons, the researchers' impressions, perspectives and reflections about comparing were also located on different levels of analysis.

One of us (Schües) participated explicitly as the philosopher in this project. In this position she experienced the ambiguity that arose from actually having two roles. For one thing, she worked as an embedded philosopher, yet she also remained faithful to her independent philosophical existence that allowed her to work on the themes that provoked her attention and urged her to reflect upon them regardless of any promises to what the project might deliver.

This ambiguity is of a different kind than the ambiguity between subjectivity or objectivity, which has been discussed by thinkers in the existential-phenomenological tradition such as Georg Wilhelm Friedrich Hegel, Jean-Paul Sartre, Simone de Beauvoir, and Maurice Merleau-Ponty. Rather, the feeling and situation of ambiguity come with the role and status that philosophy, as we understand it, must have in an interdisciplinary project. The term "embedded philosophy" means being in collaboration and conversation with other scientists and trying to intervene by aiming for conceptual clarification, by probing, sometimes even twisting the questions, by critically assessing assumptions and methods, and last but not least by reflecting about the relations between the different disciplines. Overall, an embedded philosopher does not gain knowledge *about* the science, but tries "to participate in resolving problems that scientists raise or encounter in their work" (Pradeu/Lemoine/Khelfaoui/Gingras 2021: 2–3). Thus, an embedded philosopher participates in gaining knowledge within the concreteness of the project's theme and the disciplines in question: in our case, the social sciences.

If we understand philosophy as an intellectual and communicative practice in this very specific sense of embeddedness, it becomes possible for the philosopher to understand the methodological and concrete procedures of the social sciences from the inside. These considerations do not lead to only doing philosophy about something, but also to philosophy within the frame of the social sciences and daily practices of the project. Philosophy is itself actively involved in the process of developing social theory, not only in order to understand how social theorists work methodologically and what they are doing, but also in order to interact with social scientists and to improve sociological interpretations and understandings. In this project, such work very concretely included suggesting questions for the semi-structured interview guide, participating in feedback sessions with the interviewers, and discussing the methods of interview analysis and interpretation. In classical terms, none of this may be considered as the business of philosophy; but philosophy has always used examples from concrete life as well.

A philosophical existence, as Hannah Arendt famously phrased it in her interview with Günter Gaus, amounts to a striving to understand what things are: "I want to understand." We can call this approach *critique by reflection*. It is a never-ending task because in all different historical, social or cultural contexts it exposes questions or concepts that seem questionable, unclear or surprising. The material of philosophy that is put to reflection concerns our relation to ourselves, to the Other, and to the world. That is, it is about finding presuppositions and conditions of human conduct – thinking or acting – and their criteria of validity. In short, philosophy is "concerned about the question: how do we think what" (Schües 2008). How "something" is thought or dealt with is described and reflected both in its necessary generality and its utmost concreteness. Philosophical activity may lead to the destruction of certain concepts and facts by revealing their underlying preconditions. In this ambiguous enterprise, philosophy sometimes does good service, but it can also become a disturbing factor that might not always be "useful" in the context of a defined "study".

Occupying these two roles (Schües), and seeing her in both roles, was never boring; indeed, at times it was a real struggle. One of these productive struggles had to do with the status of the *fait accompli*. It often seemed that the interpretation of interviews was supposed to show the attitudes of the interviewees and to explain how they described their practice. In this context the researchers believed that the narratives and the acts they described might reveal a sense that is already there. A philosophy of human conduct that is focused on findings and interpretation may be called, to quote Merleau-Ponty (1988: 181), a *retrospective* philosophy. To do this is not necessarily wrong. But on the other hand, the art of philosophy is to intervene in the present. A *philosophy of intervention* must regain a way of thinking that shapes the present *in advance* of the claims of empirical science, market drivers, or biopolitical forces. Therefore, the philosopher cannot be satisfied with interpreting how interviewees make sense of their practical dilemmas in prenatal diagnosis.[4] The philosopher needs to question further and must not take a position; philosophy is an activity of both – a science and a form of life.

1.4   Philosophy in a transnational perspective

In this project we are concerned with transnational and cross-cultural perspectives insofar as each participant – researcher or interviewee – is understood as a member of a state, as well as of a particular cultural and social setting. During our work it became clear that a comparison of the practices of different cultural and social settings can open up different possibilities and realities that reflect back one's own self-certainties. We learned to see our own realities differently through the gaze of the other. We sometimes noticed an unease with regard to this other reality, or rather what we take as our "reality".

Thus, comparisons and the conversations *about* the Other not only reveal interesting details about Israeli or German practices but also aspects of one's own position on the themes of life and reproduction in Israel or Germany, on Jewish tradition, on practices of family life, on German feelings about historical responsibility, on underlying concepts of the body, and so on. These discoveries would accord with the difficulty in actually defining what Jewish or

---

4   Rehmann-Sutter et al. (2012) made a similar point about "ethics" in relation to "empirical" ethics.

German philosophy is in modern times (beyond a superficial nod to Kant or Rosenzweig). Certainly conversation, understood as a kind of mindset or attitude, may take place in face of the other but also by reading the different sorts of texts that may inspire a hermeneutic dialogue with the reader.

Doing philosophy in this project also meant learning about Jewish bioethics, and re-considering German bioethics, or Anglo-American bioethics, and questioning the aspirations of a "global bioethics" (ten Have 2016). Due to historical exchanges between scholars of countries and regions, such as the long tradition of Jewish scholars living and working in Germany who ultimately were forced to leave because of the Nazi regime and who continued their work in the USA, in Israel or elsewhere, there is no clear-cut distinction between these different currents of doing philosophy or ethics. However, there are different styles of thinking and different prerequisites for what counts as good reasons, or how much a decision must rely on feelings, social habits, or strong reasoning. Some Israeli and German thinkers introduce religion into ethics, but how this is done, in a Jewish or a Catholic sense for example, shows a huge difference. It turns out, as Shai Lavi (2010) describes in his article about "the paradox of Jewish bioethics in Israel", that a traditional conservative view of life and family can cohere with the extensive use of the most modern biotechnology. Thus, what we learned is that certain positions, such as conservatism or liberalism, can be related to science and technology in very different, even opposite ways.

It soon became very clear that a comparative analysis between prenatal genetic practices in Israel and Germany must distinguish between the different levels on which these practices can be approached. Not all of them concern philosophy, and strictly speaking comparison between countries is not a philosophical matter. In contrast to a cross-cultural comparison, a transnational comparison does not compare nations as holistic entities. Rather we compare, firstly, the practices and ways of thinking of those who live in these different countries and who happen to be differently situated historically, socially and culturally. Secondly, in the transnational perspective the national affiliations of the people and their cultural and social situatedness cannot always be clearly distinguished on the basis of their positions and narratives about their decisions and feelings about prenatal genetic practices. Thirdly, we took seriously the meaning of the prefix "trans" in "transnational" – "across" – and, as explained above, considered conversation part of our methodological approach. Conversation is understood as listening and talking *across* borders. There are still different possible ways of comparing.

On the level of policy, a comparison seems more straightforward, since health governance and regulations in the healthcare system are national (see chapter 2). When it comes to the level of attitudes, experiences or justifications of the people concerned, we analyse, for instance, an interview with an Israeli woman. But how much will her narrative really tell us about Israeli practice? We often observed that some of the narratives could just as well have been told in the other country's social and cultural context. Yet we discovered tendencies and also ways of acting and justifying that were surprising or enlightening. On the third level, we may consider different ways of thinking and judging. Here we see an ambivalent tension between the local situation in which a judgment is held to be convincing, and the claim of generality in the understandings involved and in relying on certain ways of justification.

Overall, there was a lot to learn together: different understandings of the beginning of life and of human entanglement with biotechnology are always fascinating. It was also striking that Israeli and German women's different reasonings may accord with the same practice, but the same reasonings may lead to different practices. For example, we can point to the simple fact that the number of women who use NIPT is very similar in both countries, but in Germany some women hesitate to find out the foetus' genetic disposition for trisomy, while in Israel some women do not want to use NIPT because this test cannot do enough and they want to know even more. Another example: in both Germany and Israel, women care greatly about feeling secure in their pregnancy. But for most Israeli women testing provides security, because they feel that they are doing everything to avoid suffering and to protect the family; whereas many women in Germany feel that testing means times of uncertainty and waiting.

Only by bringing the whole conceptual context and historical, social and ethical horizon into the picture, can the social and philosophical understanding of prenatal practices of genetic diagnosis have a chance to emerge, but at the same time such a broad picture might dissolve the concreteness of a comparative analysis. Thus, we needed the different ways of conversation and the ongoing practice of understanding.

1.5   "Thin" and "thick" morality reconsidered

Based on this transnational philosophical perspective, and in view of Michael Walzer's distinction between a "thick" and a "thin morality" (Walzer 1994), we can better explain what we mean by conversation that goes beyond comparison. Walzer was looking at the differences between moral arguments that we use when talking to our fellow citizens and moral arguments when we are talking to (or about) citizens of foreign countries. When we are addressing others in our own country – we could replace "country" by "socio-cultural environment" as well – we use, as Walzer has called it, a "maximalist" view of morality that is "thick from the beginning, culturally integrated, fully resonant" (1994: 4). A maximalist conception of morality is full of contextual meanings that can be understood, or may even be necessary to understand and to address if one is to be respected as a competent participant of the respective realm of moral discourse. When addressing others in another country or in a foreign socio-cultural environment, we instead use a "minimalist" conception of morality. We refer to universal values, because we expect the others also in their own "thick" context to understand what they mean. A minimalist morality is therefore necessarily "thin" and consists only of those elements that can be understood *across* the differences of national traditions, while the explanation and application of thin morality within a tradition involves the "thick" morality, including tradition-specific experiences and narratives.[5] Let us look at an example:

In NIPT, a minimalist, thin approach would, for instance, merely mention the principle of autonomy and would explain its functioning and criteria. That is, such an approach would explain the right of the pregnant woman to decide about prenatal testing and to receive all the relevant information, and it may also refer abstractly to condemning discrimination against children with disability and special needs. A maximalist, thick explanation of morality, however, would look at the perspectives of the persons affected, or those living with disability who are faced with the concrete situation of decision-making and who are embedded in a particular historical, social and cultural situation. Researchers interested in a thick understanding would thus investigate *how* the principles of autonomy and its practice are historically and socially embedded. In our transnational project, the identification of a "thin morality" or "thick morality" with regard to one's own and the other country's practices is well supported by conversation.

The point of a philosophical conversation between scholars in one country and those in another is to embark on a journey that aims is to understand essential parts of the others' moral practices in a thick sense. This involves learning about the historical, political and cultural particularities, to be able to

---

5   Walzer borrowed this idea of "thickness" from Clifford Geertz (1973); see Walzer (1994, xiii).

comprehend and appreciate the ethical concerns and the sense of injustice in the other context. Conversation, however, also involves more than just understanding; it also means entering into an argumentative deliberation. Walzer was seriously engaged in social criticism, which he sees not only relevant as "internal" criticism but also across what he has called the "spheres of justice".[6] In philosophical conversation about bioethical matters – such as prenatal diagnosis and the many issues connected to it – the social criticism learned in the other sphere can be brought home and lead to a more attentive view of things that may have appeared "normal" and remained unquestioned in one's own country. Also in this regard, philosophical conversation reaches beyond a purely comparative research: its ambition is to do joint moral work from the view of the other, moral work both at home and abroad.

We believe that this resonates in some ways with Amartya Sen's point that in order to see injustices better we all need to be influenced by the opinion of foreigners (Sen 2009). Being critical of a "transcendental position", Sen refers in a transnational perspective to the approach of an "impartial spectator", which can be seen as an alternative of a social contract. The device of impartial spectator does not amount to a "view from nowhere" or a "view from above"; it invites us to imagine what someone from the position of the outside would think or do. Sen presupposes here that the impartial spectator has no personal preferences of their own in the matter of investigation. For our project comparing the social realities of prenatal genetic practices in Israel and Germany, it is interesting to consider the option of a distant perspective that may allow us to see more impartially what is going on in our own society. In order to see our sentiments from a distance, it is a great help to have such a "conversational" perspective that includes the imagination of this impartial spectator.

By trying to understand how a particular practice is assessed in another country, or in other countries in the world, conversation allows for an *interested* and *engaged* comparison. Its aim is to look at one's own customs and habits

---

6   See part III of Walzer (1994) with references to his earlier works. However, we do not fully follow Walzer's communitaristic intention in the "Spheres of Justice". For him justice is determined by the concept of community that is constituted by a common language, history and culture, which generate a collective consciousness and common institutions and sensibilities. With this approach, the concept of justice is fundamentally relativistic. Walzer's approach has a critical potential but fails when it is applied to judging the unjust practices of other countries, i.e. the Indian caste system would be as just as a democratic system.

from the perspectives of others who themselves may not actually be looking critically at us. The conversation includes these interacting perspectives of interest, and the engagement includes the sphere of the in-between (Waldenfels 2006: 109f.). The sphere of the in-between cannot be reduced to either one's own or the Other's but its establishment in conversation may allow insights into each other's practices that were not possible without it. It may bring out differences or similarities, but even more so different understandings about the differences. Hence, *different differences*.

Alluding to the notion of "difference" is essentially intended to avoid two blind alleys that are sometimes used politically to marginalise or denigrate people. The concept of difference is used in very different cultural, political or epistemological fields, and sexist or racist practices are often behind it. In our study we take the notion of difference as a concept of reflection to help us to understand the "other" in their otherness but also in their similarities, in terms of their practices of reproduction and use of prenatal diagnosis. There are epistemological and moral risks here: relativism and universalism. Clearly, both positions stand in opposition to the intention of our research: the former leads to a (perhaps even degrading) view of "THEY do it this way" and, hence, nothing more can be said politically or ethically; and the latter amounts to a disregard of or refusal to acknowledge any concrete historical, cultural or social embeddedness of human practices. Conversation and situating the differences and similarities in context and perspective would not be possible with either of these. The concept of "different differences" means that indicating some differences, for example about the use of NIPT, may in fact be understood in different ways. That is, a difference between two social practices still allows for the possibility of having the same understanding of it or, actually, a different understanding of the difference. *Conversation* may bring this out because it transforms the individual perspectives of the participants, and each participant is involved in an ambivalent way by being absorbed in the conversation and by being someone on her/his own. Of course, we all have our personal interests, motives of engagement, and moments of surprise.

2. Personal reflections

If we now describe some personal experiences and reflections as researchers, we consider them as experiences that have to do with differences and similarities, but also with proximity and distance. An ethnographer may believe that visiting a foreign country means being far away, hence at a distance; yet strangely enough, what is very different may also be very close. The stranger is your neighbour, Emmanuel Levinas would say, showing us that it is humanity, the face of the Other, that brings us this proximity.

Very different situations or practices can therefore be surprising. But they can also bring about a feeling of proximity. What we have learned is that difference and similarity might not cohere with feelings of distance and proximity. There are types of behaviour that are quite familiar to some of us, such as the way some (German) teachers look down on their pupils, or a kind of bureaucratic order that we know well and can handle but that still gives us a feeling of distance.

Each of us had some productive frictions, more or less dramatic moments when differences became surprising. Friction becomes productive when it turns one's own reaction or response towards a situation into a question and an urge to think, observe, or investigate deeper in the "phenomenon" that became questionable.

2.1 Carrying a foetus diagnosed with anencephaly to term (Yael Hashiloni-Dolev)

I wish to share a major moment of discomfort I experienced in my fieldwork. When interviewing in Germany, one of the prenatal genetic counsellors told me a story about a German Catholic woman whose foetus was diagnosed, in the middle of the pregnancy, with anencephaly, a condition that means the baby can survive only a few days after birth, with zero hope of any kind of recovery. Although this woman was fully entitled to have an abortion (not because of the foetus' condition, but because it posed a threat to her mental state), she decided not to. As a religious Catholic she explained to the counsellor that it was very important for her to carry the pregnancy to term, to give birth and hold the baby in her hands, baptise it, and have a funeral.

My emotional reaction was strong. Here I am in Germany, a country and a culture I think I am quite familiar with, yet the story I hear is shocking, exotic, and in a sense hideous to me. My first response is great sadness, but also great discomfort and alienation. I am judgmental, as I find it frightening and repulsive to carry to term a baby that is doomed to die, and to prepare for letting it die in your own arms. I think of my own pregnancies, and of this very frightening situation.

The story haunts me. When returning to Israel I meet women who had experienced late selective abortions/stillbirth. Their stories about rapid terminations, often without seeing the aborted foetus, and never with any formal goodbye ceremony or formal grieving, troubles me. I start comparing both ways of handling this painful event, which obviously have to do with religious beliefs about when life begins and with the concept of the afterlife. I see disadvantages in how such a situation is dealt with in Israel, especially in the sense of the women's psychological ordeal. What was familiar and "normal" becomes somewhat strange, and the "strange" is now understood differently. Although the story the German counsellor told me is atypical even in Germany, as a marginal case it helps me draft the borders of my field of research, and gaze from one culture to another less judgmentally and more contemplatively. It is clear that the emotions evoked in me are cultural and not simply personal or dependent on my private experience as a pregnant woman and a mother. Reflecting on my own experience and emotional reactions helps me to become a better sociologist, as I can move back and forth between the two cultures and understand their effects on the experiences and decisions of the women I wish to understand.

2.2 Elephants in the room (Christoph Rehmann-Sutter)

In the first year of the Israeli-German project on NIPT, I gave a Masters course at my University in Lübeck for psychologists on ethics and trauma. With a group of students during the Winter semester I read and discussed Dan Bar-On's extensive interview study on the memories of the Holocaust through three generations of victim/survivor families in Israel and three generations of descendants of Nazi perpetrators in Germany (Bar-On 1989; 1995). Reading these interview transcripts and comparing them was a tough experience for all of us. The interviews showed how family memories of the Shoah still affect people in Israel and Germany very deeply, even in the third generation, which is the older generation of those currently alive. However, they see the atrocities from the victims' and from the perpetrators' perspectives, which makes them see very different difficulties in their lives in both countries. Bar-On, who died in 2008, was a renowned peace researcher, promoting personal story-telling as a method for peacemaking and peacekeeping. He held the David Lopatie Chair for Post-Holocaust Psychological Studies at Ben Gurion University at Be'er Sheva, which happened to be exactly the place where our project was affiliated. This was an unplanned coincidence.

Victimhood as well as the Holocaust are, in different ways, defining elements of the Israeli identity. Meanwhile historical responsibility and the burden of guilt are central elements of German postwar identity, although in different ways in the German Democratic Republic and in the Federal Republic of Germany, until the *Wiedervereinigung* in 1989. These differences between East and West Germany became strikingly evident in another three-generation study that was conducted in German families, which we also read in the seminar and which made a deep impression both on my students and myself: *"Opa war kein Nazi"* by Harald Welzer, Sabine Moller and Karoline Tschuggnall (Welzer et al. 2002). The authors tracked stories in family members' accounts of remembered events during the time of the Nazi regime and compared how they have been retold in each generation and were substantially transformed in families over the three generations. This impressive study shows that each generation in German families has the atrocities in view, but in a different way. They all have their distinct motifs that are characteristic of the first, second and third generations, which influence how they wish to see their present role in society and their tasks in life that need to be undertaken.

Of course prenatal diagnosis has nothing directly to do with these difficult memories. But this must be lurking in the background in many different ways. How is the history of eugenics incorporated into German memories, and how is the building of a new state of Israel incorporated into Israeli ones? Is there no relation at all to prenatal diagnosis, or can we see traces of a perfectionist ideology in Israel's body politics? In German public discourse about prenatal diagnosis, references to Nazi eugenics and "selection" are abundant (Rehmann-Sutter 2021). Our Israeli team members explained to us that Max Nordau's ideas for body perfectionism around 1900 need to be seen in a context: they echoed eugenic ideas that were present in Europe and other countries at the time, including the USA, UK, Sweden, Germany and even Switzerland (which is my home country). The two countries that we had selected – Germany and Israel – are connected in a tragic way, and the reason why they are connected is not completely unrelated to the topic that we intended to study. I needed to reflect about my own perspective as a member of the German team.

I realised that here I really was confronted with the "elephant in the room" of any Israeli-German study that intends to look at biopolitics. It is actually two elephants, a different elephant in Israel than in Germany. This must be thematised somehow in any study comparing Israel with Germany, as we have now tried to do in this book. In a way I was trapped in this too-big issue. We could not deal with it adequately in our four-year study of NIPT. However, I realised that in order to see more clearly and to understand the "thick moralities" (to use Walzer's term again) on both sides, I needed at least to look at this issue and to ponder it. Otherwise it would have distorted my vision. When working on the ethics and politics of repro-genetics in Israeli and German cultures, this past is not dead, and can be obtrusive. Yet it is all very complicated.

2.3 Normality can be surprising. Facing the silence (Christina Schües)

Being interested in issues concerning the beginning of human beings, I very soon noticed that most women in Israel just self-evidently have genetic testing during pregnancy. I wondered about their urge, even for those below the age of 35, to have the foetus tested. The question seemed not to be *whether* to test but rather *what sort* of genetic testing they should choose. Thus, I realised that Israel's prenatal practice is implemented in society as normal procedure. Overall, I am not particularly shocked by medical life and death issues: seeing a severely ill newborn dying in his mother's arm may be one way of dealing with severe health problems, or the idea of the abortion of a foetus which may be understood as selection of life or the reasonable right of a woman can be the other; both ways seem to me quite understandable as long as they remain on the individual basis. And I also noticed that in parks, for instance, in restaurants or in the street, the atmosphere and relationships with children seem to be a lot more relaxed, open and affectionate in comparison to what I was used to in Germany. *Voilà!* – without having started to consider the projects' questions themselves, I was already in a mode of comparison about what seems "normal". What also startled me in the public sphere was the presence of the military and the men and women carrying weapons in everyday life. Of course, I had already heard about this and knew that the weapons are carried by young people who are doing military service. Emotionally, the image of weapons in public was surprising, if not shocking – but I got used to it quite soon. Yet, men and women carrying weapons in the streets did not allow me to forget that Israel is always in a state of emergency, in defence mode. This fact is not only due to the Shoah, but also to the present political situation. For me, the fact that I am from Germany with its history, is very present.

In Germany, "Never Again" is emphasised. It remains ambiguous what exactly is meant: *Never again war, Never again crimes against humanity, Never again crimes against Jews* – there is some room for interpretation (e.g. Sznaider 2017: ch. 2, ch. 4). In Israel, too, as I quickly learned, remembrance is important and the "Never Again" is emphasised. One day, I heard the voices around me fall silent, people stopped in consternation. This ritual is expressed physically. In April of each year, a two-minute siren wail reminds everybody of *yom hashoah*, Holocaust Remembrance Day. The Jewish people suffered the crimes of the Shoah – this must be remembered. Presumably, we are dealing with a plurality of understandings of "Never Again", both in Israel and in Germany. I feel a great shyness, almost awe, at the task of undertaking a comparative project about testing and selecting life in the face of these complexities.

I remember a discussion about one of the leading German intellectuals, Jürgen Habermas, who was invited in 2012 to give the annual Martin Buber Lecture in Jerusalem. In an interview, the Israeli daily *Haaretz* asked him for his opinion on Israeli politics. In his answer he agreed that "the present situation and the politics of the Israeli government require a political kind of evaluation," but this is not "the business of a private German citizen of my generation."[7] Somehow, at least from a German perspective or from my perspective – a person who has just formulated a kind of hesitation to judge Israeli politics or practices – this answer is understandable. Yet the fact that a public intellectual who was considered the founder of discourse ethics withdraws into the private realm here contains a political message. Commenting on the interview, Omri Boehm refers to Immanuel Kant's insistence that "understanding" needs "public use of reason" and the demand that the individual should transcend private commitments to a "standpoint of everybody else" and have the courage to think "aloud" (Kant 2013; Boehm 2015). Even though I think it is surely not always sensible to speak up or to engage in the process of judgement – regardless of whether one does or does not believe in the discourse of "universal human reason" – I also believe that taking refuge in a private position produces a silence that is eloquent (*Schweigen, das beredt ist*). Habermas is silent *as* a German: he can speak up about a huge variety of subjects as a social philosopher, but when turning to Israel's politics he can only be silent *as* a German. Before, I was certainly aware of this problem but I was not aware of its profoundness. It comes as no surprise that people, philosophers or poets become mute in the face of atrocities and human suffering. Or those who are excluded or not heard may remain silenced. But should we always be silent, or only speak *as* German or *as* Israeli? Hannah Arendt holds the thesis that "if one is attacked as a Jew, one

7   Noa Limona (2012): Interview with Jürgen Habermas. Haaretz, 10 August 2012. https://www.haaretz.co.il/magazine/1.1797148; Omri Boehm: The German Silence on Israel, and Its Cost, The New York Times, 9 March 2015 (https://opinionator.blogs.nytimes.com/2015/03/09/should-germans-stay-silent-on-israel/), accessed 12 March 2022.

must defend oneself as a Jew. Not as a German, not as a world-citizen, not as an upholder of the Rights of Man" (Arendt 1994: 12). In this perspective the "as" makes sense; but a researcher, an intellectual or academic might try to overcome the constraints that lie in a reaction provoked by being "as" a German, as someone being nationally impregnated. Saying this does not mean that scientists and their studies are not situated and embedded in a particular history and society. However, taking refuge in the private and remaining silent means remaining in a state of anxiety and also refusing communication. Realising this means for me to live the research with the ambiguity between remaining a silent listener and a speaker as well as a writer who feels challenged by the tension between one's own and the Other's, history and presence. I hoped and still hope these are good conditions for conversations.

2.4 How to Sail a Boat (Aviad Raz)

In the spirit of auto-ethnography I would like to highlight some of the signals of the conversation that in retrospect can be used to connect the dots. Just as the metaphor of conversation became embodied in the everyday intricacies of our teamwork, we spoke at the beginning of the project about the challenges of dialogue as sailing a small boat together – where each team member needs to balance their weight against the others, and if someone leans out too heavily or abruptly this might compromise the whole boat. We/I even played with the notion of the sailing boat for a while as a potential project logo, presented for example in a PowerPoint slide that I showed in our second workshop (see figure 1). This slide, captured here in its final form, is actually a multiplicity of images in a collage of layers, each layer appearing on top of the other in a manner that visually and symbolically represent the conversation between the different layers and researchers involved in the project.

When the slide presentation begins, the first figure depicts the foetus, shown in the womb, surrounded by maternal blood, with an arrow pointing to the site of placental DNA. This is the first layer, focusing on the biology of NIPT. Then, with another click, the names of various commercial companies offering NIPT appear. This is a second layer, that of the commercialisation of NIPT, which has also become a driver of its globalisation. The following layer adds the flags of Germany and Israel, for the international comparison of policies, as well as symmetrical figures of a pregnant woman and a doctor, representing the socio-empirical level of interaction. Finally, three pictures are added to the collage, representing different manifestations of culture-specific reactions to

NIPT. There is the famous "Don't Screen Us Out" poster from the UK disability advocacy campaign against NIPT, a picture from a demonstration in Germany against PraenaTest, and a picture of a modern Orthodox Jewish-Israeli couple holding a baby with Down syndrome. Each one of these pictures tells a story that is of course only part of a much larger cultural and philosophical puzzle. They all have various political undertones, which could be potentially spelled out or remain hidden. At the very outset of the project, we thus confronted the urgent need to be conversant in various fields, each with its own terminologies and expertise. This is evidently a well-known challenge in any interdisciplinary collaboration. The last part of the collage in the slide was the sailing boat, a centrepiece that is supposed to hold together all the other pieces and layers of the puzzle. The boat carries the acronym of the project, PreGGI, standing for "Practices of Prenatal Genetics in Germany and Israel".

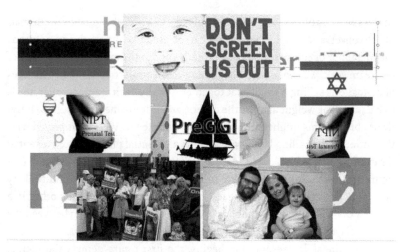

Figure 1 PowerPoint slide showing the layers of the PreGGI project with the sailing boat logo, 5 March 2018, project workshop in Tel Aviv with invited experts.

Throughout the project we participated in sailing this boat. Sometimes it was plain sailing, smooth and uninterrupted. The sociologists, philosophers and bioethicists had to learn how to be crew members. At other times, it felt like sailing against or close to the wind, with productive frictions that needed to be overcome so that the boat could sail on. An illustration of this conversational work can be seen in a PPT slide designed as a summary of an interim workshop (fig. 2). Already halfway through the project, the slide again presents the layers of different comparisons: policy, empirical-social, phenomenology, intercultural and philosophical. The order is both intended and arbitrary. Yet the fact that the philosophical comparison comes at the end of the list, while policy analysis is at the start, is intriguing – as well as open to question and interpretation.

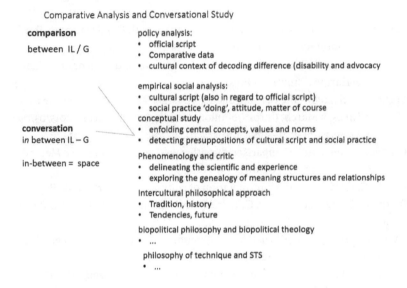

Figure 2 Summary slide entitled "skizze comparison conversation" composed at the end of a workshop, 16 March 2019 (IL= Israel, G = Germany)

In the project's third year, the metaphor of conversation was already half-routinised and semi-institutionalised, epitomised as the organising platform for the final/semi-concluding conference of the project (11–12 December 2019), defined as a "socio-philosophical platform for conversations" to initiate and support intercultural, philosophical and discursive conversations between different participants, mainly but not exclusively from Israel and Germany. And now, finally, we are conversing over the book's pages. I am moved by the per-

sonal and individually different nature of the conversation. The sailing boat has
anchored; long live the conversation.

References

Arendt, Hannah (1994): "'What Remains? The Language Remains': A Conver-
    sation with Günter Gaus." In: Jerome Kohn (ed.), Essays in Understand-
    ing, 1930–1954, Formation, Exile, and Totalitarianism, New York: Schocken
    Books, pp. 307–327.
Bar-On, Dan (1989): Legacy of Silence. Encounters with Children of the Third
    Reich, Cambridge: Harvard University Press.
Bar-On, Dan (1995): Fear and Hope. Three Generations of the Holocaust, Cam-
    bridge: Harvard University Press.
Boehm, Omri (2015): "The German Silence on Israel, and Its Cost." In: The New
    York Times, 9 March, (https://opinionator.blogs.nytimes.com/2015/03/09
    /should-germans-stay-silent-on-israel/), accessed 12 March 2022.
Candea, Mattei (2018): Comparison in Anthropology: The Impossible Method,
    Cambridge: Cambridge University Press.
Geertz, Clifford (1973): The interpretation of cultures, New York: Basic Books.
Gingrich, Andre/Fox, Richard G. (eds.) (2002): Anthropology, London: Rout-
    ledge.
Kant, Immanuel (2013): What is enlightenment? Transl. by Samuel Fleis-
    chacker, London: Routledge.
Khelfaoui, Mahdi/Gingras, Yves/Lemoine, Mael/Pradeu, Thomas (2021): "The
    Visibility of Philosophy of Science in the Sciences, 1980–2018." In: *Synthese*,
    pp. 2–3, (doi.org/10.1007/s11229-021-03067-x), accessed 3 May 2022.
Lavi, Shai (2010): "The Paradox of Jewish Bioethics. The Case of Reproduc-
    tive Technology." In: Friedemann Voigt (ed.), Religion in bioethischen
    Diskursen, Berlin: De Gruyter, pp. 81–102.
Levinas (1988) : À l'heure des nations. Paris : Éditions de Minuit.
Limona, Noa (2012) : "Interview with Jürgen Habermas." In: Haaretz, 10
    August, (https://www.haaretz.co.il/magazine/1.1797148), accessed 3 May
    2022.
Marcus, George E. (1995): "Ethnography in/of the World System: The Emer-
    gence of Multi-Sited Ethnography." In: Annual Review of Anthropology 24,
    pp. 95–117.

Merleau-Ponty, Maurice (1988): The Praise of Philosophy, transl. John Wild and James Edie, Evanston: Northwestern University Press.

Monnin, Luc (2004): "Le rêve d'un réductionniste." In: MLN 119/ 4, French Issue, Baltimore: The Johns Hopkins University Press, pp. 819–844.

Needham, Rodney (1972): Belief, language, and experience, Oxford: Blackwell.

Perrot, Adeline/Horn, Ruth (2021): "The ethical landscape(s) of non-invasive prenatal testing in England, France and Germany: findings from a comparative literature review." In: European Journal of Human Genetics, (http s://doi.org/10.1038/s41431-021-00970-2), accessed 3 May 2022.

Ravitsky, Vardit/Roy, Marie-Christine/Haidar, Hazar/ Henneman, Lidewij/ Marshall, John/Newson, Ainsley J./Ngan, Olivia M.Y./ Nov-Klaiman, Tamar (2021): "The Emergence and Global Spread of Noninvasive Prenatal Testing." In: Annual Review of Genomics and Human Genetics 22, pp. 309–338.

Raz, Aviad E./Nov-Klaiman, Tamar/Hashiloni-Dolev, Yael/Foth, Hannes/ Schües, Christina/Rehmann-Sutter Christoph (2021): "Comparing Germany and Israel regarding debates on policy-making at the beginning of life: PGD, NIPT and their paths of routinization." In: Ethik in der Medizin, (https://doi.org/10.1007/s00481-021-00652-z), accessed 3 May 2022.

Rehmann-Sutter, Christoph/ Porz, Rouven/ Scully, Jackie Leach (2012) How to Relate the Empirical to the Normative. Toward a Phenomenologically Informed Hermeneutic Approach to Bioethics. Cambridge Quarterly of Healthcare Ethics 21, pp. 436–447.

Rehmann-Sutter, Christoph (2021): "Should prenatal screening be seen as 'selective reproduction'? Four reasons to reframe the ethical debate." In: Journal of Perinatal Medicine 49/8, pp. 953–958, (https://doi.org/10.1515/jpm-2 021-0239), accessed 3 May 2022.

Scheffer, Thomas/Niewöhner, Jörg (eds.) (2010): Thick Comparison: Reviving the Ethnographic Aspiration, Leiden: Brill.

Schües, Christina (2008): "Aufgabe der Bildung: Theodor W. Adorno und Hannah Arendt." In: Rudolf Rehn/Christina Schües (eds.), Philosophie und Bildung. Grundlagen – Methoden – Perspektiven, Freiburg: Alber, pp. 136–156.

Sen, Amartya (2009): The Idea of Justice. London: Penguin.

Sørensen, Estrid (2010): "Producing Multi-Sited Comparability." In: Thomas Scheffer/Jörg Niewöhner (eds.), Thick Comparison. Reviving the Ethnographic Aspiration, Leiden: Brill, pp. 43–77.

Sznaider, Natan (2017): Gesellschaften in Israel. Eine Einführung in zehn Bildern, Berlin: Jüdischer Verlag.

ten Have, Henk (2016): Global Bioethics. An Introduction, London: Routledge.

Waldenfels, Bernhard (2006): Grundmotive einer Phänomenologie des Fremden, Frankfurt: Suhrkamp.

Walzer, Michael (1994): Thick and Thin. Moral Argument at Home and Abroad, Notre Dame: University of Notre Dame Press.

Welzer, Harald/Moller, Sabine/Tschuggnall, Karoline (2002): "Opa war kein Nazi": Nationalsozialismus und Holocaust im Familiengedächtnis, Frankfurt: Fischer.

Biographies

Kathrin Braun is a political scientist based at the Center for Interdisciplinary Risk and Innovation Studies (ZIRIUS) at the University of Stuttgart, Germany. Her main areas of study are critical biopolitics studies, the politics of biomedicine, and more recently the digital transformation of society and the chances of shaping it in a democratic and responsible way. She is also forum editor of Critical Policy Studies. Her recent publications include *Biopolitics and Historic Justice: Coming to Terms with the Injuries of Normality* (transcript 2021).

Hannes Foth was a member of the DFG project "Meanings and Practices of Prenatal Genetics in Germany and Israel (PreGGI)", located at the Institute for History of Medicine and Science Studies, University of Lübeck, Germany. He received his bachelor's degree in philosophy (major) and politics (minor subject) and a master's degree in philosophy from the Heinrich Heine University Düsseldorf, Germany. He wrote his dissertation in philosophy on *Responsibility and friendship in parent-child relationships in the adult age*. His main fields of interest include the social philosophy, (bio)ethics and politics of family relationships and their shaping through societal and technological change.

Marina Frisman is a student at the University of Lübeck, Institute for History of Medicine and Science Research, Department of Psychiatry and Psychotherapy. Her research interests focus on the background and contexts of the human psychology. One topic area includes decision making in non-invasive prenatal testing and the socio-cultural factors that influence these decisions. In her other research field she is investigating fractal dimensions as potential biomarkers of psychotic disorders in structural magnetic resonance *imaging* (MRI).

Hille Haker, Ph.D., holds the Richard McCormick S.J. Endowed Chair in Catholic Moral Theology at Loyola University Chicago. Her scholarship in bioethics centres on reproductive medicine, genetic diagnosis and gene editing, methods of bioethics, such as narrative bioethics and feminist ethics, and the history of eugenics, racism, and human dignity and vulnerable agency. Her recent books are *Towards a Critical Political Ethics: Catholic Ethics and Social Challenges* (2020) and *Unaccompanied Migrant Children: Social, Legal, and Ethical Perspectives* 2019 (co-edited with Molly Greening).

Yael Hashiloni-Dolev is a sociologist of health and illness. Formerly a member of Israel's National Bioethics Council (2013–20), she is Co-president of the Israeli Society for the History & Philosophy of Science (2018–21), and member of the Gender Equality Committee – Council for Higher Education Israel. She is a Full Professor and head of graduate studies at the Department of Sociology and Anthropology, Ben-Gurion University of the Negev, Israel. Her areas of interest include the beginnings and ends of life, new reproductive technologies, cryopreservation, gender, bioethics, family studies and contemporary parenthood.

Tsipy Ivry, Ph.D., is chair of the graduate program in medical and psychological anthropology at the Department of Anthropology, University of Haifa, Israel. She is the author of a comparative double ethnography, *Embodying Culture: Pregnancy in Japan and Israel* (2010). Her research in Israel explores the intersections of religion and reproductive biomedicine from the vantage point of rabbinically mediated assisted reproduction among deeply religious Jewish communities in Israel, and rabbinically mediated post-diagnostic termination decisions. Her current research in Japan explores the impact of the 3/11 disasters on prenatal care, with a focus on the implementation of NIPT. Her research is supported by ISF and JF grants.

Swantje Köbsell is Professor at the University of Bremen in the Department of Inclusive Education. She is a representative of German-speaking disability studies and a long-time activist of the German disability movement. Trained as a teacher for special education, she worked in several disability projects before starting her university career. Her research interests lie in eugenics/bioethics, in particular with regard to disability, intersections of disability with gender, age, forced migration, and the history of the disability movement in East and West Germany.

Sabine Könninger is a political scientist at the Philosophical-Theological University of Vallendar, Germany. Her main areas of research and interest are the politics of biomedicine and bioethics, the history of medicine and science, the politics of prenatal diagnosis, healthcare, science and technology studies, governmentality studies and interpretative policy analysis.

Burkhard Liebsch is Professor of Philosophy at the University of Bochum, Germany. His main research interests are practical, political and und social philosophy in cultural-historical perspective, philosophy of history, phenomenology and hermeneutics. He is currently working on *Kraft der Hermeneutik. Zum Werk Ricoeurs; Orientierung und Ander(s)heit* (with W. Stegmaier), and has recently published "Zur aktuellen Theorie des Krieges" (Labyrinth 2022).

Rachel Lihansky is a mother of four children and a grandmother to twelve, and she lives in Moshav Almagor in the north of Israel. She has a BA in Social Work and a MA in Education and has worked for forty years in educational services in Israel. Since the birth of her daughter Nitzan, who has Down syndrome, she has been active and involved in this field. She has written two books and has given countless lectures, interviews and support sessions on the subject. For many years, she was head of Yatid, an organisation for children and families of those living with Down syndrome, and she continues this same role for the current organisation in Israel, known as Atid. Today, she is retired from educational services but her activism and involvement with Down syndrome support is ongoing.

Tamar Nov-Klaiman is a former genetic counsellor, and currently a PhD student in the Department of Sociology and Anthropology at Ben-Gurion University of the Negev, Israel. Her areas of research include bioethics and regulatory policies in the field of reproductive technologies and biobanks.

Aviad Raz is Professor of medical and organisational sociology and Chair of the Department of Sociology and Anthropology, and Director of the Eitan Program for fostering inter-Disciplinary Excellence, all at Ben-Gurion University of the Negev, Israel. In addition to studying religious/ethnic groups and identities in contemporary Israeli society, especially in the context of health and medicine, he also focuses on the global social and bioethical aspects of medical organisations, medical sociology, and cross-cultural bioethics, especially regarding community genetics and patient support organisations.

Christoph Rehmann-Sutter is Professor of Theory and Ethics in the Biosciences at the University of Lübeck, Germany, and honorary Professor of Philosophy at the University of Basel, Switzerland. He has published widely in philosophy and ethics of biomedicine; his research interests include the philosophical foundations of bioethics and phenomenological philosophy of biology. With a hermeneutic approach to ethics and often using qualitative empirical methods, he has been working on the ethical issues of genetic engineering, medical genetics and genomics, including prenatal testing and gene therapies, transplantation, stem cell medicine and palliative care, and currently also on the ethics of climate change. Since 1991 he has published widely on the ethics of genetics in medicine. Co-edited books include *Ethik und Gentherapie* (Attempto 1995), *Disclosure Dilemmas* (Ashgate 2009) and *The Human Enhancement Debate and Disability* (Palgrave Macmillan 2014). *Stefan Reinsch* is a physician and medical anthropologist working at the Centre for Health Service Research and the University Children's Hospital Neuruppin, both at Brandenburg Medical School – Theodor Fontane, Germany. He holds an MA in social anthropology from the Institute of European Ethnology, Humboldt University Berlin, and an MD-PhD from the Charité – University Medical Centre. Since 2006, he has been conducting a long-term ethnographic study with a group of patients, caregivers and health professionals about life with cystic fibrosis, a rare chronic genetic disease. His other current research interests include medical education, professional identity formation, and rural health.

Christina Schües is Professor of Philosophy at the Institute for the History of Medicine and Science Studies at the University of Lübeck, and honorary Professor of Philosophy in the Institute of Philosophy and Sciences of Art at Leuphana University, Lüneburg, Germany. Her research aims at understanding the *conditio humana* with regard to the life sciences and their political dimensions, and concepts of inter-corporeality, vulnerability and responsibility. She combines a historical and phenomenological perspective with the belief that epistemology and anthropology must be integrated into the work of political, medical and peace philosophy.

Natan Sznaider is a Full Professor of Sociology at the Academic College of Tel-Aviv-Yaffo, Israel. Sznaider publishes mainly in English and in German. His research interests over the last few years have centred on giving a sociological account of processes of trauma and victimhood. His project has focused on Jewish politics after the Holocaust through the lens of cosmopolitan memory.

Most recently, he has researched the connections between the Holocaust and Colonialism.

Anne Weber, Dr. phil., Mag. Theol., is currently Graduate Fellow in the Faculty of Theology, Paderborn University, Germany, where she analyses the socio-ethical chances and risks of digital transformation processes. She completed her PhD in Philosophy and is involved in interreligious dialogue at the Centre for Comparative Theology and Cultural Studies, Paderborn University. Her research interests address hermeneutical questions, critical theory and gender studies, as well as biomedicine and post-growth concepts.

CPSIA information can be obtained
at www.ICGtesting.com
Printed in the USA
JSHW050322130123
36235JS00005B/33

9 783837 659887